About the aut

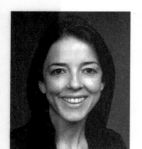

Alison Orman is a Melbourne-based writer and editor with more than 15 years experience in publishing, having worked in book publishing, magazines, television and online media. She holds a BA Communications and Master of Professional Writing, both from the University of Technology, Sydney. She is also the mother of two young children, one of whom has multiple food allergies.

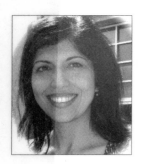

Dr Preeti Joshi, MBBS (Hons) FRACP PhD, is a specialist Paediatrician in Allergy and Immunology in the Department of Allergy and Immunology at the Children's Hospital Westmead, Sydney. Dr Joshi is involved in caring for children with allergies and teaching young doctors and other specialists about the recognition and management of allergies. She is an active member of the Australasian Society of Clinical Immunology and Allergy. She is also the mother of two young children who have food allergies.

To Noah and Lucy
AO

To Maya and Anika
PJ

THE COMPLETE AUSTRALIAN
GUIDE FOR PARENTS

Managing
Your Child's
Food
Allergies

Alison Orman

WITH DR PREETI JOSHI
from The Children's Hospital at Westmead

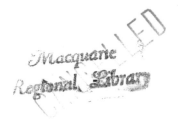
HarperCollinsPublishers

HarperCollins*Publishers*, Australia

First published in 2009
by HarperCollins*Publishers* Australia Pty Limited
ABN 36 009 913 517
harpercollins.com.au

Text copyright © Alison Orman 2009

HarperCollins*Publishers*
25 Ryde Road, Pymble, Sydney, NSW 2073, Australia
31 View Road, Glenfield, Auckland 0627, New Zealand
1–A, Hamilton House, Connaught Place, New Delhi – 110 001, India
77–85 Fulham Palace Road, London, W6 8JB, United Kingdom
2 Bloor Street East, 20th floor, Toronto, Ontario M4W 1A8, Canada
10 East 53rd Street, New York NY 10022, USA

National Library of Australia Cataloguing-in-Publication data:

Orman, Alison.
Managing your child's food allergies : the complete
Australian guide / Alison Orman, Preeti Joshi
ISBN 9780732285289 (pbk.)
Includes index. Bibliography.
Food allergy in children–Popular works.
Food allergy in infants–Popular works.
Food–Labelling–Australia.
Children–Health and hygiene–Australia.

Other Authors / Contributors: Joshi, Preeti.

618.92975

Cover design by Darren Holt
Internal design and layout by Agave Creative Group
Illustrations by Alexis Seabrook
Index by Catherine J. Page

Printed and bound in Australia by Griffin Press on 70gsm Classic White

70gsm Classic White used by HarperCollinsPublishers is a natural, recyclable product made from
wood grown in sustainable forests. The manufacturing processes conform to the environmental
regulations in the country of origin, Finland.

6 5 4 3 2 1   09 10 11 12 13

Contents

Part 3: The emotions of food allergy

Part 4: Food allergy in the future

How to use this book

Managing Your Child's Food Allergies has been written to share with you research and factual information about understanding and managing food allergy, combined with the personal experiences of other families around Australia who have already been successfully managing food allergy for some time.

This book is designed to be used as an *adjunct* to medical care and advice. There are many doctors in Australia who are knowledgeable and experienced in diagnosing and managing food allergy, including clinical immunologists, paediatricians and GPs. After your child has been formally diagnosed with food allergy by a medical professional, we hope this book will offer you further in-depth information about food allergy, as well as practical ideas for you to adopt or adapt, where relevant, in managing your child's food allergy.

The way food allergy is managed is dependant on any number of variable factors, including: the allergen (for example, peanut allergy may be managed differently from a fruit allergy), the number of allergens, a child's medical history, their age, associated medical conditions (asthma, for example), to name only some. It is important to understand that the *majority of allergic reactions to food are mild* — and not every child with food allergy is prescribed an adrenaline autoinjector (for example, an EpiPen): the first-line treatment for anaphylaxis. Accordingly, not all of the practical ideas about managing food allergy discussed in this book will be relevant or necessary for *all* children with food allergy. Read this book with your family's individual circumstances in mind.

The first part of this book deals with understanding food allergies: what is a food allergy, how the condition is diagnosed, how it is treated and what to do in an emergency. The second part of this book is about living with and managing food allergies on a day-to-day basis. We guide you through common situations such as eating out, travelling, childcare, school, social occasions and coping with the new challenges involved in the transition from childhood to the teenage years. The third part of this book deals with emotional aspects of food allergy, presenting important research findings and offering practical advice to help you and your food-allergic children live positively with food allergy. Finally, the fourth part offers hope in the form of an overview of some of the important research currently underway into the prevention and treatments of food allergy.

While we hope many parents and carers will enjoy reading this book from cover to cover, it has been written and structured in a way that makes it easy for you to access the information you need when you need it. Where medical terms are used, we explain them within the text. Where one topic is closely related to another, you will find useful cross-references included. A comprehensive index at the back of this book ensures the answers you need are at your fingertips. Dip in and out of relevant chapters when a new challenge arises and share them with family, friends and anyone who is involved in caring for your child.

We hope this book will affirm some of your own experiences of living with food allergy and act as a springboard for new ideas in managing food allergy in your family. Remember, though, there is no one-size-fits-all approach to managing food allergy. Always follow the advice of your child's doctor and dietitian to the letter, and discuss any concerns or questions with your child's doctor to ensure you receive advice specific to your child's diagnosis.

—Alison Orman and Dr Preeti Joshi

Introduction by Alison Orman

Food allergy has been described as an 'invisible' condition.[1] Children with food allergy are expected to, and (for the most part) can, live normal lives. As long as the child is avoiding their allergen, they appear to all who meet them as regular, healthy and happy children. However, behind the scenes, their condition is usually being managed in ways that impact upon the whole family and anyone who cares for them.

Food allergy is not uncommon: it is estimated that 1 in 20 children have food allergy.[2] While statistics are essential and telling for doctors and scientists, they in no way reveal the human story of families managing food allergy on a daily basis. For parents, being charged with the responsibility of keeping a food-allergic child safe, well nourished and well adjusted is no easy task. While the majority of allergic reactions are *not* severe, medical science cannot predict with absolute certainty which children will experience anaphylaxis — the most severe and potentially life-threatening form of allergic reaction — when exposed to their allergen. Families have to adapt to living with the uncertainty of food allergy and maintain constant vigilance to prevent an allergic reaction. For parents of children at risk of anaphylaxis, the knowledge that a taste of the wrong food can make their child sick — possibly even threaten their life — can, at times, be overwhelming.

The good news is, with specialist medical care, education, training and community support, along with a hopeful outlook, food allergy is very manageable. If your child has recently been diagnosed with food allergy, this book will reassure you that it does get easier. If you have already been living with food allergy for a long time, this book will provide you with advice to help you with new challenges that are bound to come your way. Whether you are new to food allergy or just want to learn more, this book will provide helpful information on all aspects of food allergy as well as encouragement and reinforcement that managing food allergies can be done.

This book was born out of my own family's experience of living with food allergy. It was a series of events that eventually led to a diagnosis of food allergy for our son, Noah. In June 2005, life at home with our new baby wasn't the way we thought it would be. Noah developed eczema on his face, stomach and back and, as regular as clockwork, after his evening 'top-up' formula feed, he would become extremely unsettled. He vomited, was itchy and uncomfortable, and would scream until very late. As first-time parents, we assumed this was just what babies did. What new parent doesn't say at some point that they have a 'chucky' baby, or a baby who won't sleep? It didn't even occur to us that there was a pattern to his distress — vomiting always after formula but never after breast milk. (We eliminated formula when he was 2 weeks old and the vomiting stopped.)

The next piece in our food-allergy puzzle presented when we noticed hives appearing on Noah's skin when friends and family kissed him after drinking milk or eating egg or dairy products. And, on one particular occasion, I had whole-egg mayonnaise on my fingers and touched his lips while trying to help him breastfeed. Within seconds, his lips began to swell and hives surrounded his mouth. We thought his skin reactions were odd, but it still didn't occur to us they might be a symptom of something potentially serious.

We didn't realise something might be wrong until I spilt a teaspoon of cow's milk on Noah's hand while I was eating cereal. He rubbed the milk into his eye and mouth, and within minutes welts appeared on his face, stomach and legs. One eye became swollen and he began coughing persistently. By this time, Noah was 5 months old. The reaction was disturbing to watch, largely because of Noah's distress, but also because of the speed at which the symptoms developed and the fact that I had no clue as to what I should do to help him. I should have called an ambulance immediately, but at the time I had no idea that milk could cause a serious allergic reaction.

Thankfully, Noah recovered and I took him to our GP. Our GP immediately suspected food allergy and referred Noah to a paediatric immunologist for review. Noah was 6-and-a-half months old when he was diagnosed with food allergies to cow's milk, egg and peanut (he has since added cashew, hazelnut and sesame to his list).

My husband and I left the office of our son's specialist with mixed emotions. We were relieved that he had been diagnosed with something specific, so we could now follow a prescribed management plan, but also confused as to what it all really meant. We understood the 'big picture' if you like — of what could happen in an emergency and what to do if it did — but we weren't really sure what to do on a day-to-day basis to keep him safe and well fed.

Over the next few months, I became increasingly nervous. I wasn't comfortable being assertive and asking people not to eat allergenic foods near Noah. When Noah started crawling, I often stayed at home instead of attending mother's group sessions that involved food because I just found it too stressful. Every time we were invited to a social occasion involving food, I felt a sense of dread.

I can see clearly, now, that when Noah was diagnosed as being at risk of anaphylaxis, my reaction was almost entirely emotional and only a tiny bit rational. I couldn't get past the fact that there was the potential for a life-threatening reaction. I knew statistically the risk of a life-threatening reaction was small, but what parent likes to think about the wellbeing of their own child in terms of a statistic? The fact that the risk was there at all was difficult to get my head around. After witnessing several of Noah's allergic reactions, mostly on my own, my response to Noah's diagnosis was fear. This was understandable, but not sustainable. I didn't want Noah or our family to become socially isolated. The biggest problem wasn't Noah's allergies but rather my own response to the diagnosis.

One of the main reasons I wasn't coping with Noah's food allergies was because I did not have enough information; my fear of the unknown was causing me to switch into over-protective-mother mode. So I made a decision to find out more. My husband and I visited several local book stores to try to find a parenting book on food allergy. To our surprise, and disappointment, there were no Australian titles to be found. I resorted to ordering books from the US — which were very helpful and comforting, but there are significant differences between our cultures, for example, our diets, special occasions celebrated, food labelling regulations, school and childcare options; the list goes on. What we really wanted was an Australian handbook for parents: something to keep on the bookshelf and dip into when we faced a new challenge or had a specific question in between appointments with Noah's doctors.

With no Australian book on offer, we fell back on our own resources. Our lovely friends Anne and Phil have four children, two of whom have food allergies, and they have been a wonderful support and the suppliers of safe recipes. I went to a library and read science-based journal articles on food allergy. I enrolled in an anaphylaxis education and training course and joined an education and support group, Anaphylaxis Australia. Noah's specialist referred us to a paediatric dietitian, who helped me work out what to feed Noah to ensure he received all of the nutrients he needed while also keeping him safe. The initial learning curve was steep, but with a team approach to Noah's allergies, life suddenly became so much easier. Noah's food allergies became far more manageable than I had ever imagined they could be.

It was accurate education and meeting other parents in the same situation that helped us, as a family, turn our attitude to food allergies in a much-needed new direction and cope with the ever-present risk of anaphylaxis. We learned to manage Noah's allergies within the (almost) normal life we wanted all of our family to enjoy. Of course, there is always room for anxiety — it fluctuates depending on the situation — and, yes, ongoing vigilance, learning from mistakes, endless cooking and planning ahead are constants, but food allergy does not loom as an all-consuming 'dark force' in our family's life. We accept food allergy as part of everyday life rather than living our life around Noah's allergies.

As I became more knowledgeable and confident in managing Noah's food allergies, I still regularly checked in book stores to see if anyone had written an Australian book on the subject. They hadn't. In mid 2006, I sent an email to Shona Martyn, the Publishing Director at HarperCollins, and suggested it might be a good idea for a book. She responded immediately and with enthusiasm, and said, 'I think you should write it.' And so I did. Researching and writing this book quickly became a full-time job over a period of three years (with 'maternity leave' in the middle, following the birth of our daughter, Lucy, in 2007).

I was able to write *Managing Your Child's Food Allergies* thanks to the expertise of a team of people. Working under the supervision and guidance of Dr Preeti Joshi (Staff Specialist in the Department of Allergy, Immunology and Infectious Diseases at The Children's Hospital, Westmead, Sydney) and in association with Anaphylaxis Australia Inc, with Maria Said at the helm, I set out to create an accurate, supportive and positive resource that would help family, friends and carers understand and manage food allergy. Where relevant, I have drawn on the professional experience and knowledge of a range of specialists from varying fields, including psychologist Olivia Keene, paediatric dietitian Barbara Dennison, the Australian and New Zealand Food Standards Agency, early childhood and education professionals, school teachers and principals, and resources from the Australasian Society of Clinical Immunology and Allergy, to name only some. My goal was to present — in 'parent speak' as opposed to medical jargon — the latest research and expert advice on the major aspects of understanding and managing food allergy in children in Australia.

In addition, I have interviewed more than 20 parents of food-allergic children from around Australia: parents of children with varying food allergies and with different challenges. Talking to other families can often help fill a void that is left when you walk out of your doctor's office. You might be armed with all the medical information in the world, but on a practical, everyday level, really useful and helpful tips often come from those who have already 'been there and done that' ahead of you. I hope you will feel comforted and inspired by the words of other parents who have generously contributed their experiences throughout the book.

My hope is that *Managing Your Child's Food Allergies* goes some way in helping to fill an information 'gap' for families living with food-allergic children. I hope that after you have sought personalised treatment and care from your child's doctor, this book might be a helpful talking point between you and your own family, friends and carers. I hope that it might direct you to helpful resources and enable you to relate to other families experiencing challenges similar to yours. Above all else, I hope that through this book you will feel inspired that your child's allergies can be managed successfully and positively. If your child sees that you and others in their life can manage food allergies in an educated, confident and optimistic way then, hopefully, they, too, will adopt a similar attitude they can then carry with them for life.

With best wishes to you and your family,
Alison Orman

Mother of Noah (4), allergic to cow's milk, egg, peanut, tree nuts and sesame, and Lucy (2), no food allergies — fingers crossed

Introduction by Dr Preeti Joshi

Being a parent is one of the greatest joys in life but also has many inherent challenges. When a child has a food allergy, these challenges are even greater as we seek to balance a normal life with keeping our children safe and healthy.

In my day-to-day work, I treat hundreds of children with food allergies. As most parents of children with food allergies know, there are many complexities involved in managing food allergy, from the initial diagnosis to avoiding foods and the possibility of recognising and treating anaphylaxis. There are many common questions I am asked by most families and I have often thought that a reliable book addressing these issues would be very useful.

There are multiple sources of information available about food allergy and many of these can be very confusing or simply wrong. It is vitally important to have clear, concise information that helps to navigate through this maze.

The purpose of this book is to provide straightforward and well-researched information about managing your child's food allergies. We have included the most up-to-date information from the most reputable medical sources. While this book does not replace a doctor or a dietitian, it is designed to supplement their advice and further explain some of the areas that may be difficult to understand. The book discusses the causes of food allergies, the tools we use for diagnoses, the symptoms and signs of allergies and how to manage allergic reactions. There is information that examines the fears that you and/or your child may experience around food allergy. Importantly, there are also practical chapters aimed at dealing with common situations, such as parties and school excursions and feeding fussy toddlers. Finally, we have discussed the most recent information about future treatments and possible cures.

As a paediatrician and specialist in the treatment of allergy and, equally importantly, a parent of children with food allergies, I am well aware of the anxieties and challenges that life-threatening food allergy can present. My role is to help children grow up and adapt to life in as healthy and happy a fashion as possible. By reading this book, I hope that families will gain confidence in dealing with food allergies and safely enjoy life's many experiences.

Dr Preeti Joshi
April 2009

Foreword by Maria Said, AAI

I'll never forget my experiences as a new mother struggling to come to terms with my son's food allergies. What I longed for then was for someone who had walked in my shoes to say, 'It's going to be okay.' And this is the message at the heart of *Managing Your Child's Food Allergies*.

In this meticulously researched book, Alison Orman and Dr Preeti Joshi — both of whom have children with food allergies — reassure parents and carers of children diagnosed with food allergy and the risk of anaphylaxis that it *is* a manageable condition. And, just as importantly, they provide practical guidance on how to approach it.

I would love to have had this book when Alex had his first reaction, more than 18 years ago. It would have helped me learn about food allergy as a concerned mum, rather than as a frightened parent who had little practical support. This easy-to-read publication would have helped me get him properly diagnosed, understand what food allergy is, and it would have supplied me with level-headed ideas on how I might approach everyday life, childcare, school, social occasions and even people who just didn't 'get it'!

All children are special; however, an increasing number of children now have extra-special needs because they are food-allergic. Many of these children also have other allergic conditions and, as a consequence, early childhood can be a series of hurdles for all concerned. A diagnosis of food allergy does impact on the quality of life of the individual and their family. The challenge for parents is that they have to learn how to care for children with food allergy while on the run. None of us were born knowing how to manage life with a child who has food allergy. We need help. We want useful answers to our many questions. We are longing to do things right. Parents often say, 'I need to know how to do this because it isn't just about a rash.'

While no book on allergy can have all the answers, *Managing Your Child's Food Allergies* helps those living with food allergy make decisions on the best way forwards. Information, guidance and support help us live life to the full: with care but not fear! This book reiterates to readers that while the risk of anaphylaxis is real, there are lots of things we can do to help keep our food-allergic children safe.

Food allergy is also a public health issue and a community concern. Although management is primarily a parental responsibility, Alison Orman gently but clearly talks about how others can — and indeed do — help. The community, be it school, childcare or other, has a crucial role to play in supporting families and helping educate and care for the child at risk of anaphylaxis while they, too, learn to care for themselves. The multi-pronged approach to management is crucial. Another powerful message this book sends is that we are all in this together.

Education of those in the community helps decrease the impact that the risk of anaphylaxis has on quality of life. We need to normalise the condition, and this book helps everybody to understand food allergy. It helps ease the fear surrounding management and the risk of a life-threatening allergic reaction.

It's a cliché to say, 'Knowledge is power' but when we are talking about allergy management, this can't be truer. Accurate information must form the basis of decisions made on management. Education is a critical part of living with food allergy in the real world, and *Managing Your Child's Food Allergies* is a credible learning tool that all parents and carers of food-allergic children should have access to.

I commend Alison Orman and Dr Preeti Joshi on this helpful book. It contains a wealth of information — including input from credible professionals and real people who live the life and speak the speak on a daily basis. It is a practical guide to management that dispels myths and focuses on what is real.

Perhaps the motto of the book could be: Be careful but not fearful.

Maria Said
President of Anaphylaxis Australia Inc

Part 1

Understanding food allergy

1

Understanding food allergy

If your child has been diagnosed with a food allergy, you and your family are not alone. In fact, your child is part of a growing trend: it has been estimated that 1 in 20 children have food allergy.[1]

Think back to when you were at school. How many children did you know who had a food allergy? Probably very few, if any. Today it is common to find Action Plans for allergic reactions taped to the walls of classrooms and staffrooms. While it is impossible to provide directly comparable food allergy statistics from decades ago (methods of research have changed considerably), scientists do have convincing evidence to suggest an escalation in the incidence of food allergy, in line with increases in allergic disease in general.

While the majority of allergic reactions are *not* severe, medical science cannot predict with absolute certainty which children will experience anaphylaxis — the most severe and potentially life-threatening form of allergic reaction — when exposed to their allergen. Uncertainty goes hand-in-hand with food allergy.

Many people still respond with disbelief when told that someone cannot eat a particular food without the risk of an allergic reaction. For those not living with food allergy, it can be difficult to comprehend that something as seemingly benign as food can cause a potentially life-threatening reaction. Many parents of food-allergic children find themselves labelled by others as over-anxious or neurotic. Although food allergy can be a serious medical condition, the perception that a food allergy somehow equates to a food preference has never entirely disappeared.

A diagnosis of food allergy can be daunting for families, especially so when they have witnessed their child experience a serious or life-threatening reaction, but with specialist medical care, education, training and community support, along with a hopeful outlook, food allergy can become manageable. Children with food allergy do have special needs, but they are needs that can be met through education and the help of others.

The first important step in education is to gain an understanding of food allergy. The information in this chapter will cover the various types of food allergy, explain the difference between a food allergy and a food intolerance, help you to become familiar with the foods usually associated with childhood food allergy and offer some insight into current theories as to why rates of allergic disease might be increasing. Even if you have been living with food allergy for some time, hopefully you still might learn something new. This chapter might also serve as a valuable resource for others involved in the life of your child who wish to understand more about food allergy.

If science isn't your thing

As the parent, relative, friend or carer of a food-allergic child, you don't *have* to understand all the medical science behind an allergic reaction or why allergic disease is increasing in order to provide excellent care for food-allergic children. If you are a little overwhelmed by some of the explanations or terminology in this chapter, a summary of the key points can be found on page 16.

What is food allergy?

'Food allergy' is often incorrectly used to describe any reaction or aversion to a food. There are many explanations as to why someone may want or need to exclude a particular food from his or her diet, including: food intolerance, disease, dieting trends, religious beliefs, ethical principles, personal preferences and psychological reasons. However, all of these are very different from being *allergic* to a particular food. So what does it really mean to be 'allergic' to a food?

A food allergy is an adverse reaction to a generally harmless substance within a food (usually a protein) which is triggered by the body's immune system. Our immune system is designed to protect us from infections and to fight illness, but in a food-allergic person, it is the immune system that actually triggers an allergic response. The immune mechanisms that a food-allergic person experiences occur in all people, but these immune responses are not normally directed against food.

There are two main types of food allergy:

1. IgE-mediated
2. Non-IgE-mediated

Sometimes people can have a combination of both types of allergy. Just to muddy the waters a little more, food intolerance is often confused with food allergy, and some people suffer a combination of the two. While the symptoms of food allergy and food intolerance can be similar, there are key differences in diagnosing, treating and managing each condition. (For further discussion of food intolerance, see pages 5–6.)

IgE-mediated food allergy

IgE stands for immunoglobulin E. This is a type of protein which is also known as an antibody — a substance our body produces in order to protect us against infection. This antibody circulates through the blood.

In IgE-mediated food allergy, the immune system produces IgE antibodies to particular proteins found in a food. These IgE antibodies then attach to mast cells as well as other cells in the body, and basophils (a type of white blood cell). Mast cells contain chemicals, including histamine. Mast cells are usually found in areas of the body where symptoms of food allergy most commonly present: the skin, respiratory tract and mucus membranes (as found in the lining of the mouth, nose, eyes and gut, for example). When a food-allergy sufferer ingests a food containing their allergen, the allergen attaches to the IgE antibodies. When this happens, the antibodies mistakenly identify the protein as dangerous, and this causes the mast cell to release masses of chemicals, resulting in allergic symptoms that can affect the skin, gut, respiratory system and cardiovascular system (heart and blood vessels). (For an illustration of an allergic reaction, see page 9.)

For example, if your son is allergic to cow's milk, his IgE antibodies will have a 'cow's milk receptor' sitting on the surfaces of his mast cells and blood cells. It is a bit like having an in-built radar that scans everything entering his body that might be cow's milk. If your son ingests cow's milk, his IgE cow's milk receptor will, firstly, recognise the shape of the cow's milk protein and, secondly, lock together perfectly with the allergen (cow's milk protein). As soon as this happens, the mast cells release their stores of chemicals throughout the body, causing an allergic response — the signs and symptoms of an allergic reaction.

Allergic symptoms in IgE-mediated allergy are commonly referred to as 'immediate onset' because they occur within minutes up to approximately 2 hours after ingestion of the offending food. IgE-mediated food allergy is diagnosed by skin prick testing or blood testing in conjunction with a patient's clinical history, or by food challenge.

As stated at the beginning of this chapter, the majority of allergic reactions to food are not severe and usually only involve symptoms of the skin and/or gut, such as hives, vomiting or tummy cramps. However, severe reactions to food are no longer rare. Anaphylaxis, the most severe form of IgE-mediated food allergy, involves the respiratory system and/or heart, and is potentially life-threatening. (See Chapter 5, Anaphylaxis, page 68.)

IgE-mediated food allergy, also sometimes referred to as 'true food allergy', is the subject of this book, and the following chapters will include detailed information on diagnosing and managing IgE-mediated food allergy.

Non-IgE-mediated food allergy

Compared with IgE-mediated food allergy, understanding of non-IgE-mediated food allergy is less clear. As with IgE-mediated food allergy, the immune system is involved, but the reaction does not involve the production of IgE antibodies.

Particular syndromes classified as non-IgE-mediated food allergy include:

- Food protein induced enterocolitis (FPIES)
- Food protein induced proctocolitis
- Coeliac disease (an intolerance to gluten)

Some of these syndromes have distinct symptoms that will alert your doctor to a diagnosis, but in many instances the presenting features can be confusing and it can take time for a doctor to make a diagnosis.

Most non-IgE-mediated food allergies are not usually associated with anaphylaxis.[2] Symptoms of non-IgE-mediated allergy usually involve the gut and can include vomiting, diarrhoea, poor weight gain, failure to thrive and abdominal pain. Unlike IgE-mediated food allergy, the symptoms are typically delayed, appearing many hours to days after ingestion of an allergen. What IgE- and non-IgE-mediated food allergy do have in common is that treatment for both involves strict avoidance of the allergen.

There is still much to be learned about non-IgE-mediated food allergy.

Food intolerance

It is not unusual for any unpleasant reaction to food to be incorrectly labelled as a food allergy when, in reality, it is much more likely to be a food intolerance. While food intolerance is not the subject of this book, it is worthwhile knowing a little about it, as some food-allergic children also suffer from food intolerance.

As previously stated, unlike food allergy, food intolerance does not involve the immune system. Food intolerance can be caused by the following:[3, 4, 5]

- Pharmacological mechanisms: reactions caused by particular chemicals in food. The chemicals can be naturally occurring, for example, caffeine; or additives, for example, monosodium glutamate (MSG)
- Metabolic mechanisms: caused by an enzyme deficiency, for example lactose intolerance
- Toxic reactions: caused by food poisoning
- Idiopathic reasons: unexplained or unknown causes

Some (but not all) of the symptoms of food intolerance are similar to those of food allergy, which adds to confusion in the community over whether someone has a food intolerance or a food allergy. Symptoms of food intolerance *can* include: hives, bowel irritation, stomach cramping/

pains, mouth ulcers, headaches, aches and pains, a feeling of being 'run down', and, in children, irritability.

Any reaction to a food for a child, whether it be an allergy or an intolerance, can range from annoying to traumatic, and the symptoms of both can be difficult to cope with. However, in general, food intolerance involves milder reactions than true food allergy and does not usually have the potential to be life-threatening.

Food intolerance is commonly diagnosed by an elimination diet, which involves cutting out 'suspect' foods from a patient's diet in a methodical way until symptoms disappear and then slowly re-introducing foods, one at a time, in an attempt to directly link symptoms with a specific food. This is done under medical supervision. Food intolerance *cannot* be diagnosed by skin prick tests or blood tests.

Some foods, such as tomato, may cause local histamine release in the skin. This results in contact irritation of the skin. For example, some people notice a red rash around their child's mouth when they self-feed with tomato but no reaction if the tomato is spooned into their mouth. In these cases, skin prick tests are usually negative and the condition resolves with time.

It is essential to know for sure whether your child has a food allergy or a food intolerance because the potential reactions and medical management of each condition are markedly different. Medical help is usually necessary to diagnose and confirm a true food allergy.

Food allergy or food intolerance: what's the difference?*

Adverse reaction to food
Any unpleasant or problematic reaction to an ingested food

Food allergy
Involves the immune system

Food intolerances
Does not involve the immune system

IgE-mediated
Involves the production of IgE antibodies

Non-IgE-mediated
Does not involve the production of IgE antibodies

May be caused by any of the following mechanisms

Pharmacological

Metabolic

Toxic

Unexplained

* This diagram is based on information sourced from: Australasian Society of Clinical Immunology and Allergy (ASCIA), 'Diagnosis and management of food hypersensitivity in childhood', October 2007, www.allergy.org.au/content/view/166/1/

'Sensitisation' and route of exposure

Q My 2-year-old daughter is allergic to peanut. Is it true that a baby first has to be exposed to an allergen before a reaction can occur? My baby reacted to her very first taste of peanut butter, so I don't understand what my doctor means when she says my baby was probably 'sensitised' to peanut prior to her first allergic reaction.

A 'Sensitisation' to a food is considered a prerequisite for an IgE-mediated food-allergic response. When the body is first exposed to an allergen, it becomes aware of the allergen, decides it is a threat and puts in place measures to protect the body from this particular allergen in case it enters again (producing IgE antibodies to a particular protein found in that food). This process is referred to as 'sensitisation'. The allergic response then happens on the body's *subsequent* exposure to the allergen in question.

Researchers are trying to understand the route of initial exposure to an allergen (the route of 'sensitisation'). They are investigating theories that it may be via means other than ingestion — for example, through breast milk, the skin or even inhalation — but no one really knows.

On a practical level, none of this is particularly helpful knowledge for a parent, because their child's allergic reaction frequently occurs on their first *known* exposure to the allergen. While it is hard not to continually question how your daughter's allergy developed, science cannot yet provide the answers you and countless other parents are looking for. The most important information you need to focus on now is how to recognise the signs and symptoms of an allergic reaction and how to treat it — ensuring you have an up-to-date Action Plan (see page 372) and always carrying any medications prescribed by your doctor, as well as becoming educated in how to prevent your daughter from being inadvertently exposed to peanut.

Allergic sensitisation

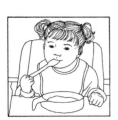

Egg protein

Plasma cell

IgE antibodies to egg

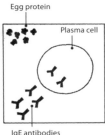

IgE antibodies to egg

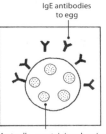

Mast cell — containing chemical mediators, including histamine

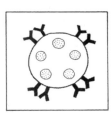

Ingestion is one way in which a child may become sensitised to an allergen. Here, baby Kate is having her first taste of egg in a bowl of custard.

When egg protein enters baby Kate's body, her plasma cells (cells of the immune system) produce IgE antibodies against the allergen: in this case egg.

The IgE antibodies against egg then attach to baby Kate's mast cells. Mast cells contain chemicals, including histamine. These chemicals are responsible for the symptoms of an allergic reaction.

These IgE antibodies against egg will stay attached to baby Kate's mast cells until she is exposed to egg again. Baby Kate is now 'sensitised' to egg.

Allergic reaction

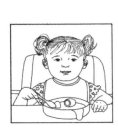

Egg protein

Egg allergen binding to mast cell

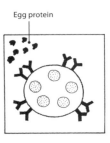

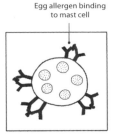

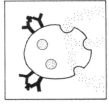

The next time baby Kate is exposed to egg, her body is already primed for an allergic reaction to take place.

The IgE antibodies against egg that are already attached to baby Kate's mast cells now mistakenly recognise the egg protein entering her body as dangerous.

The IgE antibodies — in an attempt to protect the body from something it sees as harmful — bind to the egg allergen: a perfect fit.

This causes baby Kate's mast cells to release chemicals, including histamine, resulting in baby Kate suffering symptoms of an allergic reaction.

The main offenders

Even though our diets include hundreds of different foods, possibly thousands, it is only a relatively small bunch that is responsible for most food-allergic reactions. In children, more than 90 per cent of food allergies are caused by the following:[6]

- Cow's milk
- Egg
- Peanut
- Tree nuts
- Fish
- Shellfish
- Soy
- Wheat

And while there is still a relatively small amount of data available on sesame, it is also now considered to be one of the top allergens.[7]

It is specific proteins in foods that trigger allergic reactions, so while the above list of most common food allergens is widely cited and helpful to know, it is equally important to understand that any food containing protein can cause a mild to severe allergic reaction. Examples include: rice, kiwi fruit, celery, mustard, bananas and potatoes, to name only some. So if someone you know claims their child is allergic to a particular food, no matter how strange it might sound, they need to be taken seriously.

For more information on each of the most common food allergens, see Chapter 6, Common food allergens, page 91.

Allergy is on the increase ...

Allergic disease in general, not only food allergy, is on the rise, at least in the Western world, and Australia has one of the highest prevalences of allergic disorders in the world.[8, 9] Common allergic disorders include: asthma, eczema and allergic rhinitis. One in five Australians suffers from at least one allergic condition, and it has been estimated that allergies are costing the Australian community more than $7 billion a year.[10]

As stated at the beginning of this chapter, it has been estimated that

1 in 20 children have food allergy;[11] however, it is virtually impossible to find a *universally* accepted statistic on the incidence of food allergy in children. This is due to several reasons, including: a varying definition of food allergy (some figures only take into account IgE-mediated responses, some also include non-IgE, some even include food intolerances) and consideration of the fact that many early childhood allergies commonly resolve by school age (so the different age group categories used in statistics can significantly affect the end result).

In Australia, recent studies have shown that rates of food allergy and anaphylaxis are rising. During a 12-year study period, from 1993 to 2005, the rate of hospital admissions for anaphylaxis in children under 5 years of age rose from 4.1 to 19.7 per 100,000 population, with most of the increase due to food-related anaphylaxis.[12] In another Australian study, published in 2009, admissions to hospital for food-induced anaphylaxis increased by approximately 350 per cent.[13] (Although, reassuringly, fatalities from food-induced anaphylaxis remain rare.)

Regardless of the variation in statistics reported, there is little argument that the prevalence of food allergy, like allergic disease in general, is increasing.[14, 15, 16]

... but why?

When considering why the incidence of allergies has been on the increase, it helps to understand that allergy can be influenced by two main factors:

1. Genetic
2. Environmental

— and how these factors interact with the body's immune system.

Genetic factors

In the case of childhood allergies (allergic diseases in general, not only food allergy) a history of 'atopy' in the mother, father or a sibling is a significant risk factor. Atopy refers to the tendency to become sensitised and produce IgE antibodies on exposure to an allergen and, as a result, develop symptoms of asthma, allergic rhinitis, eczema or food allergy, which are referred to as atopic diseases. Or, more simply, atopy is the genetic predisposition to develop allergic disease.

Children born into atopic families are, statistically, at increased risk of developing allergic diseases (again, referring to *any* allergic disease, not only food allergy) compared to those born into a family with no history of atopy. If there is no allergy in either parent, offspring have an approximately 20 per cent chance of developing allergic disease. If one parent is allergic, the likelihood increases to about 30–40 per cent, and if both parents are allergic it jumps again to 60–80 per cent.[17, 18, 19] (The risk is reportedly higher if the mother, as opposed to the father, has a history of allergic disease.)[20]

A child does not inherit a specific allergy from either parent, only the *likelihood* to become allergic; the allergy itself can manifest in any form. For example, if the mother of a child has eczema and the father has asthma, their child has a 60–80 per cent likelihood of developing allergic disease, but if their child does develop allergic disease, it won't necessarily be asthma or eczema.

Likewise, the severity of an allergic reaction cannot be inherited. For example, if a parent has had anaphylaxis to a particular food, insect sting, latex or medication, there is no evidence to suggest their child is at any increased risk of having anaphylaxis to anything. In fact, the child may not develop any allergies at all.

It needs to be added that while genetic factors play a role in the development of allergic disease, it is unlikely that our genetic make-up has changed over the past two decades, during which time the rate of allergic disease has increased.

Environmental factors

While there are no black-and-white answers as to why allergic disease is on the increase, a range of environmental factors can be associated with promoting and preventing allergic disease.

The most commonly cited theory to explain the increase in allergic disease is the hygiene hypothesis. Originally based on studies examining the incidence of atopic disease in 'clean' living environments compared with 'dirty' living environments, it proposes that a clean living environment in the early years of life means we are no longer exposed to recurrent infections and bacterial products, and that this lack of exposure is affecting the way in which our immune system functions. As a result, it is thought that a clean living environment might actually promote the development of allergic disease. This hypothesis has been complemented by other related studies, which have reported a lower incidence of allergic disease in: children from large families;[21] younger siblings;[22] and children placed into childcare at a young age[23] (suggesting that children in these situations are exposed to other children's germs which, in turn, may provide protection against allergy). In addition, children of farming families in Western European countries[24, 25] who were exposed to farm animals — and their bacterial products — have also been shown to have fewer allergies, as have children who grow up with household pets.[26] The hygiene hypothesis is complex and by no means proven.

Considering the rate at which allergy has been increasing in recent years, it seems unlikely that a single cause can be identified as being responsible. Research into the reasons behind increasing rates of allergic disease has been extensive, but when looking specifically at food allergy, peanut allergy has been the focus of a large number of studies to date. This is because peanut allergy is quite common, often lifelong and frequently the cause of more severe reactions.

An increase in peanut consumption is often cited as a reason behind rising rates of peanut allergy. In Australia, we only have to consider the influence of Asian cuisine on our diets, the growing number of individuals choosing vegan or vegetarian diets (where peanuts and tree nuts are often used as a significant source of protein), as well as the ubiquitous use of peanut in processed foods such as muesli bars, cereals, lollies and other popular childhood snacks. As the rate of peanut consumption has increased in the Western world, so too has the prevalence of peanut allergies, with recent studies suggesting the rate of peanut allergy in young children has doubled in the past two decades.[27, 28] However, in countries such as Israel, where peanut consumption is high very early in life, there is relatively little peanut allergy.

Closely related to this finding is research which suggests geographical and cultural factors may also play a role. The pattern of food allergy varies from country to country, and the rate of allergy is often related to food consumption trends in the relevant country. For example, mustard allergy has increased in France (France is the largest European producer and consumer of mustard);[29] in Singapore, bird's nest, a local delicacy, is the leading food allergen among children;[30] and in Israel, sesame is a major cause of food allergy in infants and young children (it is common in Israel for sesame products such as tahini to be included in the diet of infants in the first year of life).[31] As you can see from some of the above examples, it is not yet clear whether early or delayed introduction of a particular food affects the prevention or development of allergy. It may be that the timing and amount of food introduced is critical in the development or prevention of allergy.

Researchers are exploring another possible explanation for the surge in the rate of peanut allergy: the way in which Western countries process peanuts. For example, in Western countries, peanuts are usually dry-roasted while in countries with low rates of peanut allergy, such as China, peanuts are usually boiled or fried. It is believed that the high temperatures needed for dry-roasting peanuts may increase the allergenicity of peanuts more so than the lower temperatures required for boiling or frying.[32] In China (which has a peanut consumption rate on par with that of the US), peanut allergy is rare.[33]

The above is by no means an exhaustive collection of theories. Other areas of research into increased rates of allergy include: maternal diet during pregnancy (it is now generally accepted that this does not influence the development or prevention of allergy), maternal diet during breastfeeding,[34] maternal age at birth,[35] caesarian delivery and allergy[36] and the timing of introducing common allergenic foods to infants (this will be discussed in detail in Chapter 18, Allergy prevention, page 352). The barrier function of skin and the development of allergic disease,[37] exposure to pets in early life,[38] the role of sensitisation *in utero*,[39] the role of antacid medication,[40] the use of multivitamin supplements in infants,[41, 42] and the use of probiotics in preventing and treating allergic disease[43] have also been studied.

A definitive answer on why allergic disease is on the rise has not yet been found, but it seems likely that an interaction of genetic factors with environmental factors is responsible. It may well be that cures for specific allergic conditions are found before the causes are identified.

While it can be fascinating and often heartening for us, as parents, to keep abreast of scientific research into the possible causes of allergy, caution is also needed. It would be unwise to read a limited selection of research articles and then jump to the conclusion that there may be some benefit in you altering your child's current allergy management program based on something you have read. If you want to read more, then by all means refer to the endnotes for this chapter as a starting point, but always follow the advice of your child's allergy specialist to the letter. New research is being published all the time, and your allergy specialist is best placed to offer advice specific to your child's medical condition.

Too hygienic?

Q I have been reading about the hygiene hypothesis and wonder if it means my cleanliness has contributed directly to my son's food allergies (milk, egg and kiwi fruit). I am now pregnant with my second child and am wondering when he/she arrives should I consider lowering my current standards of hygiene? I feel guilty that I may have contributed to my son's allergies by sterilising his feeding equipment and dummies, and continually washing my hands and his. I thought I was doing the right thing; now I'm confused.

A This is a common concern, and the confusion is largely due to the hygiene hypothesis being taken 'out of context', so to speak. The hygiene hypothesis is based on a *style* of living — particularly the lifestyle of the Western world — as opposed to the hygiene practices of individual families. It is unlikely that a single cause is responsible for the increasing rate of allergies, but rather it is a collection of reasons associated with our style of living as well as genetic backgrounds.

There is no reason to feel guilty, and definitely no need to change your hygiene standards for your next baby; in fact, it is important you maintain them. The usual recommended practices of good hygiene for newborns are all important, indeed essential, in the prevention of avoidable illness and disease.

Understanding food allergy: a summary

- Food allergy can be a serious medical condition.
- Food allergy can be successfully managed through education and support.
- There are two types of food allergy: IgE-mediated and non-IgE-mediated. Both involve the immune system.
- Food intolerance does not involve the immune system.
- In a food-allergic reaction, the body's immune system reacts to a certain protein in a food, causing symptoms that can affect the skin, gut, respiratory system, heart and blood vessels.
- The majority of allergic reactions to food are not severe and usually only involve symptoms of the skin and/or gut.
- Anaphylaxis is the most severe form of food allergy, and is potentially life-threatening.
- Any food containing protein can cause a mild to severe allergic reaction, although the most common causes are cow's milk, egg, peanut, tree nuts, fish, shellfish, soy, wheat and sesame.
- Food allergy, like allergic disease in general, is on the increase. Food-related anaphylaxis is also increasing; however, deaths remain rare.
- It is not yet known why the rate of food allergy is rising, but it is believed that an interaction of genetic factors with environmental factors may be responsible.
- The management of food allergy is not a 'one-size-fits-all' approach. Regular review by an allergy specialist is essential in providing advice specific to your child's medical condition.

2

Diagnosing food allergy

The journey to a diagnosis of food allergy is often arduous: from observation of symptoms to suspicion that something might be wrong, to seeking medical help in order to finally pin down what is causing your child's symptoms. Many parents interviewed for this book reported that their food allergy journey began with an unsettled baby, often with eczema, runny nappies and vomiting. Others told the story of offering their child a new food for the first time and noticing a mild reaction such as hives or a rash appearing, so they simply decided to wait until their child was older before offering that food again. Nearly every parent made the observation that, in hindsight, they should have realised something wasn't right, but at the time, they knew nothing or very little about food allergy. Most were constantly reassured by well-meaning advice such as, 'All kids get eczema,' 'All kids get hives,' 'They'll grow out of it.' And while many parents reported it took years for their child to be formally diagnosed, an unlucky few were unexpectedly launched into the world of food allergy via an ambulance ride to hospital when their child suffered anaphylaxis after eating a particular food.

The pathway to a diagnosis of food allergy differs from family to family and, unfortunately, diagnosing food allergy may not be straightforward. However, on the positive side, there are steps you, as a parent or carer, can take to help your child's allergy specialist diagnose (or eliminate) food allergy as the cause of your child's symptoms.

This chapter will help you understand the signs and symptoms of IgE-mediated food allergy, offer guidance in what to do if you think your child may have a food allergy and arm you with information to help you work with your GP and allergy specialist in getting to the bottom of your child's food allergy.

The symptoms of food allergy

The symptoms of IgE-mediated food allergy are referred to as 'immediate onset' because they occur within minutes up to approximately 2 hours after ingestion of the offending food. The symptoms can involve four main organs:[1]

> **Skin:** eczema, hives (urticaria), swelling (angiodema)
>
> **Gastrointestinal system (gut):** itchy mouth, diarrhoea, vomiting, stomach cramps
>
> **Respiratory system:** persistent cough, wheezing, sneezing, runny nose (rhinorrhoea), a high-pitched noise made when breathing in or out (stridor), tongue swelling
>
> **Cardiovascular system:** a drop in blood pressure (hypotension), collapse

As stated in Chapter 1, the majority of allergic reactions to food are not severe. A mild to moderate allergic reaction is characterised by symptoms involving the skin and/or gut only. Severe allergic reactions, or anaphylaxis, are characterised by symptoms involving the respiratory and/or cardiovascular systems.

A wide range of factors can influence the severity of a child's allergic reaction to a food. Some are listed below.

- The amount of allergen ingested.
- The sensitivity of the child to the allergen in question (and a child's sensitivity to an allergen can change considerably over time).
- There is some evidence to suggest that inter-current illness may also play a role; for example, if your child is unwell with a bad cold, their reaction may be worse than usual.
- A child with underlying asthma can be at risk of a more serious reaction (involving the respiratory system).
- The form of the allergen (for example, some children react to lightly cooked egg in an omelette or quiche, but can tolerate egg in goods baked at higher temperatures, such as cakes).

- The length of delay in administering prescribed medication.
- Previous history of anaphylaxis to a particular food.
- The route of exposure — for example, skin contact with a food allergen will usually only result in a mild, skin-related response such as hives, whereas ingestion of an allergen can lead to anaphylaxis.
- In some patients, additional factors can aggravate an allergic reaction to food; these include exercise, aspirin and alcohol. (For more information on exercise-induced anaphylaxis, see page 88.)

Don't forget that many of the symptoms of food allergy are not exclusive to food allergy; they can also be involved in other medical conditions. Food allergy must be diagnosed by a doctor to exclude other possible causes and to ensure that if your child does have a food allergy, you have the appropriate medication, diet and an Action Plan (see pages 371 and 372) in place.

Help, I think my child has a food allergy ...

If you think your child may have a food allergy, you need to make an appointment to visit your GP. If your child has experienced any of the immediate-onset symptoms (listed on the facing page) after contact with or ingestion of a particular food, avoid this food in any form until you have consulted your GP for further advice. Although having said this, you must see your GP as soon as possible, because restricting a child's diet for an extended period of time is often unnecessary and can be dangerous.

In preparation for your appointment with your GP, you should, if possible:

- Document any reactions, including what foods were ingested, how much of each food was ingested, the type of reaction, how long the reaction lasted and any other important details such as medication administered. (See the sample food symptoms diary on page 21.)
- If you have a digital camera on hand, you might like to take a photo of any obvious symptoms.
- If your child's symptoms occurred after eating a packaged food, save and freeze a portion of the contents — this may be helpful for your

child's specialist in identifying the allergen. You should also save the labels of the food in question to bring along to the appointment.

- If your child's reaction occurred after eating a meal at a restaurant, call and ask to speak to the manager or owner. Explain that you need their help in knowing exactly what ingredients were used in your child's meal so you can help your doctor try to work out what your child may be allergic to.

- If you are unsure if there is a history of allergic disease in your family, for example, asthma, eczema, hayfever, you might like to call grandparents or other close relatives to check prior to the appointment.

Food symptoms diary

It can be helpful to keep a food and symptoms diary while you are waiting to see your doctor. In this diary, you would record all of the food and drinks your child consumed over a 2-week period and any suspected reaction. See the following page as an example. However, it cannot be emphasised too strongly that if your child has an immediate reaction to a food, you must remove it from your child's diet and consult your GP or allergy specialist immediately.

	Food	Symptom and the time of onset	Medication or treatment required
Date			
Breakfast	Plain wheat toast with margarine and Vegemite Glass of cow's milk	Well	
Lunch	Egg and lettuce sandwich on brown bread with butter Glass of cow's milk	Hives around the mouth and swelling of the lips within 5 minutes of tasting. Spat food out of mouth and refused to eat any more after small taste.	Antihistamine given and called our GP. Swelling and hives disappeared within 30 minutes of antihistamine. GP advised to remove egg from diet until specialist appointment. (Has tolerated milk and same bread on sandwich before, but this was first taste of egg.)
Dinner	Small portion of white fish, potato, carrot, peas Fruit salad: apple, pear, watermelon	Well	
Snacks	Glass of orange juice Plain potato chips Vanilla dairy yoghurt Rice cakes with avocado	Well Well Well Well	

Visiting your GP about suspected food allergy

When you visit your GP, he or she may conduct a physical examination of your child and will take a detailed history, asking you a wide range of questions that will probably overlap with questions an allergy specialist may also ask you. (See questions listed on page 25.)

If your GP suspects food allergy, he or she may refer your child to an allergy specialist for consultation and a clinical diagnosis. If you are geographically isolated from an allergy specialist, your GP may ask your child to take a blood test to screen for food allergens (see page 43) or may refer you to a paediatrician or dermatologist with experience in the area of food allergy.

To see a paediatrician, dermatologist or allergy specialist, a referral is essential. A referral from a GP is valid for 12 months and a referral from a specialist is only valid for 3 months. This is important to remember because the waiting list to see an allergy specialist can be lengthy, so ensure your referral is current. It is also worth knowing that some specialist allergy clinics require a referral from a specialist such as a paediatrician as opposed to a GP, so when you make an appointment with your allergy specialist, be sure to check what kind of referral you need.

Be prepared to be wrong

One of the most helpful things to bring with you to your child's appointments with a GP and allergy specialist is an open mind. No matter how convinced you are that your child is allergic to a specific food, be prepared to accept that you might be wrong.

For example, if your child displayed symptoms of an allergic reaction after a bite of a peanut butter sandwich, you may be convinced your child has developed a peanut allergy. Perhaps your child has eaten peanut butter before without any problem but this time their sandwich was made on a different bread, one topped with sesame seeds, and it may be the seed on the bread to which your child has reacted. Or perhaps your child consumed something after the sandwich, but you are convinced peanut is the problem, so you haven't worried about writing down everything else your child ate or drank prior to the reaction.

Of course, in this example a child may indeed be allergic to peanut, but the point is, you should write down *everything* your child has consumed prior to a reaction, without personal bias.

The best way to ensure an accurate diagnosis is to provide your doctor with all of the facts surrounding your child's suspected allergic reaction.

Eczema (atopic dermatitis)

Eczema, or atopic dermatitis, is an inherent condition of the skin (eczema is not just a manifestation of allergy) that may be associated with allergies. The skin is dry, with a tendency to become itchy, red and bumpy (spotty in appearance), and using soaps will make the skin even drier. When a child scratches at their eczema, the skin releases chemicals that make the skin feel itchy, so the more a child scratches, the itchier they feel. Scratching can lead to the skin cracking and bleeding, resulting in infection.

Eczema is often the first presentation of allergic disease in a child, usually appearing at around 3–4 months of age. Nevertheless, only 40 per cent of moderate-to-severe eczema is associated with food allergy. Don't lose sight of the fact that food allergy is not the cause of eczema but it may trigger eczema in some people. Other allergies, such as house dustmite, may contribute, and the skin may also be more sensitive to irritants, such as synthetic clothes and heat.

If your child has eczema, visit your GP as a starting point. It is helpful to be able to tell the doctor which foods (if any) trigger your child's symptoms and how soon after your child eats the particular food the symptoms occur. Consider keeping a food

continued

symptoms diary (see pages 20 and 21). Keeping a food symptoms diary is also very helpful if you are breastfeeding and feel your diet might be affecting your baby's skin.

If food is thought to trigger your child's eczema, removing foods from your child's diet must be carefully discussed with your doctor because there may be a risk of malnourishment or the development of more serious food allergies once the intolerance to that food is outgrown. Often, removing foods does not clear the eczema completely, and other measures will be needed.

Treatments for eczema include not bathing with soap, adequate moisturising, steroid creams and ointments as well as other medications. Discuss treatment options with your doctor.

If your child has eczema and your GP suspects food allergy, your child needs to be referred to an allergy specialist for review and testing. Bear in mind, however, that it is not always possible to confirm any or all of the triggers of your child's eczema.

Finding an allergy specialist

In Australia, 'allergy specialist' is a colloquial term for a clinician trained in diagnosing and managing allergies. Many allergy specialists have been trained in allergy and clinical immunology after their initial training as a paediatrician or physician.

The number of paediatric allergy specialists in Australia is limited (the waiting lists do vary greatly from state to state and it also depends on whether you are on a waiting list at a public clinic or seeing a specialist in private practice). A recommendation from your GP or paediatrician is usually your best bet for selecting an allergy specialist. You can also visit the website of the Australasian Society of Clinical Immunology and Allergy, which lists, state by state, the contact details of many allergy specialists in Australia: **www.allergy.org.au**

Note that there are *many* doctors in Australia who are

knowledgeable and experienced in managing food allergy, including GPs and paediatricians.

(For tips on Working with your allergy specialist, see pages 27–29.)

Visiting your allergy specialist about suspected food allergy

At the first visit, your allergy specialist will probably spend a lot of time taking down a detailed history of your child's suspected allergic reaction as well as their overall health. Questions your allergy specialist might ask you include:

- Can you describe the suspected allergic reaction?
- How long did the reaction last?
- Did you give your child any medication and, if so, what was it and in what dosage?
- What food or foods were ingested prior to your child's reaction?
- How much time was there in between your child consuming a food and the reaction taking place?
- How much of each food was ingested?
- Is there a history of asthma or allergies in your family?
- Where was your child when the reaction took place?
- Is it possible your child was stung by an insect just prior to the reaction?
- Did your child exercise after eating?
- Was your child on any medication when the reaction occurred?
- Expect questions about your child's general health, too, for example: Does your child have any chronic medical conditions? Does your child take any regular medications?

After your child's specialist has taken a detailed history, they may conduct a physical examination — including weighing and measuring your child, listening to their chest, looking in their ears and nose, and closely examining any skin conditions.

If your allergy specialist considers that food allergy is likely, a diagnostic test will probably be the next step, usually in the form of a skin prick test or a blood test. The results of your child's skin or blood test, combined with your child's medical history, is the information your specialist will use to formally diagnose your child with food allergy. From a doctor's perspective, your child's medical history is of the utmost importance, and a skin or blood test will only be used to help confirm your doctor's suspicions.

If a skin prick test is ordered, it is often done as part of the initial consultation, typically by a doctor or specially trained nurse or technician, with the results available immediately afterwards. If a blood test is ordered, your child will probably be required to visit a pathology collection centre, and the results will not be available until they have been processed by a pathology lab. If your child's skin or blood test is negative to a suspected food allergen, but your specialist still suspects your child has a food allergy, a medically supervised food challenge may be the next step (see pages 46–51 for more information).

Allergy testing is a subject of concern for most parents of food-allergic children, not just the newly diagnosed. Misunderstanding often surrounds allergy testing and what the results may or may not mean, so we have devoted Chapter 3 to the ins and outs of allergy testing, while Chapter 4 moves on to dealing with a positive diagnosis.

'My husband and I were devastated when Amelia was diagnosed [with food allergies]. We both love eating! We knew Amelia wouldn't be able to share in what we really enjoy. And also the risk to her; that this could be potentially fatal. When I was in year 12 on a school camp, a girl died of peanut allergy, so I had a very clear understanding of what could happen and how dangerous allergies can be. The reality of everyday practicality was, "Oh no", but then the advantage we could see was that, with education, it was something that could be managed.'

—Anne Frisby (Vic), mother of Amelia (6),
allergic to egg, milk and peanut,
and Hugh (4), allergic to egg and peanut

'When you discover that your child has a food allergy with the potential risk of anaphylaxis, it is a frightening and confusing time. What will we feed her? Can we still eat out socially with friends? What about other children around her as a toddler eating the very foods she is allergic to? Little children touch each other all the time and they also tend to put everything into their mouths. How will we keep her safe? What about school? When she was first diagnosed, we didn't have any friends or family with the same condition. There was no history of food allergy in the family. Why did this happen to us?'

—Jodie Bellchambers (WA), mother of Kate (9),
allergic to peanut (and previously egg)

Working with your allergy specialist

Successful doctor–patient relationships are two-way and, like any relationship in life, they often take time to develop to a level where you are comfortable. Preparing for appointments with your allergy specialist can make a big difference to the outcome: how many times have you walked out of a consult with any doctor and then remembered all the things you should have raised? The following suggestions are offered to help you make the most of your relationship with your allergy specialist.

- Prepare and prioritise questions in advance, writing them down and keeping them succinct.
- Time your questions appropriately; for example, if you are concerned about introducing a particular food into your child's diet, mention this before the skin prick test or blood test.
- If you are particularly anxious about something, be sure to raise it with your specialist early in the appointment. For example, have you been told any scary stories about food

continued

allergy? Have you read something in the press that concerned you? If you hear something that doesn't fit with what you understand about your child's allergy, make sure you bring it up at the consultation because the medical research might have changed, or it may be that it doesn't apply to your child.

- If your child has experienced reactions, try to ensure that the parent or carer who witnessed the reaction is present at the appointment to answer any questions the doctor might have.

- If you took a digital photo of the reaction, take that along to the appointment with you.

- When communicating your child's history, try to be as direct as possible and don't over-dramatise or exaggerate symptoms.

- If you have other children, try to arrange for them to be cared for by a friend or relative while you attend the appointment.

- If you have a very young child, try to attend the appointment with an extra adult so they can take the child outside to play while you talk to the doctor. Involving another adult on an ongoing basis can also help with coping with the responsibility of managing an allergy later.

- Ask for any references, written material or websites your doctor can refer you to for further information.

- Many specialists have wonderful nurses who are happy to field follow-up calls and questions from patients. If a question is outside their area of expertise, they will ask the doctor and get back to you. Ask your doctor who you can contact if you have follow-up questions.

- Remember that your appointment with an allergy specialist is to focus on your child's allergy and related health problems. While your doctor will take an interest in the general health of your child as a whole, other health issues are best reviewed by your child's paediatrician or GP.

- If you have more than one child who needs to be reviewed by your allergy specialist, be sure to make appointments for each child so that adequate time is allocated.
- Always be up front. For example, if you have inadvertently given your child a food to which they are allergic and they have had a reaction, tell your doctor — they really need to know. You certainly won't be the first parent to have made a mistake — and you won't be the last.

3

Food-allergy testing

When parents of food-allergic children get together, food-allergy testing is often discussed at length: what kind of test their child has, how their child copes with the test, and the test results. While it can be reassuring to discuss the experience of food-allergy testing with other parents, trying to compare results usually ends in confusion and can be the source of misinformation. Why? Because food-allergy tests always need to be interpreted by an allergy specialist within the context of your child's unique medical history. Food-allergy tests are less than perfect: they do not provide black-and-white answers, only useful information to help your doctor confirm a diagnosis of food allergy.

While the emotions and outcomes of food-allergy testing will be different for every family, the purpose of this chapter is to help you set realistic expectations of specific food-allergy tests. It will cover their purpose, explain how food-allergy test results are interpreted, suggest ways to prepare your child for food-allergy tests, give an overview of what's involved in a food challenge, and provide a word of warning about unconventional food-allergy testing techniques.

Of course, allergy testing practices vary from clinic to clinic and methods can change over time. Never hesitate to raise any questions or concerns you have about allergy testing with your doctor to receive advice specific to your child.

Diagnostic tests and food challenges

Food-allergy testing provides useful information for your doctor to help diagnose and manage IgE-mediated food allergies. The two diagnostic tests most commonly used in Australia are:

- Skin prick testing
- RAST blood test

Skin prick testing, as the name suggests, involves testing on the skin, while RAST involves testing blood. Skin prick testing and RAST are used in conjunction with a child's clinical history as a predictive *indicator* of food allergy — that is, your doctor will use either (and sometimes both) of these tests to assess how *likely* it is your child is allergic to a particular food, but neither test is 100 per cent accurate in predicting whether your child will experience symptoms after eating that food. The only way to be 100 per cent sure that your child is truly allergic to a food is by undergoing a food challenge. Both of the diagnostic tests will be explained in detail in the following pages, followed by an overview of food challenges.

Skin prick testing

What happens in a skin prick test

In a skin prick test, your doctor is trying to establish if your child produces IgE antibodies against a specific food protein — or, in other words, if your child is 'sensitised' to a particular food.

The way the test is conducted will vary from clinic to clinic, but below is a general outline of what you might expect to happen when you take your child to be tested.

- You and your child will be seated in a testing room or area of the clinic.
- The allergen extracts (or, in some cases, fresh foods) your doctor has ordered to be tested will be laid out on a tray ready for the test. If your child has had a reaction to a particular food, it will certainly be selected for the test. If there is no clear history but a suspicion of food allergy, the most common foods to which children react might be selected, for example, egg, cow's milk, wheat, peanut, soy — often more. If there are particular foods your family eats which you are concerned about, for example, shellfish, you should mention this to your doctor before the test. (See pages 33 and 34 for more on allergen extracts and fresh foods used in testing.)

- Skin prick tests are well tolerated by most children. The test causes minimal discomfort.
- The practitioner will choose an area of skin on the body that is suitable for testing. This is usually the inside of the forearm, leg or back. Different clinics have different preferences. The site chosen has to be clear of eczema or rashes and needs to be big enough to cover the site of the test.
- Some practitioners use a marker to write numbers directly on a child's skin to identify the allergens being tested. Other practitioners have allergens arranged in a particular order on their testing tray and this corresponds with the order in which the allergens are placed on the skin. The method varies depending on the clinic.
- Babies and young children need to be held securely by a parent or carer in a position where the practitioner can easily access the testing site.
- The skin may be cleaned with an alcohol swab (although not all practices do this as alcohol can be an irritant).
- A drop of each allergen extract is then placed onto the test site, along with a positive and negative control. (See 'Positive and negative controls: what are they?', page 35.)
- Using a sterile lancet or pricking device, the skin is lightly pricked and scratched in the centre of each drop to allow a tiny amount of the allergen to enter the skin. There are no needles involved and usually the prick doesn't draw blood — if it does, it is only a very tiny amount. The allergen drops are then carefully blotted to stop them from running into each other.
- The area is left for approximately 15 minutes (again, the time period may vary from clinic to clinic) before the results will be recorded. During this time it is essential that your child does not touch or scratch the site. Scratching can cause a local release of histamine to the skin, affecting the results of the test.

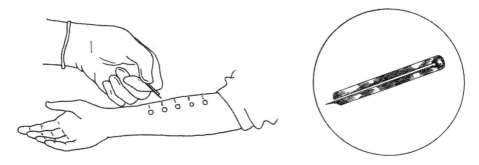

Skin prick tests can be performed on any area of suitable skin, but are commonly performed on the inside of the forearm (above, left), leg or back. A lancet (above, right) is commonly used for skin prick testing in Australia.

Scratch or prick?

When talking about skin prick testing, some people say the child's skin is scratched, others say it is pricked. So which is it? Different doctors use different skin prick testing devices, but a lancet is one of the most commonly used instruments for skin prick testing in Australia. A lancet has a tiny curled tip on the end, so the person conducting the test is firstly pricking a little bit and then scratching. So while the test is officially known as a skin 'prick' test, it actually involves both scratching and pricking.

Allergen extracts: what are they?

Allergen extracts are commercially made. An extract is obtained by separating the protein component of a food (or other allergen) via a variety of manufacturing processes that produce a pure product, free of irritants. For example, peanut allergy is tested for with peanut proteins and egg white tested with egg albumen. The protein is mixed with liquid substances to stabilise it and keep it in its liquid form. Considerable effort is made to

continued

ensure that the same amount of allergen is present in each batch of allergen extracts.

Commercially prepared extracts are not available for all foods and, for those that are, some are particularly unstable in their extracted form, especially fruit, vegetables and tree nuts. In such cases, fresh foods are often used in skin prick tests. Fresh foods are also used if a child has had a reaction to a processed food. The first step might be to take a sample of that food, crush it and mix it with saline and then perform a skin prick test.

Measuring skin prick test results

After approximately 15 minutes, the practitioner conducting the test will look at your child's skin for a response to the allergens. If your child is sensitive to an allergen, a lump that looks like a mosquito bite will appear at the site. The reaction usually consists of two parts: the central lump, which is called a wheal, and the red area around the wheal, which is called the flare.

There are numerous methods for measuring results; again, it varies from clinic to clinic, but what every practitioner will be looking for is the size of the wheal in millimetres. Some practitioners draw a circle around the wheal with a biro and then place a strip of micropore tape over the top, which forms an impression of the wheal. The micropore tape is then removed and stuck onto a piece of paper, so the result can be measured with a ruler. Other practitioners place a ruler directly onto the child's skin to measure the result.

Two measurements are taken: each axis of the wheal at 90 degrees. For example, a measurement might be 6mm on the vertical axis and 3mm on the horizontal axis (that is, measuring the diameter of the wheal). When a doctor is assessing the results, he or she will average out these measurements: in our example, 6 + 3 = 9, which you divide by 2, so the result will be 4.5mm. This process is standardised for ease of comparison.

Some practitioners also look at the size of the flares, but most are only looking for the measurement of the wheal.

Positive and negative controls: what are they?

When undergoing a skin prick test, a positive and negative control will be placed on your child's skin. A drop of saline (salt water) is used for the negative control and a drop of histamine for the positive control.

The saline control should be negative (that is, no wheal and flare should develop) in everybody unless they have extremely reactive skin, which is known as dermatographism. If your child does test positive to the saline, the size of the wheal will be measured, and this measurement will then be subtracted from the size of any positive results to food extracts. For example, if your child's skin produces a 1mm wheal to the saline control and 5mm to peanut, your child's score for peanut will be recorded as 4mm. This system is used to take into account how your child's skin is reacting to an inert substance.

The histamine control should be positive (that is, it should produce a wheal and a flare), because the reaction the doctor is looking for is, in fact, a histamine response. If a wheal doesn't form, or it is very small, then it is possible that the child has some antihistamine onboard, often inadvertently through cold and flu medications. If this is the case, the reliability of the skin prick test is reduced and may need to be repeated at a later date.

Interpreting skin prick test results

Positive results

Interpreting skin prick test results is a tricky business — especially so when they are positive. While most medical literature regards a positive skin prick test result as 3mm above the saline control, 'positive' is quite a loose term.

A positive skin prick test result means your child is producing IgE against a specific food protein — so your child is 'sensitised' to the food in question. In practical terms, this means your child may have an allergic reaction if they eat this food, but not necessarily. Many children will test positive to foods they can eat safely. In the United States, one research study into peanut allergy has suggested that 95 per cent of individuals who are 'sensitised' to peanut — so they produce a positive skin prick test — are not allergic to peanut.[1]

So, what's the point of having a skin prick test, parents sometimes wonder? The point is that a skin prick test result on its own is usually not used to diagnose food allergy, but it is a very important piece in the puzzle your doctor is trying to put together. Your doctor will carefully review your child's clinical history in conjunction with the skin prick test result. If your child has presented with a suspected allergic reaction after eating a particular food, for example, peanut, a positive skin prick test to peanut may help your doctor confirm peanut allergy. Or, if your child has presented with a suspected allergic reaction to a food but you are uncertain of what the offending food might have been, a skin prick test may be the first step in helping to identify the culprit.

It is important to understand that results of a skin prick test can mean different things at different ages and to different allergens. For example, in the case of particular allergens, including peanut, egg and cow's milk, diagnostic cut-off measurements of skin prick test wheal diameters have been defined in medical literature that predict a positive food challenge with greater than 95 per cent accuracy.[2] This means that a skin prick test result over a certain size for these allergens at a certain age can help a doctor to assess, with great accuracy, whether or not it is advisable for your child to undergo a formal food challenge. (The interpretation of cut-off points is assessed on a clinic-by-clinic basis;[3] factors such as population, type of allergen extract used and testing techniques all come into play, so cut-off measurements are not included here.)

Generally speaking, though, skin prick test results are viewed in a spectrum: the larger the skin prick test result, the greater the *likelihood* your child is allergic to that food. But again, your child's history will always be taken into account. For example, in my son Noah's first skin prick test, at 6 months of age, he tested positive to cow's milk, egg, peanut and chicken. Noah's skin prick test scores for cow's milk, egg and peanut were considered to be at the upper end of the spectrum, and he had presented with clinical reactions to both cow's milk and egg, so our allergy specialist considered it highly likely Noah was allergic to cow's milk, egg and peanut. However, Noah's score to chicken was at the lowest end of the spectrum and, taking into account Noah's age and clinical history, our allergy specialist thought it was unlikely that Noah was allergic to chicken. A food challenge to chicken was prescribed when Noah was 12 months old and it was negative. So Noah was producing IgE antibodies to chicken, but he could eat it without any problem. This is sometimes referred to as a 'false positive'.

A 'false positive' can also occur due to cross-reactive proteins in foods. Sometimes the structure of a protein in one food is very similar to the structure of a protein in another food, especially if they are members of the same food family. For example, a peanut-allergic child may also test positive to one or many other foods in the legume family; for example, lentils. This test result might mean the child is also allergic to lentils, or it might mean the child's immune system is confusing lentil protein with peanut protein, because the structure of each is so similar. If this is the case, a doctor may suggest a food challenge (see page 46) to rule out lentil allergy.

Negative results

A negative result provides very helpful information for you and your doctor as it usually means your child can safely eat the food or foods in question. Statistically speaking, if your child records a negative skin prick test result to a certain food, it is highly unlikely they will have an allergic reaction to that food: the negative predictive accuracy of a skin prick test is greater than 95 per cent.[4] So-called 'false negative' results are uncommon.

However, as always, your child's clinical history needs to be considered. For example, if your child has experienced a recent suspected allergic reaction to a particular food but the skin prick test result for this food was negative, your doctor might request a RAST test (see pages 43 and 44) or food challenge (see pages 46–51) to confirm your child is not allergic.

Risks associated with skin prick testing

Skin prick testing is generally considered very safe. For the majority of children, a skin prick test involves some discomfort (as opposed to pain), hives and associated itchiness, and sometimes minor swelling. Often, the anticipation of a skin prick test is far worse than the event.

However, like many medical procedures, a skin prick test is not completely risk-free. Severe allergic reactions, although extremely uncommon, can occur. Statistically, the risk of anaphylaxis from skin prick testing is reported as being less than 0.02 per cent.[5] Some patients are considered at higher risk than others, including young children, patients with a history of anaphylaxis, a high degree of reactivity and/or uncontrolled asthma.[6] The risk is also considered greater if fresh food is being used for the test.[7] If your doctor believes a skin prick test does pose a potential risk for your child, a RAST test will usually be prescribed, where your child will not be directly exposed to any allergens.

Remember to keep all of this in perspective. Adverse reactions during a skin prick test are *extremely* rare, and tests are always conducted by specially trained practitioners.

The value of repeating skin prick tests over time

While skin prick testing is not infallible, it is an important tool in helping your doctor to monitor your child's allergies over time. For example, if your child had an allergic reaction to a particular food some time ago, and his or her skin prick test result is increasing over time, this information may help your doctor to determine that your child is still highly likely to react to this food. If the skin prick test result is decreasing in size to a very small number, your doctor may decide it is likely that your child has outgrown his or her allergy and arrange a supervised food challenge to confirm this suspicion. Regular review and follow-up skin prick testing is critical in monitoring your child's food allergies.

Size of skin prick test results related to severity of reaction

MYTH: The higher the skin prick test score the more likely your child is to have a severe reaction.

FACT: The size of your child's skin prick test score refers to the measurement of the lump in millimetres (the 'wheal size'). The size of your child's wheal correlates with the *likelihood* of your child reacting to a particular allergen, but not the *severity* of a reaction.

For example, if your child records a skin prick score of 3 to cow's milk, this lets your doctor know your child may have an allergic reaction to cow's milk. If your child's skin test to cow's milk is 15, your child's doctor will probably consider it very likely your child will react to cow's milk.

However, while the higher the skin prick test score, the more likely it is your child will react to the food in question, at present there is no conclusive evidence to suggest that higher skin prick test scores equate to a child experiencing more severe reactions or anaphylaxis.

Likewise, if a child has a small skin prick test result, it does not mean that they definitely will not have a severe reaction or anaphylaxis. At present, there is no test that can accurately predict if a child will or will not experience anaphylaxis.

When your child has a skin prick test, don't focus on the size of the reaction recorded against your child's allergens; in isolation, these scores mean very little at all. Instead, listen closely to your doctor's interpretation of your child's skin prick test and ensuing advice, and ask questions about anything you don't understand.

Fear of skin prick tests

Q I am taking my 3-year-old for his first skin prick test next week. He is very scared of doctors so I am quite anxious about how to prepare him for the test. Should I warn him in advance? If so, what should I tell him?

A Firstly, remember that skin prick tests are not meant to be painful. Uncomfortable, yes, but not painful, and most children tolerate the tests very well. With younger children, it is often their fear of the unknown that makes the test more difficult, along with trying to keep them still.

How parents handle this situation will very much depend on the personality and age of the child having the test. There is no formulaic advice that works for everyone; however, as soon as a child is old enough to understand, it can be a good idea to tell them something simple and gentle, such as, 'We are going to see a doctor today to talk about food allergies' or 'We are going to see a doctor today to try to find out what makes you so itchy and scratchy.'

Young children have very little concept of time, so it is probably pointless in forewarning them of the allergy test too far in advance. An hour or so before the test is probably plenty of notice for little ones. But again, you know your child best. When my son Noah was 2, we didn't tell him about the test until just beforehand, but at 3, we decided to tell him the night before, so he could ask questions.

When talking about the test specifically, it may be helpful to use the word 'scratch' instead of 'prick', and do not use the word 'needle' — because there aren't any involved. When children hear the word 'prick' or 'needle' they often associate it with their own not-too-fond memories of immunisation.

You might like to tell your child they will be having a test on their skin which will involve 'little scratches' or 'little ouches', they might feel a bit itchy and then it will be all over. Reassure your child that you will be with them during the test. You also might like to arrange something fun to do together after the test, so they have something to look forward to.

On Noah's last test, at age 3, the nurse drew a pussy cat on his hand and then told him she was going to draw more pussy cats on his back. She then put a drop of water on Noah's hand and explained she was also going to give all of the pussy cats on his back a drop of 'water' (allergen extract) to drink. She then explained to him that each pussy cat was going to have a tiny scratch and it would be all over very quickly. Her step-by-step approach helped Noah to stay calm and interested in the process; it wasn't until halfway through the scratches that he became upset, and by then it was only a matter of seconds until the test was over.

With toddlers and young children, producing a token gift from your bag can work wonders, especially if it is wrapped. Timing is important, though — don't produce the gift while the test is taking place and they have to keep still. Unwrapping a surprise can provide a welcome distraction while you have to keep your child from scratching or touching the test site for the 15 minutes before the results are read.

With slightly older children, a lollipop can also be a good distraction — most children cannot cry and lick a lollipop at the same time! Of course, you just need to make sure it is a type of lollipop your child has safely consumed before, and check the label before offering it to your child.

It's probably fair to say no child is going to enjoy a skin prick test, but they are over quickly, are not really painful and provide your doctor with important information to help with diagnosing and monitoring your child's food allergy.

Preparing for a skin prick test: what you need to know

- Children pick up on anxiety from their parents. Reassure yourself that this is a safe and relatively painless procedure. If you are calm, your child is likely to be so, too.
- Children need to stop taking antihistamines prior to their skin prick test. How long depends on the type of antihistamines. In most cases it is a minimum of 48 hours, but if the child has been taking regular and quite high doses of antihistamines it might need to be a longer timeframe — discuss this with your doctor. Antihistamine can interfere with the results of a skin prick test. The reaction the doctor is looking for on the skin is a histamine reaction. In a positive test, the allergen binds onto the mast cell and releases histamine to produce the wheal and flare. If a child is taking antihistamine it blocks the response.
- When a doctor advises that antihistamine cannot be taken, this means in any form. Most cold and flu medications contain antihistamine and these interfere with test results. If you are unsure of the contents of a medication, check with your pharmacist and/or doctor.
- It is important to note that if your child has an allergic reaction just prior to the skin prick test, you should not hesitate to give your child the required dose of antihistamine. Just call your doctor's office to see if the skin prick test needs to be rescheduled. Even in busy clinics with long wait times, the doctor will often still see you and your child and

may decide to perform the skin test at a later date.

- Most other drugs do not interfere with a skin prick test, but make a point of mentioning all medication your child has been taking to your doctor before the test.
- Your child does *not* need to stop taking asthma medications unless specifically instructed to do so by your specialist.
- If your child has experienced anaphylaxis, a skin prick test needs to be delayed until 4–6 weeks after the reaction.[8] This is because when anaphylaxis occurs, there is a huge activation of mast cells and a massive release of histamine. This means the histamine from the mast cells is depleted so there is a risk of a false negative result.
- Some potent topical steroid creams (for example, cortisone), especially when applied over a long period of time, can also affect results, but it will not impact on the skin to which the steroid has not been applied. This is one of the reasons doctors choose an area of skin to test where eczema and rashes are not present. Parents should not stop using steroid creams or ointments if they are needed, as a RAST (blood) test can be performed if there is no clear area of skin.
- It is best to avoid using moisturiser on the skin prior to the test because it can make the skin test run. While there is no formal medical recommendation not to use moisturisers, it is usually better not to put them on if possible.
- Try to arrange for other children to be minded while your child is being tested. Your child really will benefit from having your undivided attention. Also, the doctor will be giving you very important information when interpreting the test results, and ideally you should not be distracted.
- If your child is young, it is invaluable if you can bring along another adult to take your child into the waiting area to play after the test, while you discuss the test results with the doctor.
- The test is over very quickly, but plan ahead for the 15-minute window of time when your child is not allowed to touch the testing site. It is a good idea to bring along a quiet activity to distract your child during this time, for example, a book or small puzzle for a young child or an iPod or game for older children.

- Ask your doctor or clinic if they have a brochure or handout outlining any information you need to know about skin prick testing procedures specific to their clinic.

Treating hives and itching after a skin prick test

Q I am taking my 5-year-old daughter for her second skin prick test in a couple of weeks' time. When she had her last test, about 18 months ago, the hives lingered on her back for about a day and a half. She had quite a large reaction to a few foods, and the hives really did seem to bother her, as she couldn't reach to scratch them. How long should these hives last and should I buy any medications to have on hand to treat her hives (assuming she still tests positive)?

A How long the hives last will vary from patient to patient. Usually they disappear quickly, but sometimes they might still be present the next day in a much smaller way. The itchiness a child may experience during a positive reaction usually passes quickly and, in the majority of cases, the hives do not require any treatment at all; however, they do bother some children more than others. You might like to apply calamine lotion or an ice-pack initially, and if this isn't enough you can try a weak steroid ointment to make it more comfortable (ask your doctor or pharmacist for the appropriate strength for your child). If your daughter's skin is really itchy and uncomfortable, she can take an antihistamine. Talk to your doctor about which antihistamine to select and the appropriate dosage.

RAST blood test

What happens in a RAST

Blood testing for food allergy is via RAST testing. Like skin prick testing, a RAST is used to identify and measure the presence of IgE specific to different food allergens. There are two types of RAST. The newer CAP RAST test is now more common. Its results are quantitative, measured in units known as kU/L. The older test, still used by some, offers semi-quantitative results, recording scores such as 1^+, 2^+ and so on.

The way a RAST test is conducted can vary from doctor to doctor, but below is a general outline of what you might expect when you take your child for a test, and what happens to your child's blood during the test.

- Your doctor will usually ask you and your child to visit a pathology collection centre for a blood test. The doctor will write up a pathology request slip to take with you, on which he or she will specify which allergens they would like to be tested.
- A small amount of blood will be taken from a vein in your child's arm.
- The blood sample, along with the doctor's request slip, will be sent to a pathology laboratory.
- At the laboratory, the serum will be separated from the blood. The serum is the part of the blood that doesn't contain cells; this is where IgE floats around.
- The serum is then placed into a tray with lines of holes that have a cap disc (in the case of the CAP RAST test) containing particular allergens at the bottom of each hole.
- Then, in very simple terms, a labelled dye is placed on top of the serum.
- The test is looking to see if, firstly, the IgE is binding to a particular allergen, and secondly — if it is binding — it then quantifies how much.

Interpreting RAST results

The results of a RAST are usually available to your doctor in a week to 2 weeks' time (sometimes more); it varies depending on the pathology lab. You will need to schedule a follow-up appointment with your doctor to discuss your child's results.

As with the skin prick test, a RAST test is only useful in detecting the presence of IgE antibodies directed towards a particular allergen. Again, like skin prick tests, the results of a RAST, on their own, are of little value; they must be interpreted by your doctor in the context of your child's clinical history.

Generally speaking, the higher the RAST result, the more likely it is that your child is allergic to the food in question — but not always. Predictive decision cut-off points of food-specific IgE antibody concentrations in children have been established for four major allergens: egg, cow's milk, peanut and fish.[9] This means that if your child has a RAST result above a prescribed level to any of these foods, there is a 95 per cent chance your child is truly allergic to the food in question.

A RAST test is often prescribed by a GP to help you and your child avoid certain allergens until you can see an allergy specialist for review and formal diagnosis.

RAST or skin prick testing: what's right for your child?

Your allergy specialist will assess your child's clinical history before deciding which test to prescribe for your child. The skin prick test is generally considered more sensitive than a RAST test, and is more commonly used. Skin prick testing has the added advantages that results are available immediately, it only involves mild discomfort, and a wide range of allergens can be tested at once (not all food allergens can be tested using RAST). However, in some cases RAST testing is recommended over skin prick testing, including:

- When a child is unable to stop taking antihistamines or other medications that interfere with skin prick testing
- In the case of severe skin conditions, such as widespread eczema
- If a child has severely sensitive skin that welts on minor trauma (known as dermatographism)
- Although very unlikely, if a doctor considers there may be a high risk of a severe reaction, he or she may wish to perform a RAST test first
- Can be used following recent anaphylaxis
- When a patient is geographically isolated from skin prick testing facilities
- A GP (or any doctor) may order a RAST test if they cannot arrange for the child to see an allergy specialist within a short period of time

Misleading RAST result

Q My child is 8 and recently had his routine review RAST test for his egg allergy. To our delight, it came back negative. Our doctor booked our son in for a supervised food challenge at the hospital to confirm he had outgrown his egg allergy and, unfortunately, he developed a rash and started to vomit after being given a small amount. Why should my son bother having this blood test — which he hates — if the results are unreliable? I feel terrible putting him through this.

A So-called 'false negative' results are uncommon, but they do happen. Remember, both RAST and skin prick tests are used to help doctors assess the *likelihood* of a food allergy in conjunction with your child's clinical history, but the only real way to find out if a child is allergic to a particular food or not is to have them undergo a food challenge.

The doctor will use the results of your son's RAST tests over time, in conjunction with his clinical history, to decide when it might be appropriate to conduct a food challenge. Unfortunately, the outcome we long for is not always the one we get.

The tests currently available are not perfect but they are, in most cases, the source of extremely helpful information for your son's doctor. It is also important to note that a RAST or skin prick test is a 'snapshot' of what is happening in your child's body at the time the test is done. Results can be affected by various factors, including your son's health at the time of the test and, in the case of a RAST, the particular lab performing the test. Your son's next RAST may well be positive on subsequent testing; or your specialist may, if possible, recommend a skin prick test on your son's next appointment, as a skin prick test is generally considered more sensitive.

Ongoing allergy tests and review by your specialist are essential, not only in managing your son's allergy but also for accessing information about the latest treatments and research developments that may become available in the future.

Food challenges

What happens in a food challenge

A food challenge is prescribed by a doctor when they believe your child may have outgrown his or her allergy or to see if a food allergy is actually present. This may be because your child's skin prick test or RAST result was negative or has, over time, decreased to a very small size. Along with the test results, your doctor will also take into account the allergen in question, your child's age and clinical history. A food challenge may also be prescribed to confirm the diagnosis of a food allergy when skin prick test and/or RAST results or history of allergy are unclear.

As already explained, there is no test that can predict with 100 per cent accuracy whether or not your child has a food allergy; the only way to discover if your child is truly allergic to a food is by a formal food challenge. Doctors do not suggest children undergo food challenges lightly; they only do so when they believe there is a reasonable chance that your child no longer has the allergy or they need to identify what your child really is allergic to.

The way a food challenge is conducted may vary from clinic to clinic, but below is a general outline of what you might expect to happen when you take your child for a food challenge.

- A food challenge involves a child ingesting a particular food to work out whether or not they are allergic to it. The challenge typically takes place in a hospital setting. 'Hospital setting' can mean your child is admitted to the hospital for a day stay or the challenge may be done in an outpatients department. Either way, you will be with your child at all times during the test.
- Generally, specially trained nursing staff will conduct the food challenge and be responsible for closely observing your child, but a doctor will always be present in the department where the test is taking place.
- In most cases, your child will not be hooked up to any medical equipment during the test, but emergency medications and specialist staff are immediately available for treatment in the event that your child does have a reaction to the food being tested.
- Initially, your child will be offered a very small, accurately measured dose of the food being tested. The food being tested is often given to the child as an ingredient in a meal they usually enjoy eating; for example, a measured dose of cow's milk might be mixed with soy drink and served with your child's favourite cereal. In some cases, the practitioner might just touch the food against the cheek or lip of your child and look for any rashes or swelling before actually offering your child the food to eat.

- If there is no reaction following the first dose, the food will be offered every 20 minutes or so (times will vary at individual clinics) in increasing amounts over a number of hours until a full serve of the food in question has been consumed. During the food challenge, the practitioner will closely monitor your child for any reactions.
- If a sign of an allergic reaction occurs to the food being tested, the challenge will be stopped and your child will be given appropriate medical treatment (if needed).
- If your child consumes a full serve of the food without reaction, they will usually be asked to stay at the hospital for at least 2 hours after they have consumed the last dose, for continuing observation.

Preparing for a food challenge: what you need to know

- A food challenge takes hours, at a minimum. You should plan to set aside the whole day to spend with your child.
- Your child should be in good health for the test. Let your doctor know if your child is unwell or has recently been unwell.
- It is essential that you let your doctor know in advance if your child has been wheezing or has asthma. If this is the case, the challenge will more than likely be postponed.
- Children taking prescribed asthma prevention medication or nasal sprays should continue on their medication.
- Your child must not take antihistamines for at least 48 hours prior to the challenge (check the specific time limit with your clinic). Remember that antihistamine is found in many medications, especially cold and flu formulations. Always let your doctor know what medications your child is taking before the test. If your child needs to take antihistamine before the test, telephone your doctor or clinic and they will advise if the challenge has to be postponed.
- Parents should point out any rashes or skin conditions the child has before a food challenge, because this is one of the key symptoms practitioners will be looking for during the test.
- You will probably be asked to bring along a food your child regularly enjoys eating in which nursing staff can disguise the taste of the food being tested. For example, if peanut is being tested, you might take

some pasta with a red spaghetti sauce. What is important to remember is that it must be a food your child not only enjoys but has eaten safely before. For example, don't buy a different brand of pasta sauce on the day of the test or bring along any new foods. The clinic conducting the test will give you specific instructions and food suggestions relevant to your child's test.

- Some clinics request that only one parent or guardian attend the challenge, usually due to space restrictions, so check with your clinic before the test.

- Most clinics will request that no other children accompany you to the hospital on the day of the test. The child being tested may be anxious and really will need your undivided attention.

- Because the test is very time-consuming, it is a good idea to bring along fun activities to occupy your child — for example, books, iPods, games, puzzles, colouring — keeping in mind that space is likely to be limited.

- It is usually fine for your child to eat and drink prior to the test (providing you only offer them foods they have eaten safely before), but it is helpful if they are reasonably hungry for the test. Again, check with your clinic.

- Children are generally allowed to drink fluids during the test, but be careful young children do not drink too much. Sometimes young children can vomit if they gulp down big drinks, and then it is difficult to tell if the child is reacting to the food being tested or has just had too much juice too fast.

- Other food-allergic children will be undergoing food challenges in the clinic at the same time. If your child is being challenged to egg, for example, but is also allergic to peanut, another child close by may be undergoing a challenge to peanut. The clinics are well supervised and the challenge foods are kept separately, so it is not a problem, but it is helpful to know what to expect before you arrive.

- Some hospitals produce a brochure or hand-out of information you need to know about food challenge procedures specific to their clinic. Make sure you request a copy and review it well in advance of the day of the food challenge.

- Last, but not least, on the day of the test bring with you your child's EpiPen and any other medications they regularly use. You will not need them during the food challenge but, very occasionally, late reactions can occur on the way home. Generally, children are observed for at least 2 hours after the last dose of food, so a late reaction is highly unlikely to occur, but you must be prepared, just in case.

What happens after a food challenge

If your child did not experience a reaction to a food during a challenge, after they have been observed they will probably be sent home with instructions to keep a record of any subsequent reactions. Some clinics provide a diary for patients to fill in. Remember, a food challenge is designed to rule out immediate-type reactions, to make sure a child is not at risk of anaphylaxis. Subsequently, though, either due to allergy or an intolerance, your child might develop symptoms, including hives (urticaria), eczema or gastrointestinal symptoms. Usually a staff member from the clinic where your child has been tested will contact you a few days after the food challenge to find out if your child has experienced any symptoms at home.

Regardless of the result of the food challenge, a follow-up appointment with your child's allergy specialist is needed. In this appointment your specialist will discuss the results of your child's food challenge, give you advice relevant to your situation and also give you the opportunity to ask any questions and discuss any late reactions which occurred at home.

If your child does react during a challenge, they may be terribly disappointed. How a child is counselled largely depends on their age and the food involved. For example, in young children, if the food being tested was one where the allergy is commonly outgrown, you and your specialist can focus on the fact that they still might outgrow the allergy and, in the meantime, the results of the challenge are helping to keep them safe: 'And we'll cross our fingers that the result will be different next time.' If the allergen is one that is often lifelong — for example, peanut — and the child is old enough to understand, then the doctor may discuss medical research that is underway to cure peanut allergy. Often parents need to be counselled more than the child.

The most important outcomes to try to achieve in your follow-up appointment with your specialist are obtaining updated information to continue managing your child's allergy and a positive message about your child's allergy relevant to your situation.

Double-blind Placebo-controlled Food Challenge (DBPCFC) and Single-blind Placebo-controlled Food Challenge (SBPCFC)

While the previous pages have outlined the most common food challenge procedures used in Australia, you may also have heard of, or read about, the Double-blind Placebo-controlled Food Challenge (DBPCFC). This test is referred to frequently in medical literature and is considered the 'Gold Standard' in food-allergy testing.[10] The DBPCFC involves a series of meals being prepared and carefully coded by an independent practitioner or dietitian who will not be directly involved in the actual test. Some of the prepared meals will contain the disguised allergen in question and some will not (the 'placebo'). Neither the child being tested nor the practitioner conducting the test will know which meals contain the allergen and which meals do not (hence the term 'double-blind').

This technique is used to eliminate both practitioner and patient bias. For example, sometimes children — especially older children — can be so fearful about consuming the allergen in question that their anxiety can masquerade as an allergic reaction during a food challenge. In other words, the reaction to the food may be psychological rather than a true food-allergy reaction.

While the DBPCFC is the gold standard for food challenges, in Australia it is most commonly used in a research setting. It is a labour-intensive and expensive test. In most clinics, if a child is particularly scared of a food challenge, they will use a Single-blind

continued

Placebo-controlled Food Challenge (SBPCFC). This means that the practitioner conducting the test is aware of which meals contain the allergen and which are placebo, but the patient is not.

If a child has no reaction during either a DBPCFC or SBPCFC their doctor will follow up with an open challenge, which may be done in a hospital setting or, in some cases, at home. It is important your child can know what they are eating and not have a reaction, be it physical or psychological.

Unconventional allergy tests and treatments

Many parents turn to complementary medicine and resort to unproven or unconventional allergy tests and treatments in the hope that trying something different might just cure their child's food allergy. While the motivation behind such a search is admirable, the results can be dangerous. It is important to understand that allergy is a science-based specialty, and any test or treatment applied to your child should be evidence-based. If you see an advertisement for a 'miracle cure' for your child's food allergy, tempting as it may be, remember the old adage that if an offer sounds too good to be true, it probably is.

It is essential that you receive an accurate science-based diagnosis of food allergy for your child, correct information on managing your child's food allergy and, if your child is at risk of anaphylaxis, emergency medications and a signed Action Plan. Important dietary advice to help your child avoid their allergens and ensure they are receiving adequate nutrition is also needed.

Unproven tests for IgE-mediated food allergy include: cytotoxic testing; oral provocation and neutralisation; vega testing; kinesiology; radionics; iridology; pulse testing; hair analysis; tests for dysbiosis; VioceBio.[11]

If you are considering an unconventional allergy test or treatment for your child, you should note that currently there are no Australian government regulations surrounding any unproven claims made in regard to such tests and treatments — it is a case of buyer beware. The Australasian Society of Clinical Immunology and Allergy (ASCIA) suggests you consider asking your prospective practitioner the following questions[12] before making any decisions:

- What is the evidence it works?
- Has such evidence been published?
- If so, where? And who reviews the publication?
- What are the risks and benefits?
- What might happen if I do not undertake this form of treatment?
- How much does it cost?
- Are there any side effects?
- What are the qualifications of the practitioner recommending the treatment?
- Why doesn't my own doctor suggest this type of treatment?
- Why can this one test or treatment detect or treat so many different problems?
- Why don't I get any Medicare (Australia) rebate for this type of test or treatment?

If you do decide to try an unconventional allergy test or treatment, it is advisable to see a clinical immunologist as well, for all the reasons outlined above.

You can read further information in regard to specific unproven allergy testing and treatments at the ASCIA website: **www.allergy.org.au/content/view/322/271/**

4

Dealing with a positive diagnosis

Hearing the news from your doctor that your child has a food allergy can be overwhelming. Some parents are disappointed, some frightened; others simply take it in their stride, relieved to finally have an explanation for their child's symptoms.

Many parents who were interviewed for this book reported feeling quite lost at the appointment when their child was initially diagnosed. They described how while their doctor was explaining the condition, they experienced information overload — often on top of trying to keep a young child still after a skin prick test. It wasn't until days after the diagnosis that they started to ask questions and really want information.

This chapter has been written for parents of children recently diagnosed with food allergy or those who are anticipating a positive diagnosis. In the first part of this chapter, we run through what your doctor may discuss with you if a diagnosis of food allergy is positive. In the second part, we arm you with some practical tips you can adopt immediately to help you manage your child's food allergies. Importantly, at the end of the chapter, we include some inspiring words of wisdom from parents who are already successfully managing childhood food allergies.

What happens if the diagnosis is positive?

At present, there is no cure for food allergy — strict avoidance of your child's allergen is the only way to prevent an allergic reaction. As such, the current approach to managing food allergies is based on three main principles:[1]

1. Knowing how to identify your child's allergen and avoid exposure
2. Knowing how to recognise the early symptoms of an allergic reaction
3. Knowing what to do when an allergic reaction happens

If your doctor or allergy specialist diagnoses your child with food allergy, they will offer advice and prescribe medications *specific* to your child's condition. In general, however, you can expect the following issues to be discussed:

- How to recognise symptoms of an allergic reaction and what to do in an emergency.
- Not all children with food allergy are prescribed an EpiPen — an auto-injector device preloaded with a measured dose of adrenaline, the first-line treatment for anaphylaxis — it will depend on a variety of factors, including your child's clinical history and the allergen in question. If your child is prescribed an EpiPen, your doctor will provide you with a signed Action Plan for anaphylaxis, a prescription for EpiPens and any other medications specific to your child's diagnosis. (See page 371 for a copy of an Action Plan for anaphylaxis.)
- Education on when and how to use an EpiPen (if prescribed) and any other prescribed medications.
- If your child is not prescribed an EpiPen, your specialist may provide you with an Action Plan for allergic reactions. (See page 372 for a copy of an Action Plan for allergic reactions.)
- Allergen avoidance measures to prevent your child from being exposed to their diagnosed food allergen, including advice about 'hidden' sources of an allergen (for example, milk as an ingredient in a biscuit), and an explanation of 'cross-contamination' (for example, the importance of using clean utensils and work surfaces to prepare your child's food).
- Diet, including recommending substitutes for particular foods that may need to be eliminated from your child's diet. Your allergy specialist may refer you to a paediatric dietitian, especially if your child has been diagnosed with multiple food allergies and/or you need advice about eating behaviour. (See Chapter 7, Feeding your food-allergic child, page 122.)

- The importance of educating others involved in your child's life.
- Any other health issues relevant to your child's food allergies, for example, asthma prevention and treatment, eczema prevention and treatment, controlling environmental allergens, such as dust mites.
- Depending on your child's allergen, your specialist may discuss the likelihood of your child eventually outgrowing his or her allergy.
- Your allergy specialist will also advise when you should bring your child back for review.

Help! Now I know my child has a food allergy

The anxiety that many parents of newly diagnosed food-allergic children experience usually relates to a combination of both practical and emotional concerns. Below we will look at ways of addressing immediate practical concerns, while emotional concerns are dealt with in detail in Chapters 15, 16 and 17 (see pages 306–348).

Practical concerns

Immediate practical concerns for families of the newly diagnosed often centre around questions such as: How will I keep my child safe? What do I feed my child? Will I remember when and how to use their medications? How do we eat out? How do I start the process of educating friends, families and carers?

In the beginning, it can feel like there is so much to learn that you don't quite know where to start. Following is a list of 20 things you can consider doing immediately to help you become 'allergy aware' and boost your confidence in your ability to keep your child safe. This list could easily consist of hundreds of ideas — and the process of learning never ends — but it is hoped these initial 20 tips might offer a positive and manageable *starting point* at a time when you are seeking direction. The more you learn about food allergy over time, the easier it will become to manage your child's food allergies.

The first 15 tips are relevant to all children with food allergy, while tips 16–20 are only relevant to children who have been prescribed an EpiPen. The following list is offered as a helpful guide only. You should always consult your child's allergy specialist for personal advice and care.

20 practical tips for parents of children recently diagnosed with food allergies

1. **Focus on the positives**

   Remember that children with food allergy can enjoy normal lives. Food allergy can be a serious medical condition but one which can be managed through education and training.

2. **Ensure you have relevant documentation and medications on hand at all times**

   Purchase all prescribed medications immediately, for example, antihistamine and EpiPens. If your child is prescribed an EpiPen, keep a copy of your child's Action Plan for anaphylaxis with their EpiPen at all times. If your child is given an Action Plan for allergic reactions, be sure to carry this with any medications your doctor has prescribed. Also remember to carry and continue any of your child's other regular medical treatments, for example, asthma medications.

3. **Learn the signs and symptoms of an allergic reaction and know what to do in the event of an allergic reaction**

   The signs and symptoms of an allergic reaction are listed on page 18 of this book. They are also listed on the Action Plan for allergic reactions (see page 372) and the Action Plan for anaphylaxis (see page 371). If you have any doubts about how to recognise any of the signs or symptoms of an allergic reaction, ask your GP or allergy specialist to explain them to you.

4. **Display your Action Plan for an allergic reaction or anaphylaxis where it can easily be accessed in an emergency**

   For example, put it up on the fridge or near your telephone. If you have an older child who may feel self-conscious about the poster being on full display, then perhaps tape it inside a pantry door or somewhere else more discreet but readily accessible. Don't forget to make copies of your Action Plan: keep one with your child's medications at all times, one at your child's school, and place a copy anywhere else where your child is left in the care of others.

5. **Communicate your child's allergy to childcare, school and anywhere else your child is in the care of others**

   If your child attends childcare or school, make an appointment with the centre manager, principal and teachers to explain your child's allergy and discuss how your child's food allergy will need to be managed. At this meeting, provide the centre or school with an Action Plan and prescribed medications. Ensure staff know how to recognise the signs and symptoms of an allergic reaction and what to do in an emergency. (More information on working with childcare centres, pre-schools and schools can be found in Chapters 11 and 12, pages 214–264.)

6. **Allocate time to learn more about food allergy**

   In the beginning, you might like to set aside an hour a week to devote to educating yourself and others about your child's food allergy. Consider watching an educational DVD, reading books, experimenting with new recipes that are safe for your child, reading food labels, attending a training course or downloading information from recommended websites. Often, allergy specialists and allergy clinics have their own website or brochures about food allergy. Be careful to visit websites recommended by your doctor, as random web searches can lead to misinformation at a time when you really need the facts.

7. **Join education and support group Anaphylaxis Australia (www.allergyfacts.org.au)**

   Anaphylaxis Australia offers regular printed newsletters packed with positive information on living with food allergies and can help you get in touch with other families in similar situations. They also have a great range of educational resources available, such as reference books, cookbooks, brochures, DVDs, information cards and more. Your child does not need to have experienced anaphylaxis to join Anaphylaxis Australia. (Also see page 326.)

8. **Talk to your child about their food allergy**

   If your child is old enough to understand, be sure to set aside some quiet time after the diagnosis, when you are feeling calm and positive, to explain to your child what their allergy is and, importantly, what your family will do to keep them safe. Consider borrowing or purchasing educational products relevant to your child's age and allergy. Children's storybooks about food allergy, aimed at children aged 3–9, can be purchased at **www.allergyfacts.org.au**

9. **Educate your child about their food allergy**

   Encourage your child to take age-appropriate responsibility for their allergy; involve your child in the process of learning. For example, remind toddlers not to share food and regularly reinforce this message. Show young children pictures of what their allergen looks like. Older children can be encouraged to help remember their medications and always ask if a food is safe for them to eat.

10. **Minimise the risks in your own home**

    Think about any changes you may need to make in your home to avoid accidental exposure to your child's allergen. For example, if your child is very young and allergic to peanut, you might want to consider removing all loose nut products from the house. If you choose to keep other nut-containing products in the house, you should move them to a cupboard young children cannot access.

    If you have a child with cow's milk allergy, be sure to label their bottle or cup clearly so it is never mixed up with another child's bottle or cup at home or on a play date.

    Think about how you organise your fridge and pantry. If your child is allergic to eggs but you still want to keep eggs in the house, store them on the bottom shelf of the fridge and your child's foods on the top shelf, to avoid cross-contamination. If you are storing any meals for your child in the fridge or freezer, clearly label them — especially when you have guests in the house. When I freeze foods for Noah, I label containers as being 'Safe for Noah' or put a red label on anything that isn't safe with the words: 'Not safe: Do not feed to Noah'. Last year our daughter became very ill all of a sudden. I took her to the emergency department and from there she was admitted to hospital for 2 weeks, and I couldn't leave her side. Knowing I had Noah's foods clearly labelled in the fridge at home gave me comfort that the grandparents caring for Noah would not make a mistake in feeding him in my absence.

    At our house, we have a 'Noah cupboard', where we keep only labelled foods that are safe for Noah. Because he is still young and has multiple allergies, this system works well for us, and it normalises eating for Noah because he can go to the cupboard and choose what he wants to eat. Having a cupboard full of safe foods shifts the focus to what he can eat rather than always having to say, 'No, that's not safe' — which we have to do frequently when we are away from home. Noah still knows to check with an adult before eating any foods, and when he is older we will teach him how to read labels, but for now it is a great system for our family. Come up with a system that works for your household and stick to it.

11. **Learn how to read labels**

Make it a habit to read every label of every food you buy for your child every time you buy it. Also check the labels of any medicines and skin-care products, which can also contain food allergens. Chapter 8, Understanding food labelling, page 146 will help you learn more about interpreting food labels. If you are ever in doubt that a food is safe, do not give it to your child.

12. **Always carry safe food you know your child likes**

Whenever you leave home, make sure you have safe food your child likes tucked into your bag. If you are caught out without safe food on hand, you may be more likely to risk buying a non-labelled food item for your child to try. There are now many cookbooks available packed with allergy-friendly recipes (see Appendix I, page 370 for some titles) and, depending on what your child is allergic to, there are some local food manufacturers who make products free from some of the most common allergens. Freeze safe treats such as muffins and cakes to have on hand so you can throw them into your bag for last-minute play dates or pull out and thaw if unexpected visitors arrive.

13. **If you are eating out, plan ahead**

It is a good idea to phone a restaurant ahead of time and see if there is anything safe for your child to eat. Always alert staff to your child's allergy and ask them direct questions about whether a meal you want to order contains a specific allergen. For example, do not ask what is in a certain meal but rather: Are there peanuts or tree nuts in this dish? Can you prepare this meal with clean utensils and away from any nut ingredients? If staff are dismissive or do not take your requests seriously, do not order a meal for your child. (Further information can be found in Chapter 9, Eating out with food allergy, page 180.)

14. **Be a positive role model**

Remember that the way you respond to your child's allergy is the way others will respond, too. If you are anxious and nervous, others may be, too. Try to be a positive role model. Offer bite-size pieces of information as a starting point and let others know how they can help, for example, by not sharing food with your child and learning the symptoms of an allergic reaction.

15. **Follow up with your allergy specialist for regular review**

Mark the date on the calendar when you need to make your next appointment and make it a priority.

16. **Always keep your EpiPen(s) in the same place**

Decide where you are going to keep your EpiPens and let everyone in your family and anyone who cares for your child know. If you have young children, be sure to keep all medications out of their reach, but never in a locked cupboard. You might choose to keep one EpiPen in a set place in the house and another in a bag you always take when you leave the house. Work out your own system, inform everyone who needs to know about it and then stick to it.

17. **Work out a system to help you remember to never leave home without your EpiPen**

For example, in the beginning, you might want to stick a reminder note on the inside of your front door or somewhere else obvious. (I found this really helpful when Noah was first diagnosed, not only for me, but also my husband, who only had to worry about the EpiPen on weekend outings, as he was at work during the week.)

18. **Ensure you are confident you can use an EpiPen in an emergency**

If you live in or near a major capital city, some allergy clinics run anaphylaxis training courses, including demonstrations of how to use an EpiPen. Consider purchasing an EpiPen trainer: a training device that functions like a real EpiPen but does not contain a needle or adrenaline (for more information see page 84). Training pens are available for purchase at **www.allergyfacts.org.au**, as is a DVD showing how to use an EpiPen. If you know a friend with food allergy, ask if you can have their next expired EpiPen so you can practise using it on an orange. Do everything you can to ensure you are completely confident that you know when and how to use an EpiPen in an emergency.

19. Know when your EpiPens expire

Mark on your calendar or in your diary when your child's EpiPens expire. You can also join the EpiClub, a free patient support program that will send you a reminder notice prior to your EpiPen expiring. Learn more at: **www.epiclub.com.au**

20. Consider purchasing some form of medical alert disc or tag

If your child has experienced anaphylaxis or is at risk of anaphylaxis, consider ordering some form of medical alert disc or tag.

● A MedicAlert brand tag enables medical emergency personnel to immediately access personalised medical information about your child. Your child's allergens are also engraved on the disc, which is a great visual reminder for others who care for your child. Learn more at: **www.medicalert.com.au**

● Other brands of medical alert tags can also be purchased from pharmacies and other providers. They are often a very affordable option.

Words of wisdom for the newly diagnosed

All of the parents interviewed for this book have been successfully managing their child's food allergies for years, but none have forgotten how hard it was in the early days of their child's diagnosis, when they had very little information or support.

These parents were asked what words of wisdom they would offer to a friend whose child had just been diagnosed with food allergies. Following is a selection of their answers. It is hoped that words of wisdom from parents who have already been down the path you are about to tread will offer some comfort and positive reinforcement that, while you will need to change aspects of the way your family lives, food allergies can be positively managed. (Most of the parents interviewed for this book have two or more children. However, due to space constraints, we have only named their food-allergic children. If you are new to food allergy, it may be reassuring to know that having a child with food allergy doesn't mean that any other children you might have are destined also to be food-allergic.)

'They just have to go through life slightly adjusted — and when you think about it, most of us have to go through life slightly adjusted for any number of reasons. For our children, food allergy is one of their reasons.'

—Jill Ahmed (SA), mother of Shana (15),
allergic to peanut and tree nuts, and Alisa (13),
allergic to peanut, tree nuts, honey and kiwi fruit

'I guess kids with any issue — any chronic condition — they develop a resilience, but as parents we worry terribly that they are missing out. In many respects, they develop far more social skills, far greater confidence and resilience because of what they have to deal with. I'd give anything for our son not to have to deal with his allergy, but he does deal with it and it makes him a very confident young man.'

—Barbara (NSW), mother of a 19-year-old son
who is allergic to cow's milk

'You may be overwhelmed at first and think there is nothing you can safely feed your child but you will find the right products. Lean on other parents in a similar situation and learn from them. Different people can come up with novel ways of doing things.'

—Angela Batten (Vic), mother of Emily (10),
allergic to peanut and tree nuts

'It will get better. When you first find out your child has a food allergy, that is the hardest bit — learning what to avoid — but it does get easier. Keep reminding yourself that there is nothing wrong with your child. These are normal, happy kids who just can't eat certain foods. Avoidance is the key. They can still do anything and become anything they want to be, they just can't eat certain foods. Be positive.'

—Jodie Bellchambers (WA), mother of Kate (9),
allergic to peanut (and previously egg)

'You will still have a life; you will make it work. You have to accept it and then re-jig your life to accommodate it.'

—Claire Bent (Tas), mother of Thomas (8), allergic to egg, peanut, tree nuts and sesame

'Both parents need to be on the same page when trying to deal with food allergy. Every time there is some dispute, for example, "Why are you ordering that muffin; it's high-risk", the child is listening to that conversation and it is causing them anxiety. Whereas if both parents are in constant agreement, it can help to downplay the issue a lot more.'

—Amanda Cheong-Duryea (WA), mother of Jason (9), allergic to peanut and tree nuts

'Our focus is on being sensible and practical. Hopefully the children will then manage their allergies in the same way in the future.'

—Anne Frisby and Phil Solomon (Vic), parents of Amelia (6), allergic to cow's milk, egg and peanut, and Hugh (4), allergic to egg and peanut

'Talk to other people. Don't do it by yourself. Call a support group. I have learned so much, received so much information, recipes, advice on certain situations. I think support groups are essential.'

—Merryn Gibbons (NSW), mother of Jessica (9), allergic to cow's milk, egg and peanut

'You can manage it, and you have just got to learn as you go. Take your doctor's advice and also know it is an evolving process; you have to deal with it one step at a time or it becomes overwhelming. I tell myself: he can still ride his bike, play soccer and tell me he loves me. It's not something you would ever choose for your child but it could be a hell of a lot worse.'

—Anne-Lii Hardy (NSW), mother of Justin (10), allergic to egg, peanut and tree nuts

'It does get better. You will come to terms with the diagnosis and go through stages of grief — including denial, anger and feelings of loss. This is all normal. But once you arm yourself with education and information, you will feel better. The more you learn about food allergy, the easier it becomes.'

—Annelise Kirkham (Qld), mother of Elly (13),
allergic to peanut and tree nuts, and Jake (8),
allergic to shellfish

'You are not alone. Seek professional help to get a proper diagnosis; this can make it easier to explain food allergies to others. Also, look for friends who really know what you are going through, who are willing to understand and help, such as an allergy support group.'

—Emilia Lie (NSW), mother of twin boys, Nathan and
Jeremy (5), both allergic to peanut and tree nuts

'It's a matter of planning ahead so your child has access to food and doesn't feel left out. Ring up people before events and explain the allergy, make sure people are aware. Most people want to help, but they need to know about the allergy. Planning is key — and making people understand the potential severity of the allergy.'

—Peta Mawson (Qld), mother of Samantha (17),
allergic to avocado, peanut and tree nuts

'Seek as much information as you can. Try not to make it a fearful thing for your child; help them to understand that they can live with allergies in the real world.'

—Katrina Meldrum (Qld), mother of David (17),
allergic to peanut, tree nuts, shellfish and soy

'The process of communicating food allergies to others is gradual and challenging. On the one hand, it takes time to educate everyone that food allergy is a serious issue. On the other hand, you also have to help them understand that, provided your child doesn't eat the wrong food and they are willing to learn how to recognise and treat an allergic reaction, it's perfectly safe for your child to visit. They needn't be afraid — food allergy is not so hard to manage. We make a huge effort to thank and reassure parents who offer to look after our son.'

—Juliet Nicholls (NSW), mother of Oliver (10), allergic to fish, peanut and tree nuts

'It's okay to be anxious; it's okay to be overwhelmed; it's okay to be angry, upset and all those emotions. But when you go through the cycle of emotions you can come out the other side and it is manageable. You can cope and live with it, and it is almost a normal life. Keep food allergies in perspective: there are a lot worse childhood illnesses out there that are far more debilitating on a day-to-day basis.'

—Tanya Paine (Tas), mother of Conrad (7), allergic to cow's milk, egg, peanut, tree nuts, soy (and other legumes), potato and latex

'Try to be as open as you can with people. Sometimes, if you say "Allergy", you can see others thinking, "What's that?" So if the opportunity comes up, I try to be very basic about it. It's important not to over-dramatise things. With some people, everything they talk about is allergies, allergies, allergies. You need to show people that, "Hey, we've got allergies, but we are just like you as well."'

—Kris Piotrowski (WA), mother of Tom (5), allergic to tree nuts, and Sam (3), allergic to cow's milk, egg, peanut and tree nuts

*'With management and education you can still have
a relatively normal life. Yes, it affects your life, but get
educated about it and know what you have to do, then
you can be safe. The more knowledgeable you are about
it, the better you will be in looking after and managing it.
And let everyone know about it, everyone who is involved
in your kids' lives.'*

—Kerry Pontin (Vic), mother of twin boys Jarod and
Samuel (7), and Mitchell (6), all allergic to peanut

5

Anaphylaxis

While the majority of allergic reactions to food are mild, in some cases a severe and potentially life-threatening allergic reaction can occur: this is called anaphylaxis.

Many children who experience food-related anaphylaxis have previously suffered some kind of allergic symptoms to the food in question, but not always: some children experience anaphylaxis on their first known exposure to a particular food. One of the most challenging aspects of anaphylaxis is its unpredictable nature.

Not every child with food allergy will experience anaphylaxis, and not all episodes of anaphylaxis are life-threatening. However, because medical science is not yet able to determine which children will or will not experience anaphylaxis, and which child is at risk of a life-threatening episode of anaphylaxis, living with the risk can be very stressful for many children and their families.

Fortunately, fatalities from food-related anaphylaxis are very rare.[1] However, medical literature reports that 90 per cent of deaths from food-related anaphylaxis are preventable,[2] emphasising just how important it is that everyone involved in the life of a child at risk of anaphylaxis is educated in preventing exposure to an allergen and knowing exactly what to do in an emergency.

Anaphylaxis can be caused by a range of different triggers, but this chapter is focused on food-related anaphylaxis. In this chapter we will explain anaphylaxis, including its symptoms, triggers and risk factors, detail how anaphylaxis is treated in an emergency situation and then outline long-term prevention and management strategies.

While no parent ever wants to see their child suffer an episode of anaphylaxis, the good news is that food-induced anaphylaxis is a treatable condition.

What is anaphylaxis?

Anaphylaxis is the most severe and serious form of allergic reaction. It is rapid in onset and potentially life-threatening. Anaphylaxis is frequently referred to as a 'systemic' or 'multi-system' reaction because it often involves more than one body system: specifically, the respiratory and/or cardiovascular system. In the majority of cases, skin and gut symptoms are also involved. In food-induced anaphylaxis, symptoms usually occur within minutes up to approximately 2 hours after ingestion of an allergen but it can occur up to hours later.

Children do not have 'anaphylaxis'. They have an allergy and may then be diagnosed as being 'at risk' of anaphylaxis.

The symptoms of anaphylaxis

Anaphylaxis is characterised by any one or more symptoms involving the respiratory system and/or cardiovascular system. These symptoms include:[3]

- Difficult or noisy breathing
- Swelling of the tongue
- Swelling or tightness in the throat
- Difficulty talking and/or a hoarse voice
- A wheeze or persistent cough
- Loss of consciousness and/or collapse
- Young children may become pale and floppy

In most cases, less dangerous symptoms associated with generalised allergic reactions appear before anaphylaxis. These symptoms usually involve the skin and/or gut[4] and include:

- Swelling of the lips, face, eyes
- Hives or welts
- A tingling mouth, abdominal pain, vomiting

In approximately 90 per cent of cases of anaphylaxis, skin or gastrointestinal symptoms appear first. It is uncommon for respiratory and/or cardiovascular symptoms to appear before skin and/or gut symptoms, but it does happen.

It is important that all carers of children at risk of anaphylaxis not only learn to recognise the symptoms of anaphylaxis but also understand that:

- Not *all* symptoms listed above will necessarily occur during anaphylaxis: any *one* of the symptoms involving breathing difficulty or the heart requires emergency treatment (see page 74)
- Symptoms can present in any order
- Symptoms can develop and progress rapidly
- If a child has previously experienced anaphylaxis, the symptoms of subsequent severe allergic reactions won't necessarily present in the same way

What triggers anaphylaxis?

Anaphylaxis can be caused by a range of different triggers.

Food

In studies examining children presenting to hospital emergency departments with anaphylaxis, food has been identified as the most common trigger.[5] While ingestion of cow's milk, egg, peanut, tree nuts, fish, shellfish, soy, wheat and sesame[6] are commonly responsible for food-induced anaphylaxis, many different foods can trigger anaphylaxis.

Medication

Any medication (prescribed, over-the-counter and herbal medicines) in any form (for example, tablet, liquid, intravenous) can trigger anaphylaxis.

Insect venom

In Australia, stings from the honeybee, jack jumper ants and wasps are common causes of insect venom-induced anaphylaxis.[7]

Medical procedures

In a hospital setting, some medical procedures are also associated with anaphylaxis, including local and general anaesthesia, blood transfusions and contrast media used for special types of X-ray.

Other

Other triggers of anaphylaxis include latex, exposure to cold, and exercise — either by itself or in association with eating a particular food. (See 'Food-associated exercise-induced anaphylaxis', page 88.) Sometimes anaphylaxis occurs where no trigger can be identified; this is known as 'idiopathic' anaphylaxis.

Touch reactions and anaphylaxis

Q My 6-year-old daughter is allergic to peanut. The other day at the park another child who had been eating a peanut butter sandwich grabbed my child's arm, leaving a smear of peanut butter on her skin. Within minutes, hives appeared on her arm, and she started to scratch. Soon after, a large welt appeared around one of her eyes and then began swelling to the point where it was half-closed. I gave her antihistamine and washed her skin and hands and the reaction subsided but it gave us a terrible fright. Is it possible for her to have anaphylaxis from touching peanut butter?

A There is currently no scientific evidence to suggest anaphylaxis can occur from casual skin contact with an allergen. In a recent study conducted at Sydney Children's Hospital, peanut butter was applied directly to the skin of 281 children who were peanut-sensitive (that is, they had returned a positive skin prick test to peanut) and none experienced a systemic reaction — including those who had previously suffered anaphylaxis from ingesting peanut.[8]

If your daughter has skin contact only with peanut butter, she may experience hives — not only at the site but sometimes even more widespread skin reactions. However, if your daughter touches the peanut butter with her hand and then places her hand in her mouth, rubs her eye, or puts a finger up her nose, then there is a chance of a more severe reaction. Because a large welt appeared around your daughter's eye, as well as the swelling, it is possible she may have rubbed the peanut butter into her eye. While the risk of anaphylaxis from skin contact alone with an allergen is highly unlikely,[9] if an allergen actually enters the body, then there is a risk of a more widespread reaction.

Parents have every reason to be worried if their child is exposed to an allergen, but an allergen touching the skin alone should not cause anything other than a skin reaction. In the event of inadvertent exposure, the allergen should be washed from the child's skin immediately, the child's hands washed thoroughly, and any skin reactions should be treated as per advice from your doctor. The allergen should also be removed or disposed of to prevent any further exposure.

How common is anaphylaxis?

The true prevalence of anaphylaxis is not known — it is frequently under-recognised and under-treated[10, 11, 12] — but it is no longer considered rare.[13, 14] A recent study by the American College of Allergy, Asthma and Immunology concluded that anaphylaxis (from any trigger, not just food) had affected up to 2 per cent of the population, with the largest number of cases occurring in children and adolescents.[15] An Australian study examining parent-reported allergy and anaphylaxis in South Australian children found that 1 in 170 pre-school children had suffered at least one episode of anaphylaxis.[16, 17]

There is some research to suggest that food-induced anaphylaxis is a growing trend in young children. A recent Australian study investigating hospitalisation trends for anaphylaxis, angiodema (swelling) and urticaria (hives) reported a steep increase — 5.5-fold over a 12-year period — in the incidence of hospitalisation for food-related anaphylaxis in children aged between 0 and 4 years.[18] These findings were comparable to trends reported in research studies in the United Kingdom.[19, 20]

Thankfully, while the rate of anaphylaxis is increasing, fatalities from anaphylaxis (from any trigger) are rare, with an estimated rate of one death in every 3 million members of the population per year.[21, 22]

The time-pattern of an anaphylaxis episode

There are three terms used in the medical world to classify the time-pattern of an anaphylaxis episode: 'uniphasic', 'protracted' and 'biphasic'.[23]

Most anaphylaxis episodes respond well to prompt medical emergency treatment, with symptoms resolving completely and without recurrence. These reactions are classified as 'uniphasic'.

However, in some episodes, symptoms may not resolve and may even worsen when the adrenaline wears off; ongoing medical treatment could be required. These cases are classified as 'protracted' anaphylaxis.[24]

In other cases, a patient appears to recover completely from the initial episode of anaphylaxis only to experience a recurrence of symptoms — without any further exposure to the allergen. This usually happens within 6 hours of the initial episode (although it can be later), and sometimes the subsequent reaction can be more severe than the initial reaction.[25] These are classified as 'biphasic' reactions, also commonly referred to as 're-bound' reactions.

There is currently no way of predicting what time course an episode of anaphylaxis will follow. Up to 20 per cent of individuals experience biphasic or protracted symptoms,[26] and fatal reactions have been reported following premature discharge from hospital emergency departments,[27] so it is essential that an ambulance is called immediately in the event of anaphylaxis, and that the child is closely observed in hospital for an appropriate time period (usually a minimum of 4–6 hours).

Who is at risk of anaphylaxis?

As stated in Chapter 3, Food allergy testing, as yet there is no test that can predict which food-allergic children will or will not experience anaphylaxis. However, while food-induced anaphylaxis can occur in anyone, your child's allergy specialist will carefully consider the following risk factors (as they apply to your child) in prescribing emergency medications (such as an EpiPen).

- A history of previous anaphylaxis.
- Asthma, especially uncontrolled asthma.
- The allergen itself: for example, the risk of a severe reaction to peanut,

tree nuts or seafood is generally considered higher than for other allergens. Given that anaphylaxis can still happen with any food, however, your child's clinical history will always be closely assessed.

- Possibly having a previous significant reaction to a very small or trace amount of an allergen.
- Your child's age: for example, the risk of fatality is higher in adolescents and young adults.[28]
- Access to emergency medical care.

> *'When something like anaphylaxis happens on an idle Tuesday afternoon and blindsides you, it changes you. To see your child experience anaphylaxis out of the blue when you are just in the supermarket doing a bit of food shopping — and to the extent that Tom suffered [after helping himself to a loose cashew nut from a display]; where your 3-year-old looks as though he has gone a few rounds with Mike Tyson — and there is absolutely nothing, not a thing you can do, you feel amazingly helpless. Many people do not understand the gravity of anaphylaxis — and the difference between allergy and anaphylaxis.'*
>
> —Kris Piotrowski (WA), mother of Tom (5), allergic to tree nuts, and Sam (3), allergic to cow's milk, egg, peanut and tree nuts

Emergency treatment of food-induced anaphylaxis

Adrenaline

Anaphylaxis is a medical emergency, and early administration of adrenaline (known as epinephrine in the US) is the first-line treatment.

Adrenaline is the 'fight or flight' chemical our body releases naturally in situations of danger or threat, giving it a surge of energy to enable us to either stay and fight the danger or take flight for survival. In the case of food-induced anaphylaxis, adrenaline helps the body fight against the most dangerous symptoms of anaphylaxis (those involving the heart and respiratory system). The adrenaline works by reversing the effects of the symptoms of anaphylaxis. In simple terms, it reduces swelling of the throat and causes dilation of the airways, so the allergy sufferer can breathe again; it causes contraction of the blood vessels so their blood pressure is raised, and it makes their heart pump faster, also raising blood pressure. It also rapidly resolves skin symptoms, especially redness.

Adrenaline must be given as soon as any of the symptoms of anaphylaxis appear (see pages 69 and 70). An ambulance must always be called. Further doses of adrenaline and other medications may need to be given, and ongoing medical observation of your child in hospital is essential. In Australia, in a first-aid situation, adrenaline is most commonly delivered in an EpiPen. A new auto-injector device, the Anapen, is likely to be available soon. (See page 90 for more information on the Anapen.)

The EpiPen

An EpiPen is a self-injectable device that contains a preloaded, single measured dose of adrenaline. The EpiPen is available in two different strengths:

1. EpiPen Jr (0.15mg adrenaline) — usually prescribed for children aged 1–5.
2. EpiPen (0.30mg adrenaline) — usually prescribed for children 5 and above as well as adults.

While the manufacturer of the EpiPen recommends an EpiPen Jr (0.15mg) for children with a body weight between 15 and 30 kilograms,[29] the Australasian Society of Clinical Immunology and Allergy recommends an EpiPen (0.30mg) for children weighing over 20 kilograms.[30] Your allergy specialist will prescribe the appropriate EpiPen for your child. If you have a child who is nearing 20 kilograms in weight, check with your allergy specialist about when you need to move them to the higher-dose EpiPen (another reason why regular review by your child's allergy specialist is so important).

The following illustration of an EpiPen is for educational purposes only: it is not to scale, and your child's EpiPen may differ slightly. Ensure you read the instructions for your child's EpiPen. Always follow your child's individual Action Plan for anaphylaxis. Speak with your doctor if you have any questions.

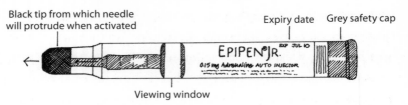

Black tip from which needle will protrude when activated

Expiry date Grey safety cap

Viewing window

Grey safety cap: The grey safety cap needs to be removed before the EpiPen can be activated.

Black tip: When the EpiPen is activated, the needle will shoot through the black tip into the outer thigh of the person being injected.

Viewing window: This enables you to check that the adrenaline inside the pen is clear. If it turns cloudy or dark, the pen needs to be replaced immediately. When an EpiPen has been activated successfully, the viewing window should display red.

Expiry date: The expiry date needs to be checked regularly.

Needle: After the EpiPen has been successfully activated, a fine needle will be visible.

How to give EpiPen or EpiPen Jr*

Instructions for use of an EpiPen and an EpiPen Jr are the same.

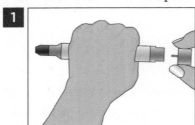

1

Form fist around EpiPen and **PULL OFF** grey cap.

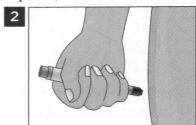

2

Place black end against outer mid-thigh (with or without clothing).

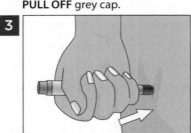

3

Push down **HARD** until a click is heard or felt and hold in place for 10 seconds.

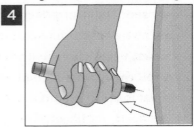

4

Remove EpiPen and be careful not to touch the needle. Massage the injection site for 10 seconds.

* ASCIA Action Plans for Anaphylaxis and Allergic Reactions are reproduced with permission from the Australasian Society of Clinical Immunology and Allergy (ASCIA). These are available to download from the ASCIA website **www.allergy.org.au/content/view/10/3/** or can be ordered as hard copies by emailing **education@allergy.org.au**

What to do after using the EpiPen

- Call an ambulance:[*] 000 in Australia.
- Lay person flat and elevate legs. If breathing is difficult, allow to sit but do not stand.
- Contact family/carer.
- Further EpiPen doses may be given if no response after 5 minutes.

[*] Medical observation in hospital for at least 4 hours is recommended after anaphylaxis.

Calling an ambulance

Protocols for calling an ambulance are different depending on what state or territory you live in, but below are some general tips to consider when calling an ambulance in Australia.

1. Call '000' and ask for an ambulance. You can also call '112' from mobile phones where the service is out of range.
2. If your call is not answered immediately, do not hang up; your call will be answered.
3. When explaining the emergency, use simple language; for example: 'My child is having a severe allergic reaction and has food allergy. We have used an EpiPen.'
4. The operator will probably ask you several questions; try to remain calm and answer questions briefly and accurately. Speak slowly and clearly and listen carefully.
5. Try to provide accurate location information; for example, in addition to your address, naming the nearest cross street or mentioning a landmark is also helpful.
6. Do not hang up: follow the instructions offered by the operator while you are waiting for the ambulance.
7. If other capable adults are with you where the emergency is taking place, send someone outside to wait for the ambulance and to direct ambulance officers to the child experiencing anaphylaxis.
8. Ring '000' again if the child's condition worsens and you are still waiting for an ambulance.

continued

If someone else is caring for your child in your home, in addition to knowing the symptoms of an allergic reaction, how to use an EpiPen and how to follow your child's Action Plan, ensure they know:
- Where your telephone is and how to use it
- Your address and nearest cross street
- Your telephone number, which the operator will almost certainly ask for in case they need to call back

'My daughter is pretty brilliant with her brother's allergies. She really watches over him. Because we are on 6 acres, if they are out playing in our big backyard and something happens, she knows what signs to look for and to come and get help straight away. I have also taught my daughter how to dial "000" in an emergency.'

—Tanya Paine (Tas), mother of Conrad (7), allergic to cow's milk, egg, peanut, tree nuts, soy (and other legumes), potato and latex

Disposing of an EpiPen

Once an EpiPen has been used, it needs to be disposed of carefully. Place the used EpiPen, needle-end first, back into the plastic EpiPen carry tube (all EpiPens come in these tubes) and screw the cap back on tightly. Put it out of reach of children until you can take it to an outlet such as a pharmacy or your GP where staff can safely dispose of sharps for you.

EpiPens cannot be reused. Once you have used an EpiPen be sure to replace it immediately.

Accidental EpiPen injection: what to do

If a carer accidentally injects themselves while trying to administer the EpiPen to a child with anaphylaxis, the focus needs to remain on the child. If a second EpiPen is available, it should be administered to the child, as per the child's Action Plan, and an ambulance must be called immediately. If a second EpiPen is not available, call for an ambulance immediately — tell the operator the child is having a severe allergic reaction and you do not have adrenaline; also try to lie the child flat and elevate their legs. If the child is vomiting, or breathing is difficult, allow them to sit but not stand.

After the child experiencing anaphylaxis has been cared for, the person who has injected themselves should seek medical help as soon as possible. If someone has injected themselves in a 'terminal' area of the body — for example, a finger or toe — they should call an ambulance or go to the emergency department of the nearest hospital, because blood circulation will be lost in these areas and there is a risk that a finger or toe could be lost. If someone has injected themselves inadvertently in another area of the body, for example, the thigh, then it is not an emergency but they should still visit an emergency department for a check-up, just to be safe. If the person who has injected themselves has an underlying heart condition, they should call an ambulance or visit the emergency department of a hospital as soon as possible, regardless of the site of injection.

Ongoing education and training in how to use an EpiPen is the best insurance policy for preventing accidental injections.

> '*I thought I knew what I was doing with the EpiPen until I did the training course at the Royal Children's Hospital in Melbourne. Then I realised I had no idea. Now I know what I need to do.*'
>
> —Justine Sayers (Vic), mother of Esme (5), allergic to cow's milk, egg, peanut and tree nuts, and Fred (2), allergic to cow's milk, fish and sesame

Storing your EpiPen

- EpiPens should be labelled with your child's name. A copy of your child's Action Plan should always be kept with the EpiPen. Specially designed wallets and belts can be ordered for storage of EpiPens (available at **www.allergyfacts.org.au**).
- If you have more than one child who needs to carry an EpiPen, ensure you clearly label each child's EpiPen in a distinct way; this is especially

important if you have children who require different strength EpiPens. Clear labelling will prevent confusion in an emergency.

- EpiPens should be kept in a safe but easily accessible location, never in a locked cupboard. Once you decide on a location for your EpiPens, stick to it and let everyone involved in the life of your child know about it.

- EpiPens must be stored in the plastic tube provided with your EpiPen at room temperature. Never leave an EpiPen in a car or anywhere in direct sunlight or heat, and never put an EpiPen in the fridge.

- Regularly check the 'window' of the EpiPen. The solution inside the pen should be clear. If the solution has discoloured or appears cloudy, you should replace the EpiPen immediately.

- Note the expiry date of your EpiPen and put a note in your diary to remind you when it needs replacing. EpiPens do not have a long shelf-life, usually only between 12 and 18 months. An expired EpiPen may not be effective in an emergency so it is essential you remember to replace your EpiPens in advance of the expiry date. Consider joining the EpiClub, a free patient support program that will send you a reminder notice prior to your EpiPen expiring. Learn more at: **www.epiclub.com.au**

> *'The EpiPen is in one bag, where I also keep nappies for my younger children, and sunscreen, and we take it everywhere. It is not a "gender-specific" bag, so my husband can feel comfortable carrying it; it's a travel bag, and it also fits on the handle of the pram. We never leave the house without the bag. We also keep antihistamine in there, and a lot of dairy-free, egg-free and nut-free snacks!'*
>
> —Anne Frisby (Vic), mother of Amelia (6), allergic to cow's milk, egg and peanut, and Hugh (4), allergic to egg and peanut

Purchasing EpiPens

In Australia, EpiPens are available under the Pharmaceutical Benefits Scheme (PBS) by authority prescription, but only for patients considered at significant risk of anaphylaxis. This means the cost of the EpiPen is subsidised by the government, making it a far more affordable and accessible medication. Authority prescriptions need to be issued in consultation with a clinical immunologist, allergist, paediatrician or respiratory specialist, or after a patient has been discharged from hospital or an emergency department following treatment with adrenaline for anaphylaxis.[31] A maximum of two EpiPens may be prescribed under the PBS for children aged under 17 years of age, and a maximum of one EpiPen for anyone aged 17 years and above.

When your doctor hands you the script for your child's EpiPen, have it filled immediately. Not all pharmacies carry EpiPens in stock (owing to their short shelf-life); many pharmacies only order them in when a script is presented, so you will have to come back to the pharmacy to collect the EpiPen when it arrives (usually the following day, but it may vary depending on where you live).

At present, anyone can purchase an EpiPen without prescription from pharmacies, but only at full cost (over AUD$100 per EpiPen). If an EpiPen expires or is used, another EpiPen can be purchased under the PBS.

PBS listings and conditions can change, as can the cost and regulations surrounding the supply of medications. Always consult your child's specialist about obtaining appropriate medications for your child.

Being 'empowered' to use an EpiPen

Research shows that EpiPens are under-used in emergency situations. In an Australian retrospective study, it was found that an EpiPen had been used in only 29 per cent of anaphylaxis cases (in children who experienced recurring episodes of anaphylaxis), despite an EpiPen being on hand and in date at the time of the emergency.[32] In an American study on parental use of EpiPens for children with food allergies, more than 45 per cent of parents reported they would feel 'outright uncomfortable in administering EpiPen to their child'.[33]

There are many reasons why EpiPens are under-used, including:
- Failure to recognise symptoms of anaphylaxis
- Forgetting how to use the EpiPen
- Using antihistamine first and adopting a 'wait-and-see' approach
- Fear of hurting a child
- Fear of adverse side effects of adrenaline

In the American study mentioned above, researchers concluded that 'empowerment' directly correlated with increased comfort in parental use of the EpiPen.[34] In simple terms, this means that parents who felt psychologically equipped to cope with a potential crisis such as anaphylaxis were more likely to actually use the EpiPen.

So how do parents go about empowering themselves to cope with a potential emergency situation? Education and support are key to ensuring you feel prepared, both technically and emotionally, to manage anaphylaxis, including administering an EpiPen during an emergency.

Below are some helpful pointers to help you on your way to 'empowerment':

- If you have an EpiPen you must also have a personalised Action Plan for your child. The symptoms of anaphylaxis are listed on this plan: learn them off by heart. (See also pages 69 and 70.) If you are still worried you will not recognise the symptoms, talk to your GP or allergy specialist, who can further explain symptoms to you.
- Do everything you can to become comfortable in using an EpiPen. Enrol in an EpiPen training course if you have access to one, or ask your allergy specialist for a training DVD. EpiPen trainers are invaluable (see the box on pages 84 and 85). Save expired EpiPens and practise using them on an orange. Consider having an emergency drill in your home from time to time, to practise how you might respond in an emergency.
- Once you are confident in your ability to use an EpiPen, don't become complacent. For example, you might mark a date on your calendar every 3 months where you will pull out your EpiPen trainer and run through your child's Action Plan. Ongoing and regular education on using an EpiPen will help you maintain your confidence.
- Ensure you visit your child's allergy specialist on a regular basis; they can help with ongoing education in use of the EpiPen and in managing any other health-related issues relevant to your child.
- Understand that adrenaline is the *only* drug that can help your child in the case of anaphylaxis — there is no alternative — so you must use it when any one of the symptoms of anaphylaxis is apparent.
- Time is of the essence. Never adopt a 'wait and see' approach. Even if

in doubt about the seriousness of your child's symptoms, still use the EpiPen and call an ambulance. EpiPens may be injected through light clothing, but ideally you should inject directly into skin.

- While it is true to say most needles hurt a bit, you will not harm your child by administering an EpiPen. EpiPens are administered in the mid-thigh area because there is a large muscle mass there, so it is extremely unlikely you can hit anything other than muscle.

- The adverse side effects of a therapeutic dose of adrenaline are usually temporary. Side effects can include pallor, tremor, anxiety, fear, restlessness, headache, dizziness and palpitations;[35, 36] however, the life-saving benefits of administering adrenaline far outweigh any possible side effects.

- Joining a support and education group such as Anaphylaxis Australia can help with furthering your education about anaphylaxis and how to avoid and prepare for emergency situations. The more you learn about anaphylaxis and how to manage it, the more confident you can become.

The golden rule: if in doubt, use the EpiPen

Failing to administer adrenaline or delaying the administering of adrenaline can place a child at risk of a fatal reaction. While deaths from anaphylaxis are rare, individual studies of fatal food-related anaphylaxis have documented that adrenaline was not usually administered after the initial onset of symptoms or exposure to an allergen.[37, 38]

You will not harm a child by administering an EpiPen unnecessarily, but you might be placing a child at risk of a fatal reaction if you hesitate or fail to use an EpiPen as soon as any one of the symptoms involving breathing difficulty or the heart appear. (The symptoms are listed on pages 69 and 70.)

Remember, if a child is having an allergic reaction and you are in doubt as to whether they need adrenaline, always use the EpiPen and call an ambulance.

'We have had three close calls for each of our boys. My husband and I did an anaphylaxis management course at the Royal Prince Alfred Hospital in Sydney early last year. Since then we are more confident in when to administer the EpiPen. We will not hesitate any more.'

— Emilia Lie (NSW), mother of twin boys, Nathan and Jeremy (5), both allergic to peanut and tree nuts

EpiPen trainers

An EpiPen trainer is, as the name suggests, a training tool for people to learn how to use an EpiPen. A training pen looks and functions like a real EpiPen but does not contain a needle or adrenaline.

For many people, the thought of having to give someone an injection — especially a child — is daunting. A training pen gives others the opportunity to see and feel just how easy administering an EpiPen is. It can really help in taking away the fear of using an EpiPen.

A training pen is also handy for ongoing practice sessions. Most of my extended family live interstate, so when they come to visit I always spend some time demonstrating with the training pen and running through the symptoms of anaphylaxis, when to give the EpiPen and how to call an ambulance. Most family members have done formal anaphylaxis training courses, but that was some time ago, so practising with the training pen from time to time, in conjunction with referring to Noah's Action Plan, is essential to ensure everyone feels confident they can handle an emergency situation if it occurs while Noah is in their care.

Training pens can be purchased via **www.allergyfacts.org.au**

After you purchase a training pen, remember:

- Never store a training pen with your real EpiPen; this can create confusion in an emergency. We keep our EpiPen trainer in a filing cabinet drawer, along with other information relating to

Noah's allergies, such as spare photocopies of his Action Plan and documentation given to us by Noah's allergy specialist.

- You might like to place a piece of coloured duct tape around your training pen to avoid confusion with a real EpiPen or find some other permanent way of making it very clear it is a training pen only.

Antihistamine or EpiPen: which to use when?

Q My child is allergic to cow's milk and egg and has been diagnosed as being at risk of anaphylaxis. Our doctor has prescribed antihistamine and an EpiPen. I am a bit confused about when to use the antihistamine. Do you always administer antihistamine before an EpiPen?

A The answer is a definite no: you do not always administer antihistamine before an EpiPen.

Antihistamine is effective in reversing the symptoms of a mild to moderate allergic reaction, for example, itching, swelling and skin rashes; however, antihistamine on its own will not prevent anaphylaxis nor will it be effective in treating it: adrenaline must always be considered the first-line treatment for anaphylaxis.

Let's look at two fictional scenarios to further explain the usage of each medication.

Scenario 1: Three-year-old Isabel is allergic to cow's milk and has been diagnosed as being at risk of anaphylaxis. At her childcare centre, a staff member suspects Isabel's face has been wiped with a milk-contaminated face cloth but isn't entirely sure. Hives appear down the side of Isabel's face, and she is scratching at the hives but still playing happily. No other allergic symptoms are apparent. In this situation, Isabel's carer would administer antihistamine as per her written Action Plan and keep monitoring Isabel's symptoms. If any of the symptoms of anaphylaxis as listed on Isabel's Action Plan were to appear, Isabel's carer would need to administer her EpiPen immediately and call an ambulance.

Scenario 2: Fourteen-year-old William is allergic to peanut and has previously experienced anaphylaxis to peanut. A relative has baked a special 'safe' cake for William, as per a recipe given to her by William's mother. Within minutes of eating his special cake, hives appear around William's mouth, his lips begin to swell and he starts to wheeze. In this situation, William's mother must assume the cake was somehow contaminated and immediately administer the EpiPen and call an ambulance. Even though William has skin symptoms, his breathing difficulty must be addressed immediately, and the only effective treatment is adrenaline in the form of his EpiPen. In this scenario, it would be dangerous to give antihistamine first, as it would cause a delay in administering adrenaline.

Remember, if a child is experiencing an allergic reaction and any one of the symptoms of anaphylaxis is present, the EpiPen must be administered immediately, as per the child's Action Plan, and an ambulance called.

Long-term prevention and management of anaphylaxis

When anaphylaxis occurs, as you have just read, it requires urgent medical treatment, but at all other times preventing exposure to your child's allergens and education in how to deal with potential emergency situations are the most important factors in long-term management.[39]

The current approach to effectively preventing and managing anaphylaxis is based on the following key steps.[40, 41]

1. Identifying the allergic trigger

If your child has experienced a suspected allergic reaction to a food, they should always be referred to an allergy specialist to ensure the allergic trigger can be identified. As covered in Chapters 2 and 3 (see pages 17 and 30), an allergy specialist will conduct a physical examination of your child, spend a lot of time taking a detailed medical history and then consider a skin prick test, blood test or food challenge to help confirm the diagnosis.

2. Education on avoiding exposure to your child's allergen

Once your child's allergen or allergens have been identified, children, parents and carers need to be educated in how to avoid exposing the child to the allergic trigger. This involves understanding how food allergens can be present as 'hidden' ingredients, the risk of cross-contamination in the preparation of foods, and the fact that food allergens may also be present in a range of other products, such as medications, skin-care products, alcohol and pet foods. (See Chapters 6, 7 and 8 for more information.) Referral to an accredited paediatric dietitian with experience in IgE-mediated food allergy is also often recommended.

3. Carrying a personalised Action Plan for anaphylaxis with your child's EpiPen

Any child who has experienced anaphylaxis or who has been identified as being at risk of anaphylaxis by their allergy specialist will be prescribed an EpiPen in conjunction with a personalised Action Plan for anaphylaxis. The Action Plan will list your child's name, date of birth, allergic triggers, emergency contact details of parents and carers and a photograph of your child. The plan also outlines the symptoms of allergic reactions, when to administer an EpiPen (including illustrations of how to use an EpiPen), how to call an ambulance and space for any other additional instructions specific to your child's condition. Action Plans are signed by your child's allergy specialist and a copy should be carried with your child's EpiPen at all times.

It is important to use the Action Plan as published by the Australasian Society of Clinical Immunology and Allergy. Some parents choose to write unique Action Plans for their children, but this can cause confusion in an emergency situation, especially if they are too long, the instructions are not expressed clearly enough, or the instructions differ from what carers have been taught in official anaphylaxis training courses. (See Appendix 2, page 371, for a copy of the ASCIA Action Plan.)

4. Regular review by an allergy specialist

Ongoing and regular review by your child's allergy specialist is essential in managing food allergy and the risk of anaphylaxis. Many childhood food allergies are outgrown, new allergies can develop, and your child's doctor also needs to know about any new health issues which might be relevant to your child's food allergy, for example, asthma. Regular review also means your child's Action Plan will be updated, you will receive ongoing education about using your child's EpiPen and it is a great prompt for you to ensure all of your child's medications are up to date. Seeing your specialist on a regular basis can also help with managing anxiety, as it gives you the opportunity to talk to your child's doctor about any recent reactions your child has experienced and any worries you might have. Your doctor can also keep you up to date with new research and development findings, which can be encouraging for both parents and older children. At the end of every appointment with your specialist, always ask when you should make your next appointment.

Food-associated exercise-induced anaphylaxis

There are two forms of food-associated exercise-induced anaphylaxis. The first occurs following the ingestion of a *specific* food prior to exercise (usually within 2–4 hours); the second — which is unusual — occurs when someone ingests *any* food prior to exercise.[42] (It can also occur when the trigger food is eaten after exercise[43] but this is more uncommon than when it is ingested prior to exercise.)

It is the association of food with exercise that causes the reaction, so the patient can eat the specific food without reaction (providing they do not exercise afterwards) and can exercise without reaction (providing they do not ingest the specific food beforehand). Wheat is one of the foods most commonly associated with this syndrome,[44] but other foods implicated include other cereals, celery, nuts, seafood, fruit and some vegetables.[45]

While the true prevalence of food-associated exercise-induced anaphylaxis is unknown,[46] it is considered rare — and rarer still in children. It is typically diagnosed in young adults and is twice as common in female patients as it is in male patients.[47] A skin prick test is often used to help diagnose the trigger food.

The importance of education: learn the three A's

Anaphylaxis triggered by food commonly occurs without warning and often in a community setting.[48] This means non-healthcare professionals, such as parents, friends, co-workers, childcare workers and teachers, are often responsible for recognising the signs and symptoms of an allergic reaction and administering emergency medication.

Sending out the right messages to those involved in the lives of our food-allergic children is critical. Anaphylaxis Australia Inc is working hard to educate not only those living with severe food allergy but also the larger community — including workplaces, the hospitality industry, airlines, childcare centres and schools, to name only some — in the importance of being 'allergy aware'.

Their message is simple: being allergy aware means ...

Awareness

Learning about food allergy and taking severe allergies seriously.

Avoidance

Understanding that people with severe food allergies must avoid their allergen in any form to prevent a severe allergic reaction.

Action

Knowing the signs and symptoms of a severe allergic reaction and knowing how to respond, including the use of an adrenaline auto-injector (EpiPen) in the event of anaphylaxis.

The process of education in becoming 'allergy aware' is gradual, but in doing so, Anaphylaxis Australia aims to build Knowledge for Life.

For more information on anaphylaxis education and advocacy, visit **www.allergyfacts.org.au**

Stop press: the Anapen

During the preparation of this book, a new adrenaline auto-injector called the Anapen was registered for marketing in Australia by Link Pharmaceuticals, an Australian-owned pharmaceutical company. The mechanism of the Anapen is different from that of the EpiPen, which means if the Anapen is adopted by doctors and patients, anyone caring for children at risk of anaphylaxis will need to become educated in using both the EpiPen and the Anapen. For more information on the functionality of the Anapen, visit **www.anapen.com.au**

At the time of going to press, June 2009, the Anapen is not yet available for sale and all Action Plans and education and training are based on administering adrenaline in an EpiPen. Watch this space.

6

Common food allergens

In Australia, eight foods are responsible for more than 90 per cent of food allergies: cow's milk, egg, peanut, tree nuts, fish, shellfish, soy and wheat.[1] More recently, sesame has also joined the list of most common allergens.[2]

It seems a pretty small list, but many of these allergens are ingredients in a wide variety of foods children regularly consume. Any parent who is asked to start eliminating a couple or more of these foods from their child's diet is initially left wondering: what on earth will I feed my child?

In this chapter, we offer an overview of each of the common food allergens, including: research findings about the prevalence of each allergy, the odds of a child outgrowing their allergy and possible clinical cross-reactions with other foods — that is, allergies to related foods. (For information on cross-reactivity see page 96.) At the end of the chapter we will also look at some other less common but often talked-about allergens.

Cow's milk (dairy)

Cow's milk is the most common allergen in infants and young children, estimated to affect 2–3 per cent of infants in developed countries.[3, 4] A child with IgE-mediated cow's milk allergy is allergic to specific proteins found in milk — for example, whey and casein — so all dairy products and any other products where milk is present need to be strictly avoided (although recent research has shown that some milk-allergic children can tolerate extensively heated milk).[5] When you are explaining your child's milk allergy to others, be sure they understand that *all* dairy products are off-limits.

Outgrowing cow's milk allergy

Research surrounding the age at which many children outgrow cow's milk allergy varies, but it is commonly cited that around 80 per cent of infants will outgrow their allergy by the age of 3.[6] A recent study from a specialist centre reported that cow's milk allergy may be far more persistent than previously thought, finding 79 per cent resolved by 16 years of age in this specific hospital-based group.[7] (See also 'Statistics and the likelihood of your child outgrowing a food allergy', page 101.) The good news here is that children developed tolerance well into their teenage years, whereas previous studies have suggested that if cow's milk allergy continued into school years, a child was less likely to ever outgrow it.[8] The findings of this study emphasise how important it is to have your child reviewed by an allergy specialist on a regular and ongoing basis.

Possible clinical cross-reactions

Mammalian milks: Proteins similar to those found in cow's milk are also present in milk from other mammals, for example, goat's milk and sheep's milk, so all mammalian milk and their products need to be strictly avoided if a child has been diagnosed with cow's milk allergy[9] (the exceptions being mare's milk and camel's milk, although they are not recommended).

Soy: Approximately 1 in 5 children allergic to cow's milk will also have a problem with soy.[10] Most allergy specialists will routinely test a milk-allergic child to soy before recommending soy formula or soy drink (depending on the age of the child) as an alternative. If your child is allergic to cow's milk, be sure to check with your child's allergy specialist before introducing soy.

A word on beef: A small percentage of children allergic to cow's milk are also allergic to beef;[11] this is thought to be due to the similarity between some of the proteins in both milk and beef. In most cases, beef allergy only produces mild reactions, such as an increase in eczema, and research suggests that cooking beef can also reduce its allergenicity.[12] As always, if in doubt, talk to your child's allergy specialist. The majority of children allergic to cow's milk can safely enjoy eating beef.

Cow's milk allergy and infant formula alternatives

Q My 6-month-old daughter has recently been diagnosed with cow's milk allergy. I am still breastfeeding her but am wondering, when I do decide to wean her, which formula should I use?

A You will definitely need to call your allergy specialist to discuss this. There are several options, but the one most suitable for your daughter will depend on her clinical history and the age at which you decide to wean.

Alternative formula options used to replace cow's milk formula in cow's milk-allergic infants include the following.[13]

1. Soy formula

Soy formula is made from soybean and does not contain any milk proteins. Several brands are available from most supermarkets and pharmacies. However, as mentioned earlier in this chapter, 1 in 5 children allergic to cow's milk are also allergic to soy. Soy formula is usually only recommended for infants aged 6 months and above. You should always check with your allergy specialist before offering a milk-allergic child any soy products.

2. Extensively hydrolysed formula (EHF)

To produce extensively hydrolysed formula, enzymes are added to cow's milk to break down most of the proteins that cause symptoms in children with cow's milk allergy. Extensively hydrolysed formula is usually the first choice for most infants allergic to cow's milk, but some children may still react to this, in which case an amino acid-based formula (see below) is prescribed. If there are concerns surrounding whether or not your infant will tolerate EHF, your allergy specialist may conduct a skin prick test using a drop of the formula. Extensively hydrolysed formula is available by prescription only; it is listed under the Pharmaceutical Benefits Scheme.

3. Amino acid-based formula (also called 'elemental formula')

Amino acid-based formula is usually prescribed for infants and children with food allergies who cannot tolerate either EHF or soy. Amino acids are commonly referred to as the 'building blocks' for all proteins. The amino acids in these special formulas are synthetic, or 'man-made', meaning they do not come from animal protein or soy protein. Amino acid-based formula is only available on prescription; it is listed under the Pharmaceutical Benefits Scheme.

Amino acid-based formula is known to have an unpleasant taste, so it can be difficult to introduce to older babies. If it is prescribed for your baby and you are struggling to get them to take it, don't be disheartened: a paediatric dietitian may be able to help you. Paediatric dietitians not only specialise in dietary knowledge but also eating behaviour. (See 'How to find a paediatric dietitian', page 125.)

As an aside, it is also worth mentioning here some of the *unsuitable* formulas for cow's milk-allergic infants, including: goat's milk formula as well as rice, almond or oat milk formulas. Most children who are allergic to cow's milk are also allergic to goat's milk: the proteins in goat and other mammalian milks are very similar and have a high chance of causing a reaction in a cow's milk-allergic baby. Rice, almond and oat milk formulas are not, strictly speaking, 'milk', and lack protein and many vitamins and minerals found in a cow's milk-based formula. They may be recommended when your child is older.

While there will be an option available for your daughter, it cannot be overemphasised just how important it is for you to consult your allergy specialist to ensure you choose one that is safe and best suited to her individual requirements. If you intend to continue breastfeeding indefinitely, it is still a good idea to discuss the issue with your doctor early, as sometimes doctors recommend special formulas be introduced in a small quantity, for example, on your baby's breakfast cereal, at a young age to get them used to the taste for whenever they are weaned further down the track.

Avoiding milk mistakes

Cow's milk, soy drink and other milk alternatives are all very similar in appearance, so you need to work out ways to ensure your child consumes the correct drink. For example, if your child uses a bottle, clearly label your child's bottles so they are never given the wrong one, especially if you have other children in the house who do drink cow's milk or cow's milk formula from a bottle. It is very easy to grab the wrong bottle in the middle of the night when you are sleep-deprived. Use a plastic storage tray or basket and place your milk-allergic child's clearly labelled bottles in this section of the fridge only.

Another problem specific to the fridge is the potential for contamination of foods from dairy products. We once had a yoghurt spill that meant I had to throw out all of the foods on the shelves beneath. Since then, the top shelf of our fridge is labelled 'dairy-free' and Noah's foods are kept on this shelf only, so there is no risk of anything leaking or dripping onto his foods. We often have visitors staying with us, so labelling the top shelf has worked really well in avoiding mistakes by house guests who are not used to living with food allergies.

Lactose intolerance versus cow's milk allergy: what's the difference?

There is often confusion in the community about lactose intolerance and IgE-mediated cow's milk allergy when they are, in fact, entirely different medical conditions.

A person with cow's milk allergy is allergic to proteins present in cow's milk. If a cow's milk-allergy sufferer ingests cow's milk, it triggers an immune-system response, which may result in mild to severe allergic symptoms, including anaphylaxis.

A person with lactose intolerance is unable to digest lactose (milk sugar) because of an enzyme deficiency. If a person with lactose intolerance ingests a food containing lactose, depending on the quantity consumed, they may experience symptoms including a sore tummy and diarrhoea. Their reaction, however, is not an allergy. For some children, lactose intolerance is permanent, but for most it is a temporary condition that often occurs after the bowel has been damaged by gastroenteritis.

A child with cow's milk allergy usually needs to avoid all dairy products and any food containing milk as an ingredient (although some milk-allergic children can tolerate extensively heated milk).[14] A person with lactose intolerance does not need to avoid all dairy products, they just need to choose 'lactose-free' products.

Cross-reactivity: what is it?

When someone is allergic to one substance (say, a food or a pollen), they may also react to another substance that has similar proteins. This may be clinically relevant, meaning the allergen triggers symptoms on exposure, or it may result only in a positive skin prick test or RAST, indicating that someone is 'sensitised' to a particular substance but not necessarily allergic. Cross-reactivity is especially relevant in seafood, tree nuts, latex and some fruit and vegetable allergies, as well as in pollen allergies.

From a parent's point of view, cross-reactivity is interesting to know about, but importantly, remember that anyone can have an allergic reaction to any food. The only way to find out if a food is problematic for your child is by consulting an allergy specialist.

Egg

Egg is one of the most common allergens in children, estimated to affect 1–2 per cent of young children.[15, 16] A child with egg allergy is allergic to proteins in egg. The proteins responsible for egg allergy are most commonly found in egg white, but some of the proteins in egg yolk can also trigger allergic reactions. If a child is diagnosed as being allergic to either egg white or egg yolk, they will generally be advised to avoid both, as cross-contamination is almost inevitable.

Some children are allergic to egg in all forms while others can tolerate egg that has been cooked at a high temperature, for example, in cakes, but not raw or lightly cooked eggs. This is because cooking can reduce the allergenicity of some proteins found in egg. If your child is allergic to egg, never feed them egg-containing foods in any form unless you have discussed this with your allergy specialist.

Outgrowing egg allergy

It is commonly cited that the majority of children with egg allergy will develop tolerance by school age;[17] however, a recent study, again from a specialist allergy centre, reported that the rate of tolerance may be much slower, finding that 68 per cent of cases resolved by 16 years of age.[18] (Also see 'Statistics and the likelihood of your child outgrowing a food allergy', page 101.) Regardless of the rate at which tolerance develops, most studies seem to agree that the majority of patients with egg allergy are likely to develop tolerance by adulthood.

Possible clinical cross-reactions

Avian eggs: Patients allergic to hen's egg are usually advised to avoid all avian eggs, for example, duck and quail, because the proteins are so similar.

A word on chicken: The vast majority of children allergic to egg will not be allergic to chicken meat, and less than 5 per cent of egg-allergic children will produce a positive skin prick test to chicken.[19] Remember that a positive skin test result does not always mean a true allergy, so check with your allergy specialist if you are worried about your egg-allergic child eating chicken.

Egg replacement

Cooking without egg can be a challenge but it soon becomes a way of life. The first few egg-free cakes I made were sunken disasters but after much experimenting my repertoire now includes numerous cakes and loaves that taste really good. Most children love cooking, so it's also a great way to have fun with your kids.

Anaphylaxis Australia Inc suggests the following for replacing eggs in a recipe: *continued*

To substitute for two eggs, mix together:

3 tablespoons water

3 tablespoons oil (always choose an oil that is safe for your
   child)

2 teaspoons baking powder (always check ingredients)

To substitute for one egg, halve each amount.

The above is just one suggestion for replacing egg; have fun experimenting in the kitchen. At our house we bake mixed berry and banana cake and we find that extra mashed banana is enough to bind the mixture without any egg replacement at all. Commercially available egg replacements are also available and are often kept in the health food aisle at the supermarket. As always, check the ingredients on every label of every product before you buy it.

The success of cooking without egg often depends on what you are cooking. For example, trying to make something that is very much egg-based, such as an omelette, is not going to work, but with baked goods such as cakes, you may be surprised at just how good the finished product can be. As a general rule, trying to substitute any more than two eggs in a recipe is not recommended. A list of recipe books written specifically for people with food allergy is featured in Appendix 1, page 370.

Noah's dairy-free, egg-free, nut-free cup cakes are a favourite of his classmates and teachers at pre-school. After his third birthday celebration, all the staff asked me for the recipe and could not believe it was missing so many of the usual ingredients.

Egg allergy and immunisation

Q My daughter is allergic to egg and is due for her MMR (measles, mumps and rubella) immunisation. Some of my friends from mother's group have told me they have heard it is not safe for an egg-allergic child to have this immunisation. I searched on the Internet and found conflicting views, which has only confused me further. Can you please clarify this issue for me, and let me know if there are any other immunisations where egg allergy is a cause for concern?

A The best way to answer your question is to handle it in three parts, dealing with MMR first, followed by other immunisations — as well as anaesthetics — and then a final and very important word on immunisation and food allergy in general.

MMR

The current measles vaccine (given in MMR) is safe to give to children with egg allergy. Contrary to urban myth, the vaccine is *not* grown in hen's eggs; it is grown on something called a chick-embryo fibroblast, which is an embryonic cell (this cell will grow into a chicken later on, but it is not actually part of the hen's egg at this point, so egg protein is only present in infinitesimal quantities).

A study published in the *British Medical Journal* in 1994 involved administering the MMR vaccine to 54 children who had not previously been vaccinated and were allergic to egg. All 54 children received the MMR vaccine as an injection and none of the children had an adverse reaction (either immediate or delayed).[20]

In the past, it was thought that the measles vaccine posed a risk to children with egg allergy, and skin prick testing to the vaccine was sometimes conducted prior to immunising an egg-allergic child: it was a long-debated subject in medical journals. This is no longer the case, but knowing this history might help to explain why you were reading conflicting views on the Internet. (As an aside, it is only natural for concerned parents to want to go searching for answers, but the Internet can be a source of misinformation. If you ever have any questions in relation to your child's food allergy, you should contact your allergy specialist, who will take into account your child's individual history and specific allergies.)

Other immunisations

The influenza and yellow fever vaccines are both grown in hen's egg cultures, meaning a small amount of egg protein is present in both, and there is a risk that a child with egg allergy — especially if they have experienced a severe reaction in the past — may have a reaction to either of these immunisations. Neither of these vaccines should be given to an egg-allergic child except under the supervision of an allergy specialist.

The Hib immunisation (Haemophilus influenzae type b) is different from the influenza immunisation, and is safe for egg-allergic children.

Anaesthetics

If your child is having an anaesthetic of any kind, you must alert your child's doctor and anaesthetist about their egg allergy because some anaesthetic agents contain small amounts of egg lecithin. However, it is extremely unlikely that an egg-allergic child will suffer an adverse reaction to these drugs.

An important final word on immunisation

Although uncommon, any vaccine can cause anaphylaxis in a child, regardless of whether or not a child has food allergy. Immunisation should always take place in a safe environment where resuscitative equipment and adrenaline is available. If you have any concerns about your child being immunised, discuss them directly with your GP and/or allergy specialist. New vaccines are added to the immunisation schedule from time to time, so not all may be covered in this book. As a general rule, whenever your child is due for an immunisation of any kind or is prescribed any medication, you should always remind your GP or immunisation centre staff of your child's allergies *before* your child's treatment.

Statistics and the likelihood of your child outgrowing a food allergy

In the previous pages we have included statistics on outgrowing allergies to IgE-mediated cow's milk and egg allergies based on recent studies. It's important to have some perspective that these studies are based on children attending tertiary referral centres, that is, seeing highly trained specialists. This means the patients in these studies probably have complicated cases of food allergy, so the statistics may not correlate in the general population — no one knows for sure. Still, they are useful to consider, and if the trend is right, it means many parents (myself included) won't lose hope when their child hasn't outgrown milk or egg allergy by school age and will be encouraged and motivated to ensure their child is reviewed and reassessed on a regular basis.

Statistics aside, your allergy specialist will be tracking the trend of your child's skin prick test or RAST results over time to help assess how likely it is that your child will outgrow specific allergies.

Peanut

The peanut, by botanical definition, is not a nut: it belongs to the legume family, along with soy, lentils and peas. Legumes are grown in the ground while tree nuts, no surprise, grow on trees. Peanut allergy is very common in childhood, occurring in approximately 1 in 50 children.[21] It is commonly diagnosed in early childhood, usually with the child's first known exposure to peanut, but it may also occur for the first time in adulthood. Not all allergic reactions to peanut are life-threatening, but peanut — along with tree nuts — is responsible for the majority of fatalities from food-related anaphylaxis.[22]

A person with peanut allergy is allergic to certain proteins found in the peanut. The most prevalent (and well studied) proteins in peanut that are responsible for triggering allergic reactions are known as Ara h 1, Ara h 2 and Ara h 3. Your child may be allergic to one, two or all three of these proteins.

Outgrowing peanut allergy

Peanut allergy will be lifelong for the majority of children, but research indicates about 20 per cent of children do outgrow peanut allergy.[23] However, if a child is still allergic to peanut by the time they reach adolescence, it is generally considered likely that the allergy will be lifelong.

Possible clinical cross-reactions

Tree nuts: Research indicates approximately 25–35 per cent of peanut-allergic individuals are also allergic to at least one tree nut[24, 25] — for example, cashew, walnut, pistachio, hazelnut — even though tree nuts are from a separate botanical family. It is usually recommended that young children allergic to peanut also avoid all tree nuts: not only because of the increased chance of tree-nut allergy, but also because peanuts and tree nuts are frequently processed together, making cross-contamination a real risk. It is also difficult for children to distinguish one nut from another. Your doctor may suggest performing an allergy test and food challenge to individual tree nuts as your child grows older. The risk of a child with peanut allergy developing tree-nut allergy also increases over time, so your doctor may test for tree-nut allergies at 1–2 yearly intervals if your child has peanut allergy.

Other legumes: While it is common for children with peanut allergy to produce positive skin prick test or RAST results to other legumes, only a tiny percentage of these children are actually allergic to other legumes. See 'Peanut allergy and other legumes' below.

Peanut allergy and other legumes

Q My 3-year-old son has peanut allergy. We currently avoid all peanut- and tree-nut-containing products. I understand that peanut is a legume, and I'm wondering if this means I also need to avoid introducing all other legumes?

A Many children allergic to peanut will also have positive skin prick test results to other legumes, but they won't necessarily be allergic to those other legumes. While the peanut is a member of the legume family, the cross-reactivity between peanut and other legumes is, statistically, very low, only about 5 per cent,[26] although lupin (see below) is thought to be the exception.

While the vast majority of children who are allergic to peanut can safely consume legumes, some allergy specialists will skin prick test for certain legumes, for example, chickpea, before allowing it to be introduced into the diet. Talk to your son's allergy specialist before introducing other legumes into his diet, just to be safe. As always, your specialist will consider your son's unique clinical history and may want to run a skin prick test for other legumes before giving you the okay.

Lupin: another allergenic legume

The *Medical Journal of Australia* (MJA) recently reported three cases of lupin allergy.[27] Lupin is a member of the legume family and looks like a round, flat yellow bean. It has been widely used in Europe for some time in flour and bran, mostly in manufactured food goods, but is not, as yet, a common ingredient in food in Australia. It is mainly found in specialty breads, usually in health food stores.

Lupin has been associated with triggering anaphylaxis and, while the cross-reactivity between peanut and other legumes is very low, lupin is thought to be the exception, with research suggesting the risk may in fact be high.[28] However, in the three cases reported in MJA, none of the patients had peanut allergy, so it can also occur in patients with no history of peanut allergy.

Lupin is not an ingredient included in the mandatory allergy warning system on food labels: this means that while it may be listed as an ingredient on the label of a manufactured food, there is no lawful requirement for it to be identified in unlabelled products, such as bread and loose bread rolls.

The authors of the MJA article suggest that lupin allergy needs to be considered by doctors in the case of unexplained food allergy and that lupin should be added to the list of allergens

continued

requiring compulsory allergy-warning labelling, in order to avoid inadvertent ingestion.

If you suspect your child may be allergic to lupin, make an appointment with your child's allergy specialist for review and testing. If your child is allergic to peanut, they should avoid products containing lupin because the chance of clinical cross-reactivity is so high.

To read the article, visit: **www.mja.com.au**

The recurrence of peanut allergy

Even if your child is one of the lucky 20 per cent to outgrow peanut allergy, you may not be out of the woods just yet. Research indicates that peanut allergy may recur, and while there is still no hard evidence, scientists suspect that limited or zero consumption of peanut after the child has outgrown the allergy may increase the risk.[29] If your child has recently outgrown peanut allergy, talk to your allergy specialist about whether or not your child should make a concerted effort to include peanut in their diet on a regular basis, and whether or not they still need to carry an EpiPen until they have proven they can safely consume peanuts over a period of time.

Tree nuts

'Tree nut' refers to any nut that grows on trees, including: almond, Brazil, cashew, hazelnut, macadamia, pecan, pine, pistachio and walnut. As already stated in the peanut section above, tree nuts are from a different botanical family to peanuts, but do share some similar proteins.

Tree-nut allergy is often diagnosed in young children, usually with the child's first known exposure to a particular tree nut, which is frequently between the ages of 2 and 4. Tree-nut allergy is not as common as peanut allergy, but still affects approximately 1 in 500 children in Western communities.[30]

Outgrowing tree-nut allergy

Tree-nut allergy is, in the vast majority of cases, lifelong, but a 2005 study produced some encouraging results, finding that 9 per cent of children allergic to tree nuts do, over time, outgrow their allergy (and the study included children who had suffered a severe reaction to a tree nut in the past).[31] Two other important findings of this study were: firstly, in children who are allergic to both peanut and tree nut, those who outgrow their peanut allergy may have a higher chance of also outgrowing their tree-nut allergy; and secondly, children who are allergic to more than one or two different tree nuts seem less likely to outgrow their tree-nut allergy. The importance of this study for parents is to understand that a tree-nut allergy is not always lifelong, so regular review and testing of your child by an allergy specialist is essential. Your child might just be one of the lucky ones!

Possible clinical cross-reactions

Other tree nuts: If your child is allergic to one tree nut then they will usually be advised to avoid all tree nuts, because there is a high chance they will be allergic to at least one other tree nut. Tree-nut-allergic individuals are also advised to avoid peanuts due to the high chance of cross-contamination with tree nuts in food processing and packaging. They may be able to ingest peanut later in life, providing the source is uncontaminated, for example, peanuts eaten directly from the shell.

Coconut and nutmeg as allergens

Q My daughter is allergic to cashews, so we avoid all tree nuts and peanuts. Do we also need to avoid coconut and nutmeg? I have heard conflicting opinions from other parents.

A People with tree-nut allergy generally do not need to avoid coconut or nutmeg (unless they have had a previous reaction to either of these foods or have been advised to do so by their allergy specialist).

Despite the word 'nut' appearing in coconut and nutmeg, neither are tree-nut or peanut products. Coconut is actually the seed of a fruit, and nutmeg comes from the seed kernel of a tropical tree.

Having said this, anyone can be allergic to any food, regardless of whether or not they have tree-nut allergy, and cases of allergy to coconut have been reported. Research suggests there may be a higher rate of cross-reactivity between walnut and hazelnut with coconut, but coconut allergy is considered relatively rare.

As always, if you are ever in doubt as to what food is safe for your child to consume, contact your allergy specialist before introducing the food to your child.

Fish

Fish allergy is far more common in adults than in children; it is estimated to affect approximately 0.5 per cent of the population.[32]

Looking at fish from a food-allergy perspective, a group from The Children's Hospital at Westmead, Sydney, has classified fish with bones and scales into six groups:

Group 1	shark, flake and sweet William
Group 2	sardines, pilchards and anchovies
Group 3	salmon, pike and trout
Group 4	cod, hake and haddock
Group 5	tuna, mackerel, snapper, pink snapper, perch, barramundi, bream, flathead and whiting
Group 6	sole, flounder, halibut

© The Children's Hospital at Westmead, Sydney Children's Hospital, Randwick & Kaleidoscope, Hunter Children's Health Network — 2005–2008. Reproduced by kind permission.

This classification can be really helpful when a doctor is deciding which fish your child may or may not be able to safely eat. (See more under 'Possible clinical cross-reactions', page 107.) It should be noted, however, that some children react to only one type of fish.

As with egg, cooking and canning fish can alter the allergenic proteins, so some people who are allergic to fresh fish can safely eat tinned fish,[33] but as always, discuss this with your allergy specialist.

Outgrowing fish allergy

Studies on fish allergy have been limited, but it is generally considered lifelong — although in one Swedish study a small number of children did outgrow their fish allergy.[34, 35] As with most things in the world of allergy, there are always exceptions.

Possible clinical cross-reactions

Other fish: If your child is allergic to one fish, there is a high risk they will also be allergic to other fish;[36, 37] this is because the allergy sufferer is usually allergic to a particular protein that is found in various species of fish.

Looking at the classification chart from The Children's Hospital, Westmead on page 106, the further away one group of fish is from another group, the less likely it is that your child will be allergic to fish in both groups.

If your child is allergic to a certain type of fish, your child's allergy specialist may be able to look at including other 'groups' of fish when testing your child. Children with fish allergy do not necessarily have to avoid all fish, but if your child is allergic to one particular fish, do not introduce any fish or fish products into your child's diet without consulting your allergy specialist, and be extremely cautious about the risk of cross-contamination. (See 'Cross-contamination: a very real issue for fish and shellfish allergy', page 108.)

A note on shellfish: There is no research to suggest clinical cross-reactivity between fish and shellfish, so many people who are allergic to fish can safely eat shellfish and vice versa, because the proteins are quite different. Regardless, fish-allergic patients will usually be routinely tested for shellfish allergy and vice versa. If your child is allergic to fish but can safely eat shellfish, you still need to be aware of cross-contamination issues. (See 'Cross-contamination: a very real issue for fish and shellfish allergy', page 108.)

Cross-contamination: a very real issue for fish and shellfish allergy

If your child is diagnosed with fish or shellfish allergy but is given the okay by your allergy specialist to eat specific types of fish or shellfish, you need to be *very* cautious and aware of the high risk of cross-contamination, especially in restaurants, fish markets and seafood retail outlets. If the same pair of tongs is used to handle all types of fish and shellfish, or staff wear the same pair of gloves in handling different types of fish and shellfish, or it seems likely that different types of fish and shellfish have had some kind of contact in their storage, display, handling or cooking (for example, fish and prawns may be cooked on the same BBQ plate), your child could be at risk of an allergic reaction and you should not give that food to your child to eat. Always make your child's allergy known to any supplier or server of fish and shellfish products; ask questions about cross-contamination; and always carry your child's Action Plan and emergency medications in case of inadvertent exposure to an allergen.

Fish food and fish allergy

Q My teenage daughter is allergic to scaly fish. When she was quite young she experienced anaphylaxis after eating fish fingers. Her school is very proactive about keeping her safe and they have just contacted me to see if it is safe for her to attend science lessons in a laboratory where there is a fish tank containing fish. Members of her class will also be responsible for feeding the fish and cleaning the tank.

A It is not a problem for a person allergic to fish to be in the same room as pet fish in a tank, unless they intend to handle or eat the fish, of course!

However, be aware that some fish food contains seafood, so considering your daughter has had a severe reaction in the past, it is probably best to play it safe and not have her handling fish food or cleaning the tank, unless your allergy specialist has checked the ingredients in the fish food and tells you it is safe for her to do so.

It is encouraging that your school is being so forward thinking and checking with you in advance of placing your daughter in this classroom.

Shellfish

Like fish allergy, shellfish allergy is far more common in adults than in children; it is estimated to affect approximately 1 per cent of the population.[38]

The term 'shellfish' is commonly used to refer to seafood invertebrates (meaning those without a backbone), as opposed to only those with a shell.

From a biological viewpoint, these invertebrates are classified into four main groups:[39]

- crustaceans (for example, prawns, crab, lobster)
- molluscs (for example, scallops, oysters, mussels)
- cephalopods (for example, octopus, squid, calamari)
- gastropods (for example, sea snails and slugs)

Outgrowing shellfish allergy
Studies on shellfish allergy have been limited, but it is generally considered a lifelong allergy.[40]

Possible clinical cross-reactions
Other shellfish: Children who are allergic to one type of shellfish have a very high chance of reacting to other members from the same group. For example, if your child is allergic to one member of the crustacean family, such as prawn, it is likely they will also be allergic to other members of the crustacean family, for instance crab and lobster.[41] Shellfish from the other groups may not be a problem for your child (but will be for some); regardless, many doctors advise any child allergic to one type of shellfish to avoid all shellfish, because the risk of cross-contamination is so high. After review and testing, your child's allergy specialist will discuss with you what your child can and cannot eat.

Soy

The soybean is a legume; other members of the legume family include peanut, lentils and beans. A person with soy allergy is allergic to proteins found in the soybean. Soy allergy is commonly diagnosed in infancy and, as mentioned in the section on cow's milk allergy, about 1 in 5 infants allergic to cow's milk also cannot tolerate soy[42] — although an infant may have soy allergy independent of cow's milk allergy.

Avoiding soy is harder than most people imagine because it is present in such a large variety of processed foods. Although it should be noted that research indicates soy oil[43] and soy lecithin (an emulsifier), both commonly listed as ingredients in processed foods, are *usually* safe to consume for children with soy allergies, always check with your child's allergy specialist.

Outgrowing soy allergy

Soy allergy is common in infancy but usually resolves by the pre-school years.[44]

Possible clinical cross-reactions

Other legumes: The vast majority of children with soy allergy will not be allergic to other legumes (only 5 per cent),[45] including peanut. However, even though the chance of a child with soy allergy having another legume allergy is low, the chance of their RAST or skin prick test result being positive to another legume is high, because the proteins are very similar. (See 'Cross-reactivity: what is it?', page 96.) Remember, a positive RAST or skin prick test result does not necessarily mean your child is allergic to the food in question. Your child's allergy specialist will work with you to let you know what legumes your child can safely include in their diet.

Wheat

A person with wheat allergy is allergic to one or more proteins found in wheat. If a wheat allergy sufferer ingests wheat, it triggers an IgE-mediated response, which commonly results in mild symptoms such as hives and aggravation of atopic eczema. It can, in some individuals, trigger a severe allergic reaction but it is uncommon. Wheat, however, is one of the foods most commonly associated with food-associated exercise-induced anaphylaxis (see page 88).

Outgrowing wheat allergy

Wheat allergy commonly resolves by the pre-school years.[46]

Possible clinical cross-reactions

Other cereal grains: If your child is allergic to wheat they won't necessarily be allergic to any other cereal grains: only 20–25 per cent of children with wheat allergy are allergic to other cereal grains.[47, 48] Talk to your allergy specialist about what other cereal grains are safe to include in your child's diet.

Wheat alert: playdough and some glues contain wheat

Commercial playdough and home-made playdough usually contain wheat, as do some craft glues (sometimes called 'wheat paste'). If your child is allergic to wheat, always check the ingredients of their craft materials at home, childcare or school, especially with young children, who love to put anything and everything into their little mouths.

Wheat allergy, coeliac disease, gluten intolerance, wheat intolerance: what's the difference?

IgE-mediated wheat allergy is often confused with wheat intolerance, gluten intolerance and coeliac disease. Below is an explanation of each of these four terms.

IgE-mediated wheat allergy: This has already been described in this chapter, so to recap briefly, it is an immune system response involving the production of IgE antibodies. The symptoms are usually immediate in onset and, in rare instances,

continued

can result in anaphylaxis. Wheat allergy is most often diagnosed in babies and toddlers and is usually outgrown; true wheat allergy is not considered common in the general population. IgE-mediated wheat allergy is diagnosed through RAST and skin prick testing in conjunction with close examination of a patient's clinical history.

Coeliac disease: Coeliac disease is a permanent autoimmune disease. A person with coeliac disease has an immune system that reacts to gluten, so when they eat gluten (found in wheat, rye, oats, triticale and barley) their own immune system damages tissue in the body. IgE antibodies to gluten are not produced in this disease.

Coeliac disease is frequently confused with gluten intolerance (see below), but coeliac disease is a specific immune system response to gluten. Coeliac disease is diagnosed through specific pathology with biopsy, as well as other related blood findings.

Coeliac disease sufferers need to exclude gluten in all forms from their diet to prevent damage to the small bowel and, in children, to also prevent growth issues.

For more information on coeliac disease visit the website of The Coeliac Society of Australia Inc: **www.coeliacsociety.com.au**

Gluten intolerance: Gluten intolerance is a broad term that encompasses any kind of sensitivity to gluten — where a person experiences adverse symptoms following the ingestion of gluten (found in wheat, rye, oats, triticale and barley). Some people who are labelled 'gluten intolerant' will have positive test results to coeliac disease (see above), a permanent autoimmune disease, but many people who are gluten intolerant do not have coeliac disease.

There is no definite pathology used to diagnose gluten intolerance in patients who do not have coeliac disease; gluten intolerance is usually diagnosed through an elimination diet.

Wheat intolerance: Wheat intolerance refers to a condition where a person is sensitive to wheat, experiencing a variety of symptoms — either gastrointestinal or related to mouth ulcers and fatigue — following the ingestion of wheat. As with gluten intolerance, it is very difficult to prove in testing and no one really knows why these reactions to wheat occur.

People with wheat intolerance are sensitive to wheat itself as opposed to gluten. People with wheat intolerance can usually consume other gluten-containing foods without any problem. Wheat intolerance is more easily recognisable in adults than in children.

Spelt and kamut

Q My 18-month-old has eczema and is allergic to peanuts and wheat. I have recently visited an organic health food store and asked them what wheat-free products I could try for my baby. Staff recommended spelt or kamut pasta. What are these two grains and is it safe for me to feed these to my child?

A Spelt and kamut are ancient types of wheat grain that many people claim are more digestible and less allergenic than regular wheat. These claims, however, are not necessarily true, and any child diagnosed with IgE-mediated wheat allergy must eliminate spelt and kamut products from their diet.

You may also come across products containing 'triticale', which is a cereal grain produced by crossing wheat and rye. Products containing triticale are not safe for anyone with wheat allergy. Couscous and semolina are also made from wheat and are not safe to include in the diet of anyone with wheat allergy.

If you are ever offered an unusual grain product in a health food shop, check with your allergy specialist or dietitian before offering it to your wheat-allergic child.

Sesame

Sesame allergy appears to be growing in prevalence in Australia. While studies on sesame allergy are limited in comparison to the other top allergens, in a review study at the Royal Children's Hospital in Melbourne from the period 1990–96,[49] the number of children sensitised to sesame was higher than the number of children sensitised to any one tree nut. The study also reported that sensitisation to sesame was occurring early — in children under 2 years of age.

A 2005 American study reported sesame allergy is growing globally, finding a significant increase in sesame allergy, mostly in developed nations, over the past 50 years.[50] There is speculation that sesame allergy may be rising in line with the increase of sesame into our diets through popular foods such as tahini, bread and grissini coated in sesame seeds, and sesame oil in cooking, but no one knows for sure.

Sesame seeds come in several different colours. If your child is diagnosed as being allergic to sesame, they need to strictly avoid all sesame products, regardless of the colour of the seed involved (for example, black sesame seeds are often sprinkled on top of Turkish bread and are just as allergenic as the pale coloured ones normally found on top of hamburger buns).

Outgrowing sesame allergy

There is no research as yet to suggest the odds of a child outgrowing sesame allergy, but it is commonly cited that allergies to seeds tend to be lifelong.[51]

Possible clinical cross-reactions

There may be cross-reactivity with other foods, including other seeds, but more research is needed in this area.

Other seeds and sesame allergy

Q My son is 12 and is allergic to sesame seed and peanut. Our allergy specialist has recently told us he suspects both allergies will be lifelong. To date we have been avoiding all seeds, not just sesame, simply because I have found it easy to do so. Now that it seems likely my son will have these allergies for life, I'd like to know if it is necessary to avoid all seeds or only sesame.

A Allergy to seeds other than sesame has been reported (mustard, poppy and pumpkin to name only some), and there is the possibility of someone having a reaction to any seed, but sesame allergy is the most common of all seed allergens.

Individuals allergic to sesame are not routinely advised to avoid all seeds, but you should check with your son's allergy specialist in case there is anything in your son's clinical history to suggest he may be allergic to any other seeds.

If you are given the green light for your son to include other seeds in his diet, you still need to be aware of cross-contamination, especially in bakery goods. The last loaf of bread I purchased that was labelled 'May contain traces of sesame' (which I purchased for other family members, not my sesame-allergic son), contained at least 30 sesame seeds — I stopped counting at 30 — on the bottom of the loaf.

Always buy labelled products, read all labels carefully every time you buy a product (no matter how many times you have bought it before), and pay close attention to 'May contain statements' in regard to sesame, as it may *really* contain sesame.

Other allergens

So far in this chapter we have focused on the nine most common allergens, but it is also worth mentioning some other 'often-talked-about' allergens: fresh fruit and vegetables, latex and food additives. An overview of each is provided in the following pages.

As already emphasised in Chapter 1, any food can cause an allergic reaction, so just because a food hasn't been included in this chapter, it doesn't mean it can't cause an allergic reaction. If you think your child may be allergic to a more unusual food, visit your GP, who will refer you to an allergy specialist for testing and diagnosis.

Fresh fruit and vegetables: oral allergy syndrome

Although uncommon, some children do experience allergic symptoms after eating certain fresh fruits and vegetables, commonly referred to as 'oral allergy syndrome'.

Oral allergy syndrome, as the name suggests, is a food-related allergic reaction involving oral symptoms. It usually occurs in individuals who suffer from seasonal allergic rhinitis or conjunctivitis,[52] and symptoms include itching and swelling of the lips, tongue and mouth after eating certain fruits and vegetables or nuts (usually raw).

The allergy occurs due to cross-reactivity between pollens. So someone who is allergic to a particular protein found in a certain pollen may also react to that same protein when it is present in a food. In Australia, plantain pollen (plantain is a common garden weed) sensitisation can occur and this protein can cross-react with fruits such as melon, orange, kiwi fruit and tomato.

Oral allergy syndrome is not usually dangerous and the allergenic protein in the food is often destroyed in cooking, so many of these allergy sufferers can safely and comfortably eat the offending food if it has been cooked.

Although rare, severe reactions — including anaphylaxis — can happen, especially if someone exercises soon after eating significant quantities of their allergic trigger (See 'Food-associated exercise-induced anaphylaxis', page 88.)

Skin prick tests using fresh food extracts are usually used to help an allergy specialist diagnose oral allergy syndrome. How this condition is managed depends on the severity of symptoms. If your child is experiencing any allergic symptoms after ingesting raw fruits, vegetables or nuts, you need to make an appointment to see an allergy specialist. (It is helpful to bring a small sample of the fruit or vegetable to your appointment for your doctor to use in the test.)

Fresh fruit and vegetables: other allergies

It should also be made clear that the above information is related to fresh fruit and vegetables in oral allergy syndrome, and that fresh fruit and vegetables, especially kiwi fruit, can also cause IgE-mediated allergies that can result in severe reactions. As always, if you think any food has triggered an allergic reaction in your child, consult your GP or allergy specialist for further investigation.

Latex allergy

Latex obviously isn't a food, but is worth including here because some individuals with latex allergy may also have food allergy. Below is an overview of the different types of latex allergy, followed by an explanation of the connection between latex and food allergy.

What is latex allergy?

Latex, also referred to as 'natural rubber', is derived from the milky sap of the rubber tree (*Hevea brasiliensis*).[53] Natural latex can be found in a wide variety of popular consumer products, including elastic in some nappies, infant dummies and toys. However, latex-allergic reactions most commonly occur following exposure to 'dipped' latex products, such as gloves, party balloons, swimming caps and condoms.

There are two types of allergic reactions to latex:[54]

1. Immediate reactions: As with food allergy, this is the most serious type of reaction, which can result in symptoms ranging from hives and facial swelling, to breathing difficulty. Anaphylaxis is the most serious form of reaction to latex. In immediate reactions, the patient is allergic to proteins in the latex, so their immune system produces IgE antibodies to particular proteins found in latex. Immediate reactions to latex are not common and mainly occur in hospital populations, for example, healthcare workers, people who have undergone numerous surgical procedures and children with spina bifida.[55] In the general population, the number of children with immediate reactions to latex is very low.

2. Allergic contact dermatitis: This type of reaction is delayed (typically 12–48 hours after initial exposure to latex) and involves irritation of the skin, or 'contact dermatitis', causing symptoms such as dry, rough skin.[56] It does not involve the production of IgE antibodies. This kind of allergic reaction is not life-threatening but treatment is still recommended to avoid more serious allergic reactions from developing. Allergic contact dermatitis reactions to latex are far more common than immediate reactions.

As with food allergy, if you suspect your child may have an allergy to latex, visit your GP, who can refer you to an allergy specialist. Allergy specialists can do a RAST or skin prick test to help confirm a diagnosis. If your child has had a reaction to something specific, for example, hives at the mouth while blowing up a balloon, or after exposure to some other product containing natural rubber latex, write down details of the reaction, including the item, symptoms, how long after exposure to the item the symptoms developed and any medications used to treat the reaction.

Latex allergy and food allergy: what's the connection?

Some children who are allergic to latex may also experience allergic symptoms after eating certain foods, especially banana and avocado, and less commonly kiwi fruit, strawberry, passionfruit, plum, tomato or other fruits.[57] This is sometimes referred to as the 'latex–fruit syndrome'. These reactions usually occur because the proteins in the plants of these foods are very similar to the allergy-causing proteins in latex. The symptoms on eating the food tend to be limited to an itching sensation in the mouth. A child with latex allergy will generally be screened for food allergies by their allergy specialist. Not all children with latex allergy need to avoid these foods.

If your child has latex allergy, you should discuss the necessary precautions and medications with your child's allergy specialist.

Food additives

Try Googling 'food additives': you could be reading various and conflicting opinions and studies for years on end. This book is not about food additives, but they are worth mentioning here to make it clear that reactions to food additives are usually distinct from IgE-mediated food allergy.

Food additives are substances that are added to food for purposes such as colour, flavour or preservation. Some food 'additives', for example, amines, occur naturally in many foods.

While food additives are held responsible for symptoms in many children and adults, the true rate of adverse reactions to additives is low. A number of symptoms and signs have been linked to food additives in some individuals and these will be outlined below, but keep in mind that this is not an exhaustive list. In medical terms, reactions to food additives are generally classified as an intolerance, while true allergic reactions to additives are considered rare.

Asthma and food additives

Sulfites and monosodium glutamate (MSG) are the most common substances linked with asthma, although less than 5 per cent of asthmatics will have additive-induced symptoms. If you suspect that your child's asthma is exacerbated by additives then they need to be formally assessed by their specialist.

Other symptoms of additive intolerance

Symptoms such as rashes (for example, hives and eczema), abdominal pain, vomiting, diarrhoea, swelling and, very rarely, anaphylaxis have been linked to additives. Sulfites, food colourings, MSG, benzoates, nitrates, nitrites and amines are the most commonly considered substances. Anyone who reacts to these additives usually won't have a positive skin prick test because they do not produce IgE antibodies to the additive.

If your child's history is suggestive of an additive intolerance, your doctor may recommend a period of time where you carefully exclude additives, followed by additive challenges. The challenges may be conducted under controlled conditions, using capsules that contain a small portion of the suspect additive, with parents asked to record their child's symptoms during the challenge period.

Behavioural problems in some children have also been linked to food additives. If your child's behaviour is causing concerns, it is important that you see a doctor, so they can take a thorough history and examine your child. Many people think that food additives are the cause of behavioural problems, but this is not always the case when formal assessments are performed, so other causes must always be investigated.

Part 2

Managing food allergy

7

Feeding your food-allergic child

Feeding a child with food allergy can, initially, be stressful and hard work. Parents of food-allergic children are often faced with numerous feeding challenges, including: trying to find alternative sources for allergenic foods they have to eliminate from their child's diet; the child's resistance to trying new foods, and other eating behaviour issues; anxiety over whether their child's diet is nutritionally balanced and provides enough kilojoules; and, in some children, growth problems. Although not every child with a food allergy needs to be under the care of a paediatric dietitian, they can be a godsend in providing help in all of these areas — and more.

This chapter covers the role of a paediatric dietitian in helping food-allergic children and their parents, when to see a dietitian, how to find and work with a dietitian, as well as listing the essential food sources a child should be aiming to eat every day. We also look at the essential nutrients provided in common allergens and some of the recommended substitutes, as well as practical ideas about encouraging positive eating behaviours.

We are grateful for the assistance of Barbara Dennison, a paediatric dietitian working in food allergy at the Children's Hospital in Westmead, Sydney, in preparing the information in this chapter. Her professional expertise, generosity and positive outlook are inspirational.

The role of a paediatric dietitian

If your child has multiple food allergies, it can be especially challenging to ensure they are gaining all the energy and nutrients they need. A paediatric dietitian can help you to identify appropriate food options that are safe for your child to eat, as well as put together an overall balanced, healthy and safe diet for your child to enjoy at different stages of their development. A dietitian can also be a source of wonderful allergen-free recipes and, importantly, help with behavioural issues around eating.

When to see a paediatric dietitian

There are many reasons why families with food-allergic children commonly seek help from a paediatric dietitian:

- When two or more allergens need to be eliminated from a child's diet.
- When a child has to eliminate, or won't eat enough, foods containing a key nutrient, for example, calcium.
- Growth issues: for example, if a child is growing consistently along a height percentile line but is dropping off significantly on their weight percentile line, it may be an indication that a family needs to seek advice.
- The family is having difficulty providing a special diet and needs further education and help.
- When the parents are highly anxious.
- Fussy or difficult eating behaviours in a child.

In terms of knowing how well your child is doing, food consumption and growth are helpful indicators, but energy levels are also telling. If your child is eating enough of the right foods, they should be satisfied after a meal and have good energy levels to enjoy playing and exploring their world.

In summary, if you are concerned about your child's diet, growth or eating behaviour or you feel your family is not coping with providing a special diet, you should make an appointment with a paediatric dietitian via a written referral from your GP, paediatrician or allergy specialist. (See 'How to find a paediatric dietitian', page 125.)

What you can expect to be discussed in an initial appointment with a paediatric dietitian

A paediatric dietitian consultation for a child with food allergy may involve discussion of:

- Your child's growth history
- Your child's diagnosed allergens
- The nutritional adequacy of their existing diet and any changes needed
- Alternative nutritional sources for the foods you need to eliminate from your child's diet
- Any behavioural issues around food

In addition, a dietitian will also answer any questions you have that are specific to your child, provide you with resources for sourcing special foods and products and how to prepare them, help you understand what to look for on food labels, recommend websites and books with appropriate recipes, and supply other information in regard to the practical management of living with food allergy.

Follow-up appointments may be required, depending on the family's situation and whether or not a child is failing to thrive. For many families, a one-off visit when the child is initially diagnosed with food allergy can educate and empower parents in managing their food-allergic child's diet, and they only need to see the dietitian again if growth or behavioural issues emerge further down the track, or possibly if additional food allergies are diagnosed.

Many children outgrow their food allergies, and when this happens some parents find the process of normalising eating a real challenge. A discussion with a dietitian at this time can also really help.

Preparing for an appointment with a paediatric dietitian

Planning ahead for an appointment with a paediatric dietitian will help you make the most of your allocated time. Following are some practical tips you might like to consider when preparing to see your child's dietitian.

- Ensure you discuss any specific questions you have about your child's allergies with your allergy specialist *before* you see a dietitian. For example, is it safe for your child to consume products with 'May contain' statements?
- The dietitian will want to see your child to assess how they are growing, but trying to hold a reasonable discussion with one or more young children in a small room can be a bit of a challenge. You will be hearing a lot of information, and having to tend to your child will probably mean you won't absorb as much information as you need to. Consider bringing along your partner, a friend or a relative to take your child outside so you can concentrate.
- Be sure to bring along your Child Health Book, in which your child's growth is recorded.
- Bring along, or send when making the appointment, a written referral from your allergy specialist or GP, explaining the results of your child's allergy tests and which foods they need to eliminate from their diet.
- It may be useful to record what your child is eating and drinking over a 2- to 3-day period, especially if those days are representative of what your child usually eats and drinks. A dietitian will also be interested to know when your child is sleeping and waking, the time they are eating and drinking, and the approximate amounts of the foods they are consuming.
- Prepare a list of the key questions and concerns you would like to discuss with your dietitian.

How to find a paediatric dietitian

There are many kinds of dietitians working in Australia, but ideally you need to make an appointment with a paediatric dietitian who has experience in IgE-mediated food allergy.

Your allergy specialist, paediatrician or GP is the best person to refer you to a suitable dietitian. My son's dietitian has worked with his allergy specialist for a long time and this has ensured we have received advice consistent with our specialist's approach to managing Noah's allergies. When Noah was initially diagnosed with multiple food allergies, the information and support we received from our dietitian boosted our confidence in managing both Noah's allergies and nutritional needs. I'll always remember the feeling of relief, as the parent of a newly diagnosed child, of coming away armed with written information on alternative food sources and some simple recipes and advice on how to stock our pantry with staples. With this practical assistance I was able to feed my baby with confidence and even enjoy experimenting in the kitchen.

When you ask your doctor for a referral to a dietitian, it must be a *written* referral which makes it clear what foods your child needs to eliminate from their diet. It is not the role of a dietitian to interpret RAST or skin prick test results — as a positive skin prick test or RAST does not necessarily mean a food needs to be eliminated; your dietitian *really* needs to know how your doctor has interpreted your child's test results.

If your child has any dietary deficiencies that have already been identified (iron or calcium, for example), it would be helpful for your doctor to include this in the referral letter along with any relevant blood results. It is also important to tell the dietitian if your child has been prescribed any medications or supplements.

If you live in a remote area, don't let distance deter you from seeking help: some dietitians are willing to conduct consultations over the phone combined with email. Check with your allergy specialist, paediatrician or GP.

Consultation with a paediatric dietitian can be arranged through a public hospital or you can visit a dietitian working in private practice. Some dietitians in private practice will offer concessions for patients in financial difficulty, and most private health funds offer rebates for private consultations, so check with your insurer.

If you do choose to search for a dietitian on your own — which is not recommended, as you really need to find a paediatric dietitian who has specialised knowledge in IgE-mediated food allergies — ensure they are an Accredited Practising Dietitian (APD), and also ensure they are communicating with your referring doctor.

What every child should be eating: the daily 5

Children should grow; it is what distinguishes them from adults. In order to grow and thrive children need to be eating a healthy and balanced diet. It sounds straightforward but, as most parents know, achieving this can be the source of constant frustration and worry.

So what should a child — with or without food allergies — be eating on a daily basis?

Keeping it very simple, Barbara Dennison recommends that parents should be ensuring their children include a variety from each of the following five food groups every day:

- Protein (such as meat, chicken, fish, cheese, yoghurt, legumes — dried beans and peas, lentils — and nuts). Most children need a palm-sized serve of meat, fish, chicken or legumes once or twice a day. 'Palm-sized' refers to a serve that covers the child's palm completely and is as thick as their hand.
- Carbohydrates (starchy foods such as wheat, potato, rice, pasta, cereals).
- Vegetables — 3 to 5 serves a day. A serve is about the amount the child can hold in their cupped hand.
- Fruit — 2 serves a day.
- Milk, cheese or yoghurt — 3 serves a day. A serve is a cup of milk, a slice of cheese, a tub of yoghurt.

In addition, from a general health viewpoint:

- Foods need to be low in saturated fat, and the overall intake of other fat-containing foods needs to be moderate. Foods are considered low in saturated fat if they have no more than 1.5mg saturated fat /100g.
- Keep foods low in salt, preferably: it is advised to not add salt to food for babies under 1 year of age. Where possible, choose foods which are not salty and add only small amounts of salt in cooking for children over 1. High fat and salt foods such as potato chips are 'sometimes' foods, not daily options.
- The intake of sugar-containing foods should be moderate. In practical terms this means that kids drink water in preference to juice or cordial;

have savoury snacks not sweet ones; have a small serve of something sweet at the end of a meal but not between meals; have lollies and chocolate infrequently — once a week, not daily.

A word about calcium

Children who have to avoid good sources of calcium such as cow's milk, cheese and yoghurt do need to ensure they are getting enough calcium from other sources. Some — but not all — soy, rice or other cereal drinks are calcium-fortified; you will need to check the labels. It is essential that whatever milk alternative is being used, your child is getting the amount of calcium they need for strong bone development.

Daily calcium requirements are:

	Children	Boys	Girls
1–3 years	500mg		
4–8 years	700mg		
9–13 yrs		1000–1300mg	1000–1300mg
14–18 yrs		1300mg	1300mg

Source: Nutrient Reference Values for Australia and New Zealand, Including Recommended Dietary Intakes, 2006, Department of Health and Ageing.

Calcium checklist

If you are concerned about your child's calcium intake, use the below checklist prepared by Barbara Dennison to help you calculate the amount your child consumes each day and compare it with the amounts recommended above. If you think your child is not obtaining enough calcium, talk to your doctor or dietitian, who may recommend a supplement as an interim measure.

Food	Calcium content*	Quantity consumed	Calcium consumed (mg)
soy/rice drink with added calcium — 100ml*	120mg		
soy yoghurt ** — 200g (1 large tub)	300mg		
soy cheese ** — 20g (1 slice)	60mg		
soy ice-cream ** — 2 scoops	120mg		
soy custard** — ½ cup	150mg		
tofu** — 60g (2 cubes)	14–190mg		
salmon with bones — ½ cup	400mg		
sardines — 1 small tin	230 mg		
breakfast cereal with added calcium**	Check label		
broccoli — ½ cup	20mg		
Other			
TOTAL			

* Calcium content of foods can vary between brands; check the label.
** Check all ingredient lists carefully as they may contain cow's milk protein.

A word on rice and other cereal drinks

Calcium-fortified rice drinks are often substituted for cow's milk, soy drinks and formula in food-allergic toddlers and children (never infants less than 1 year of age). Most are low in protein and other nutrients (there is, however, a chickpea-derived protein-fortified rice drink).

continued

> Any child who is using calcium-fortified rice drink (not protein-fortified) as a substitute for cow's milk, soy drink or formula needs to include in their diet a daily extra serve of an alternative source of protein, for example, egg, meat, fish, chicken or legumes. There have been documented cases of severe malnutrition in children whose parents have put them on calcium-fortified rice drink without including additional sources of protein.[1]
>
> Other cow's milk substitutes have been made from almonds, oats or other grains, nuts, seeds and legumes. They may or may not be suitable alternatives. If your doctor recommends your child needs to drink a cow's milk substitute, choose one which has at least 120mg calcium/100ml and is fortified with Vitamins A and D. Ask your doctor how to ensure your child will receive adequate levels of protein and other nutrients. Your doctor will ideally refer you to a paediatric dietitian.

How much food is enough?

The quantities a child needs to consume from each of the five groups outlined on page 127 varies depending on factors such as the child's age, whether or not they are growing appropriately and, importantly, their appetite: not all children need the same volume of food. Some children eat like sparrows while others — like my own two little ones — seem to be bottomless pits.

One parent's idea of how much a child should eat can be vastly different from another's. I used to laugh when my husband served our children dinner because the portions he dished out were enormous: as much as he would eat. His idea of an appropriate quantity was related to his own appetite rather than theirs. So how much should a child be eating? The only person who can answer that is your child: it's their job to let you know when they have had enough. (See, 'Who's the boss of the dinner table?', page 131.)

Who's the boss of the dinner table?

Many parents report feeling defeated by their children at meal times, and wonder how their toddlers can seemingly rule the roost at such a tender age. In truth, neither party should be aiming to be the boss of the dinner table.

According to Barbara Dennison, it's helpful for parents to understand that while they have a clear role to play, so do children. It needs to be a joint effort, with each party understanding their responsibilities.

It is the job of parents to choose the 'what' and the 'when'. So parents need to choose a balanced and healthy array of foods to offer their child from the 'top 5' food groups, and then decide on eating times — ideally three meals and two small snacks a day.

The child's job is then to choose the 'if' they want to eat and 'how much' they eat.

Parents have to try particularly hard to ensure they allow children to play their own role, instead of trying to control every aspect of their toddler's eating.

Adequate nutrition when common allergens are eliminated from a child's diet

Many of the most common food allergens (as listed in the table on pages 132–33) form the basis of the diet of most Australian children. When one or more of these foods have to be eliminated from a child's diet, it can mean that a child is at risk of missing out on certain key nutrients. Their overall intake of kilojoules, or energy, may also become inadequate.

Below is a simple table outlining the key nutrients supplied by the nine most common food allergens (note that although scaly fish and shellfish are grouped together in the table, they are normally regarded as separate allergens, likewise peanuts and tree nuts), as well as a list of foods that may be used to substitute for these common food allergens (depending on a child's individual allergies, as some children are also allergic to substitute options).

Substituting foods in the diets of children who have only one or two allergies is often quite straightforward, providing you receive advice appropriate to your child from your allergy specialist or dietitian. However, things can become more complicated when a child has multiple food allergies or other health conditions besides food allergy, for example, diabetes or coeliac disease. Sometimes supplements are needed in addition to food substitutions to ensure your child is obtaining the right amount of nutrients and kilojoules. A dietitian will always review your child's food allergies and diet within the context of your child's overall health and how they are growing.

The following table is designed to offer an 'at-a-glance' overview of the impact of eliminating a major allergen from a child's diet. A word of caution, however. The amount of nutrients offered in the substitute food may not match what is found in the allergenic food. Always discuss substitution options for your child's allergen with your child's allergy specialist and/or paediatric dietitian.

Common allergen	Key nutrients	Possible alternatives
Cow's milk	Energy, protein, calcium and other vitamins	Calcium-fortified soy drinks (which contain the equivalent amounts of energy, protein, calcium and other vitamins); calcium-fortified rice or other cereal drinks (which contain the equivalent amounts of energy and calcium, but are lacking in protein and other vitamins)
Egg	Protein and other vitamins	Meat, fish, chicken and legumes
Wheat	Energy, carbohydrate, fibre and B vitamins	Rice, corn, rye, oats and other less-used grains, such as quinoa (pronounced keen-wah), millet, amaranth and buckwheat
Soy	Energy, protein, minerals and vitamins — and calcium, if it is in the form of a calcium-fortified soy drink	Cow's milk and calcium-fortified rice or another cereal drink (although some rice and cereal drinks contain insufficient protein and some other vitamins)

Scaly fish and shellfish	Energy, protein, iron, zinc	Meat, fish, chicken, egg, legumes
Peanuts and tree nuts	Energy, protein and fat	Peanut and tree nuts are generally not considered core food selections in Australia, but other good sources of protein include meat, fish, chicken, legumes and egg
Sesame	Energy, protein and fat	Like the peanut and tree nuts, sesame is not generally considered a core food selection in Australia, but other good sources of protein include meat, fish, chicken legumes and egg

How drinking can affect eating in children

How and when throughout the day drinks are offered to a child influences how much and how well they eat. But first a word about what drinks are offered. Breast milk or an infant formula is the appropriate main drink for babies under 1 year of age and provides all their nutrition until 4 to 6 months of age. By the time an infant is 1 year old, food provides about half their nutrition, while breast milk or formula provides the other half. In practical terms, this translates to about 500–600ml of milk per day.

Apart from milk, water is the best drink to offer to your baby from about 6 months of age. Initially they won't drink much, but it is a good idea to get them used to the experience, which becomes more important in the second year of life.

From about 8 to 9 months, milk is best offered at the end of each meal, not before, and water can be offered between meals. This pattern is good to keep up as the child grows and it helps to ensure they have an appetite for food at meal times. Children from about 1 year of age, often before this time, don't need bottles of milk throughout the night. In fact, this is one reason why children refuse their meals: they are simply not hungry.

Juice, cordial and fizzy drinks are best not given as an everyday drink. Keeping them for special occasions means you have something to celebrate with.

Bottle or cup?

It is good to get an infant drinking from a cup rather than a bottle from around 1 year of age. This means they will most likely drink no more milk than they need, will have the appetite for food at meal times and won't need a bottle to go to sleep.

Some children with food allergies also suffer from eczema, and the itchiness may disturb their sleep. Parents can easily get into the pattern of feeding breast milk or milk to comfort them back to sleep — so tempting when it is 2am and you are sleep-deprived! Once you are sure that you have done all possible to manage the eczema well, try to break the habit by giving smaller and smaller amounts of milk each time they wake or simply replace the milk with water. The initial protests will quieten if you consistently give water and not milk. A visit to your allergy specialist can be a huge help in learning to manage the skin better so that your child (and you!) sleep soundly.

Fussy eating habits

Most parents of toddlers at some point become bothered, to put it mildly, about their child's eating habits, especially if their child has experienced, or is experiencing, growth issues, or if the parent has a tendency to feel anxious about food and their child in general.

Children with food allergies may become fussy eaters — especially in their second year of life — for any number of reasons, including early negative experiences of food in the form of allergic reactions, picking up on parental anxiety, and restrictions placed on usual toddler eating behaviours. For example, most toddlers enjoy sampling food off other people's plates and trying new foods when eating out, but this 'free-ranging' is strictly off-limits for many food-allergic children.

Some of the fussy habits of children are actually heightened by the behaviour of us, as parents. Many of us (myself included) are guilty of chasing a child around the house with a bottle, cup or spoon, trying to encourage them to eat, usually to no avail — in fact, it makes the situation worse.

So what can parents do to manage fussy eating habits, especially in toddlers? Barbara Dennison offers the following practical tips.

- Children need to understand that there are set times for eating and times for not eating: the 'not eating' times are for children to enjoy doing the normal things that kids do — playing, going to the park, visiting friends. Where eating is an issue, this 'not eating' time is freeing for a child and allows their natural, in-built healthy appetite to develop. Establishing set meal and snack times — ideally three main meals and two small snacks a day— is important for the wellbeing of the whole family.

- Closely related to the above point, ensure your child is actually hungry when you are expecting them to eat. If your child is given a late afternoon tea and then offered dinner a short time later, they are unlikely to be interested. If your child is really hungry and asking for food near to a meal time, bring lunch or dinner forward instead of offering them a snack that might put them off their main meal.

- Once you have established a pattern of eating and not-eating times, this allows parents to pull back on their anxiety. Everyone in the family needs a break from food, and the 'not eating' time enables this. With a regular eating pattern established and decreased anxiety at the dinner table, a child's in-built hunger will often drive an increased food intake.

- At meal times, food is best offered before a drink. After the meal, milk is given in a cup. (See 'How drinking can affect eating in children', page 133.)

- Between meals, water is the best drink, not juice or milk. Free access to water between meals means your child will still have an appetite for the next meal.

- Night feeds of breast milk or milk or juice are not necessary for older babies and toddlers. It can ruin their appetite for breakfast and, if feeding frequently throughout the night, can result in decayed teeth.

- Do not automatically offer your child a breastfeed or bottle of milk on waking after they are around 9 or 10 months old. Get them into the pattern of food before milk or any drink. This may mean that breakfast needs to be eaten earlier than you would normally prefer to eat it but it starts the day on the right foot.

- Eat with your children around a table. Try not to focus on your child and how well they are eating or not eating. Talk about ordinary things at the table, with only an occasional glance or positive comment about their eating such as, 'I like the way you are eating your peas, Holly.' Try to adopt a relaxed approach and don't let your child see that what or how much they eat matters to you. However, when your child is eating well, be sure to praise their behaviour.

- Let your child feed themselves, with appropriate assistance according to their age. Don't force spoons into their mouth, and don't threaten to punish your child for not eating. Remember that the experience of eating needs to be positive and pleasurable to ensure your child enjoys eating and, as a consequence, looks forward to meal times and eats well.

- Try not to ask your child open-ended questions about meal selections; for example, instead of asking, 'What would you like for breakfast?' you might say, 'Would you like Vegemite or jam on your toast?' In this example, you have decided your child is going to eat toast, but you are still allowing your child to have some choice in what they eat for breakfast.

- If your child won't eat a meal, cover it and keep it aside. If they are hungry later, offer the meal again or only a healthy alternative, such as a banana or a sandwich. The message is: if your child has refused their meal, that's okay, just don't allow them to eat unhealthy or 'treat' foods if they complain of being hungry later on. You don't want to give your child an incentive to keep refusing their main meal!

- At dinner time, try to take a step back in your own mind and ask yourself, 'Has my child eaten something from each of the top 5 groups today?' If the answer is yes, just think, 'Tick, I've done well today, and it doesn't really matter if my child isn't interested in eating something I wanted them to eat tonight.' Has your child had an allergic reaction today? No? Great. Don't beat yourself up unnecessarily. Only sweat the big stuff.

Encouraging your child to try new foods

When you have a child with food allergy, it can seem easy to stick to a small array of foods you know your child enjoys and you are confident are safe. Parents may claim their child is fearful of new foods, but sometimes it is the parent who is fearful, and they unwillingly transfer their own anxiety onto the child. Toddlerhood is a time of life for exploring the world in all kinds of ways, and your child should also be exploring and enjoying the world of food.

Barbara Dennison has a clear philosophy on food:

Food sustains us, but it also enriches our lives enormously, so when a child's food selection has to be restricted it can mean they miss out on a lot of things socially, especially the pleasures of sharing food. The adverse effect is that children can become fearful of food, which can impinge on their overall nutrition and also have psychosocial consequences.

Many parents of children with food allergies become fearful of trying new foods. It is like they are on railway tracks. So long as they are on the tracks they feel safe. It is really important to keep the window on the world of food opening further and further, as much as possible, within the constraints of the food the child needs to avoid. Parents need to branch out and push themselves, and keep on pushing, resisting what may be a natural reluctance. Sometimes, for those with children who have very serious food allergies, it is very difficult to be brave, but working with a paediatric dietitian can help parents to keep broadening their child's diet.

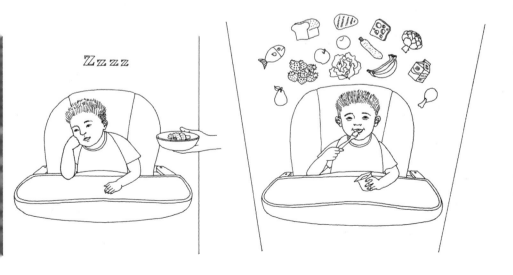

Below are some practical tips to help you encourage your child to try new foods.

- When trying a new food, place a small sample of the new food on the child's plate next to a familiar food you know they are happy to eat. For example, if you would like your child to try peas, you might place a solitary pea on the side of their plate and tell your child, 'That's a pea. I'd like you to taste that tonight.' Then leave them to get on with their job — eating their meal. If they do pick up the pea and taste it, praise their behaviour. 'Great, you ate the yummy pea.' If they don't eat the pea, don't make a fuss. 'You didn't taste your pea today. Oh well, we will try it again tomorrow.' So you are responding in a positive way, but also letting them know they are not off the hook.

- Don't give up. If your little customer is uninterested in your offerings, keep trying. According to Barbara Dennison, it may take up to 10 exposures to a new food for a child to become interested (that's right, *10* or more!). Going back to the pea example, if you offer the pea for the second night, you might prompt your child to pick up the pea, and then ask, 'What does it feel like?' If they squash it between their fingers and drop it onto the floor, great: consider that progress. The next night they might lick their fingers after squashing the pea, and you might ask them, 'What does it taste like?' Keep the atmosphere positive and relaxed, and keep offering new foods.

- Let your child help in food preparation. They might stand on a stool and help at the kitchen bench, washing, chopping, stirring, mixing, peeling (whatever is age-appropriate). Involving your child in the process can inspire them to want to taste what they helped prepare. They may even sample a raw vegetable at the bench as they 'help' but refuse it raw or cooked at the dinner table.

- Having food in the middle of the table that children can share often encourages a child to try something new. For example, you could put a glass of carrot sticks in the middle of the table. They might like to use the carrot stick to eat their mashed potato or to dip into a sauce or gravy. Allowing children to help themselves to communal food can help to relax things, give the child a sense of control and encourage them to explore new foods.

- Star charts can sometimes be useful for older children (around the age of 3 to 4) who do not want to try new foods. So you might say, 'I'd like you to try one pea tonight, and then you can stick a star on your chart.' Then the next night you might ask them to try two peas. What is important to remember is that young children need immediate rewards to change their behaviour. So you still might reward them at the end of the day, but with something that doesn't cost money — perhaps reading a book to them that you have set aside as 'the reward book', playing a game of snakes and ladders together, collaboratively building a construction from blocks, kicking a ball at the park before bedtime, or inviting a friend over to play. In this way you are setting clear expectations and praising their behaviour.
- When possible, try to make some meals that are safe for the whole family, so you can encourage normal toddler eating behaviour such as tasting food from your plate.
- Location, location, location. Sometimes taking a meal outside or to a special spot can work wonders. We often have a picnic lunch at the park or under our outdoor table, which my two call 'the cave'. Trying a new food on a 'picnic' can seem a lot more exciting to a young child than having it at the dinner table. When I give my two the choice of where they want to eat their snack, they seem less fussy about what I actually give them to try.
- Sometimes changing the way you present a food or drink can make it more appealing. For example, Noah went through a phase of losing all interest in drinking his soy drink. However, when I offered it to him in a small jug and asked him if he would like to pour his own soy drink into a teacup, his face lit up and he started to drink it again without fuss. The next time he went off his soy drink, I asked him if he would like to try plonking an ice cube into his soy drink and then give it a stir with a straw — he still drinks his soy drink with an ice cube, and loves it.
- If you have visitors, they can help: monkey see, monkey do. For example, in our house, when Noah's older cousins come to stay, Noah will try what they are eating without fuss, even if it is something he has refused to try for me. Noah now happily eats rice for the simple

reason that one of his cousins eats it, and raw carrot thanks to another cousin.

- Ask another family member to relieve you from dinner duties when they can. In our house, Dad serving dinner on a weekend is a novelty, and sometimes a change of routine can take the focus off what's on their plate and lead to interest in trying something from Dad's (safe) plate.

- Reading about new foods in books and listening to music about foods can also help. My kids love fruit salad courtesy of The Wiggles, spaghetti ('like Steve *Moneghetti*') thanks to a Peter Coombes CD, watermelon because of Justine Clarke and baby spinach thanks to the book *The Little Pea*. Positive messages from other sources can encourage young children to want to try new foods.

- Take your child to the fruit and vegetable shop and involve them in the shopping process. Let them help you push your trolley or put items in the basket and hand over the money to pay. When you are in the shop, ask them if they would like to try a new vegetable or fruit today (in a shop where just about any choice they make is going to be a good one!).

- Children love digging and gardening, so try involving them in caring for a veggie garden, watering a lemon tree or, if you don't have an outdoor area, an indoor herb pot. Some towns have community food gardens where children can visit and taste the produce. Children can be tempted to taste new foods when they are involved in picking the produce and learning about where it comes from. They are not only tasting food but really exploring food — flavours, textures, colour, smells — and understanding where the best foods come from.

- Different strategies will work for different families. Above all else, remember that food should be about pleasure not punishment. Come up with your own creative ideas, try to pull back on your own anxiety and let your children enjoy eating and exploring safe foods.

'I don't have time ...'

Some parents reading this chapter might be uttering under their breath, 'Sure, but who has time to go to such lengths? I'm flat out just getting a meal on the table and spending some time with my children before they go to bed.'

In between work, managing your child's allergies and all of the other commitments a parent has, it can seem a drag to add more chores to the list. When my second child, Lucy, was born, Noah became a fussy eater. I was so tired from feeding Lucy at night I just stuck to the same meals — whatever worked and could get me some sleep. When I returned to work, it was harder still, because by then he had become even fussier, refusing all vegetables and most meats.

I didn't want him living on chicken and fruit exclusively, and I was also worried about his reluctance to try new foods. I wasn't spending enough time encouraging him to explore food and I was becoming openly frustrated with his food refusal at a time of day when I was exhausted. I began to dread dinner time.

I made the decision to put in the extra effort and put into place the advice of a paediatric dietitian. On the weekends, I cooked up meals I knew Noah liked and froze them to have on hand on the days when I was working. This way, when I was tired I could offer him a meal that I knew he would eat and then only have to deal with preparing a small portion of something new for him to try on the side of his plate. I got Noah more involved in the kitchen whenever I could — spreading toppings on his toast at the breakfast table, chopping banana with a plastic knife, stirring and tipping in ingredients in baking, sitting up on the kitchen bench and chatting to me while I was chopping vegetables.

On days when I wasn't working, I started packing our lunch and taking it to the park and having morning or afternoon tea outside, or on a rug inside if the weather was bad. Noah made far less fuss over foods served on a picnic than if I offered them at the

continued

dinner table. I started to take him shopping with me to the fruit and vegetable shop. We introduced a star chart for vegetables and within weeks he was eating broccoli and carrot again. I made a conscious decision to relax at meal times and stopped trying to force him to eat. When I did that, it was no longer a game to him, and he started to eat more widely and with far less fuss (*most* of the time).

With a relaxed mood at the dinner table, I slowly introduced some great new healthy foods — salmon, brown rice, white fish, lamb shank stew (with veggies!), cucumber, plums, strawberries, to name only some. Noah is still adamant about what he does and doesn't like, but the difference is I no longer attempt to force him to eat something he really doesn't like. I am just happy he is now prepared to give a new food a go, gradually broadening his diet, and that I have learned to back off and let him get on with his very important job of enjoying his meals.

Yes, it does take extra effort and time to be relaxed about food, to go the extra mile to incorporate changes to the way you and your children manage meal times, but the difference is, with some effort upfront, your meal times will become far more relaxed and enjoyable in the long run. Once your child becomes less fussy, you can also start making one meal the whole family can eat rather than separate meals to cater for selective taste buds — that part I really enjoy.

Encouraging older children to try new foods

The majority of information in this chapter is aimed at younger children, but older children can also have quite strong resistance to trying new foods. They may have also had strong reactions to foods in the past or have been on extremely limited diets for quite some time. Changing their behaviours can be an even bigger challenge, but the principles are the same as those for young children.

- Explain to your child that they are going to be trying a new food. Name it. Ask when they think they could try it. Negotiate options such as when, in what form and the time of day this food will be tried.

- Provide the food at the agreed time in a small quantity alongside the usual food eaten.

- Resist the urge to get too excited about this event. Don't build up the event, hover or look anxious as the food is eaten. If appropriate, touch the child's arm and say 'good work', 'well done' or something similar once they have put the food in their mouth, whether or not it is eaten. A low-key approach which acknowledges that they have done something which was difficult for them works better than bringing out the cheering team.

- Sometimes even an older child responds well to a star chart with rewards which won't break the bank or be too demanding on you as a parent. Sometimes a week of trying the new food, followed by a reward, is the way to go.

- Involving a dietitian can also help. For example, a dietitian can explain to an older child why new foods can be beneficial. It might mean, for instance, that they can eat out or stay at a friend's place more easily.

Shopping for new foods

Shopping for alternative foods for your newly diagnosed food-allergic child can be a daunting prospect. When starting out, write a simple shopping list of staples you want to find before you hit the supermarket. For example, you might go hunting for an appropriate bread, flour, milk alternative, butter/spread, cracker, pasta, ice-cream and treat food.

Make sure you have done your homework on how to understand food labels (see Chapter 8, Understanding food labelling, page 146) and arrange to go to the supermarket on your own, so you won't feel rushed and can concentrate on reading labels. Every time you go shopping you can add new items to your grocery wishlist, and each time you shop you will be adding to your skills as an 'allergy shopper'.

Before you go to the supermarket, you might like to research some products online. Some food companies display food labels

continued

for their products on their websites, which is really helpful when you are trying to research suitable products. Of course, you will need to re-check the label on the product before you buy it, but it can help to save some time if you do some research before you shop.

I learned the hard way that you should only buy new foods in small quantities — no matter how excited you are when you find a tasty-looking safe food for your child, there is no guarantee they will actually eat it.

Importantly, once you have found a safe food and your child enjoys it, remember that you have to check the label every time you buy the food, as ingredients can change at any time.

Cooking new foods

Cooking without key ingredients can be a challenge. My initial baking efforts without egg were awful: I needed a conveyer belt running from my oven straight to the bin.

Putting in time in the kitchen experimenting is the only way to discover which recipes work and which don't. There are a lot of recipes that claim to be allergy-free and tasty but really aren't tasty at all. (Of course, on my own part I will admit that lack of talent has also been an issue.)

Keep a display book or plastic folder in your pantry in which you can store recipes you try that a) work and b) your child actually enjoys. Over time you will build an incredible resource.

A friend of mine, Anne, is a superb cook and happens to have children with similar food allergies to Noah. She has been the provider of most of Noah's favourite recipes. Recipe swapping is a popular pastime of many parents of food-allergic children: share your knowledge with friends and family.

Appendix I at the end of this book (see page 370) lists some allergy-friendly recipe books you might be interested in tracking down. However, don't dismiss regular cookbooks: once you get the hang of substituting ingredients, you can often adapt regular recipes with great success, too.

When you do get going in the kitchen, stay positive and remember:

- Only make small quantities of new foods and try not to be frustrated if your child doesn't like something you spent what feels like an eternity making.
- Be prepared for failure when cooking with new ingredients. When even the birds reject your offerings, you know it is really bad.

8

Understanding food labelling

Shopping for a child with food allergy can be tricky, especially if your child is allergic to several foods. Parents of food-allergic children rely on products being accurately labelled to ensure they can prevent their child from experiencing an allergic reaction. However, identifying which foods contain an allergen is not always as straightforward as it might seem. Many foods have several alternative names that are not in everyday use, for instance, and you need to recognise the ones that you must avoid.

Initially, there is much to learn — and there is no escaping the reality that shopping will take extra time, energy and patience. Finding foods that are safe for your child is only one part of the equation; you also have to find foods they actually enjoy eating. Over time, though, as your knowledge expands, label reading and sourcing new and safe foods will become a normal part of your daily routine.

With food labelling, as with most areas of food allergy, education is essential. Parents need to be able to interpret food labels and understand exactly what is (and isn't) contained in the foods they are buying for their food-allergic child, in order to keep them safe and well nourished, and encourage them to enjoy the pleasure of food.

In the first part of this chapter we will explain the labelling of allergens under the *Australia New Zealand Food Standards Code*, examine how to interpret important allergen information on a food label, provide an overview of the latest industry development in the voluntary labelling of trace allergens, explain how to lodge a complaint about a mislabelled food and, importantly, let you know how to keep up to date with food recalls. In the second half of this chapter, we list a broad range of lesser-known food names that may alert you to the presence of a common food allergen on a food label, and for each of the most common food allergens, we provide a list of products that often contain them. We thank Food Standards Australia and New Zealand (FSANZ) for their kind assistance in preparing information for this chapter.

Food labelling in Australia

Australia New Zealand Food Standards Code

Food labels convey important information to consumers about the contents of packaged food products. It is a legal requirement of any food company, importer or retailer doing business in Australia to comply with labelling regulations specified in the *Australia New Zealand Food Standards Code*.[1]

The regulation of food labelling specified in the *Food Standards Code* is governed by Food Standards Australia New Zealand (FSANZ): an independent statutory agency established by the *Food Standards Australia New Zealand Act 1991*. FSANZ is responsible for the safe supply of food in Australia and New Zealand and ensuring that consumers are well informed.[2]

In December 2001, Standard 1.2.3 of the *Food Standards Code* — 'Mandatory Warning and Advisory Statements and Declarations' — came into effect. In simple terms, this Standard made it a legal requirement for the following common food allergens and their products to be identified on a food label:

- Milk
- Egg
- Crustacea (the specific name of the crustacean must be declared; for example, prawn)
- Fish
- Peanuts
- Soybeans

- Tree nuts (excluding coconut, but the specific name of all other tree nuts must be declared; for example, walnut)
- Sesame

As well as:

- Cereals containing gluten and their products, including wheat, rye, barley, oats, spelt (for those with coeliac disease).
- Sulphites in concentrations of 10mg/kg or more, must also be declared (sulphites above this limit can trigger asthma in some asthmatics).
- Foods containing royal jelly (a bee product) must contain a warning statement, as people may be unaware of the severe health risk posed to some by this allergen. Royal jelly has triggered severe allergic reactions, especially in asthmatics and allergy sufferers.

All of the above must be identified on the food label of a packaged good if they have been *added* to a food product as an ingredient, no matter how small the amount.

The *Food Standards Code* is a long and comprehensive legal document, which may be accessed online at **www.foodstandards.gov.au/thecode/** Below we will answer some frequently asked questions about the *Food Standards Code* in regard to allergen labelling.

As always, keep in mind that information changes and legislation is amended from time to time. If you have any questions about food labelling under the *Food Standards Code*, you should contact FSANZ (**www.foodstandards.gov.au**), and if you are ever in doubt as to the safety of a food product for your child, call the manufacturer to ensure the food is safe before offering it to your child. Otherwise, do not offer that food.

Common questions about allergen labelling under the *Australia New Zealand Food Standards Code*

Q. Do mandatory allergy declarations apply to all packaged foods?

A. Yes. Under the *Food Standards Code* all packaged foods are required to carry a label which will indicate the presence of the most common food allergens (as listed on page 147 and above), if they have been added to that food as an ingredient.

Q. Do allergens on a food label have to be expressed in 'plain English'?
A. No. The *Food Standards Code* does not specify wording to be used to declare the presence of an allergen on the label of a packaged food. Complex and unfamiliar terms can be used. For example, 'casein' may be used to indicate the presence of milk, 'ovalbumin' may be used to indicate the presence of egg. Parents of food-allergic children need to become familiar with a wide range of terms used to indicate the presence of an allergen. (Allergen identification terms for the most common allergens can be found on pages 166–179.)

Q. Does the *Food Standards Code* specify where on the label the presence of an allergen needs to be indicated?
A. All packaged foods containing *more* than one ingredient are required to display a list of ingredients, and the presence of an allergen must be declared in the list of ingredients. However, if a product contains only *one* ingredient, a list of ingredients does not need to appear on the packaging, but the allergen must be included in the name of the product.

For example, on a packet of salted peanuts, a list of ingredients must be included on the packaging, stating that the product contains peanuts and salt. A packet of unsalted peanuts (with no additives) is not required to include a list of ingredients on the packaging, but must include the allergen in the name of the product; for example, 'Australian Unsalted Peanuts'.

The *Food Standards Code* does specify that text used to indicate the presence of an allergen is legible (for example, it cannot be in a position where a wrap-around label might overlap and cover up text indicating the presence of an allergen), however, the name of a product or the list of ingredients can appear anywhere on the packaging. Carefully read all text on food packaging to ensure you don't miss any important notices in regard to the presence of an allergen.

Q. Does the *Food Standards Code* cover labelling requirements for possible traces of allergens being present in a product, for example, statements such as 'This product may contain traces of …'?

A. No. The *Food Standards Code* only covers the labelling of allergens when they have been added to a food product as an ingredient. Voluntary allergy advisory statements, such as 'This product may contain traces of ...', relate to trace amounts of an allergen *possibly* being present in a food product due to cross-contamination. For example, if a tub of plain vanilla ice-cream is made on the same line as a nut-flavoured ice-cream, there may be trace amounts of nuts in some of the tubs of vanilla ice-cream, despite a manufacturer's best efforts to clean equipment between the production of different flavours. A vast array of voluntary allergy advisory statements can be found on food products — for example, 'Made on the same equipment as products containing X', 'Made in a facility that also produces X', 'Made on the same line as X' — but these statements are placed on a label at the manufacturer's discretion. (For information about Voluntary Incidental Trace Allergen Labelling see pages 155–157.)

Q. Does the mandatory labelling of food allergens apply to imported goods, or only those made in Australia?
A. The labelling and safety requirements of the *Food Standards Code* also apply to imported products. So imported foods must, for example, be stickered with a food label that complies with the *Food Standards Code* — with the common allergens listed, regardless of the quantity added to the food. It is also a legal requirement for the name and address of the company importing the product to be present on the package, so consumers can contact the importer for information about the product.

Having said this, be aware that while most mainstream importers comply conscientiously with labelling regulations, in practical terms there is an additional risk of errors in translating the names of ingredients. As well, there may be some smaller importers who simply do not comply with regulations but who have not, as yet, been caught out by authorities.

So in summary, the same allergen labelling regulations apply to all packaged goods sold in Australia; however, it is probably safer to stick with local products. (See page 155 for an explanation of how to identify goods made only from Australian ingredients.)

If you do decide to buy an imported product for your food-allergic child, it is a good idea to call the importer and confirm the ingredients on the stickered label.

My own experience is that mistakes sometimes happen with the labelling of imported foodstuffs. I once called an importer about biscuits that appeared to be safe for my son, but on checking I was told the product contained milk and traces of nuts: the correct stickers hadn't yet arrived, so packets had gone into retail outlets with incorrect information.

Q. What about unpackaged goods: does a consumer still have the right to know if an allergen is contained in goods at a delicatessen?

A. Yes, a consumer still has the right to know. Allergen declarations are required for unpackaged foods, by either a declaration on or in relation to the display of that food, or, when asked, staff must provide consumers with accurate information either verbally or in writing.

Again, just because a regulation stipulates something should happen, it doesn't mean it always will. When requesting information from staff, you are trusting that they are very knowledgeable about the produce they are selling — which may or may not be the case — and asking them to provide important information in what is often a very busy and distracting environment. In addition to these pitfalls, environments such as delicatessens are high-risk for cross-contamination; for example, cold meats may be sliced on the same equipment as cheese.

For children at risk of severe allergic reactions, it is safest to stick to labelled, packaged foods and learn how to interpret food labels. However, you could also consider trying to educate your local deli or food supplier about food allergy. You could ask them to slice cold meat (from a new roll) on a clean sheet of paper or plastic, using a knife just out of the dishwasher.

The golden rules of eating packaged foods

1. Read every label of every food every time you buy it. Ingredients can change unexpectedly for any number of reasons, including seasonal availability, supply chain issues, costs, different packet sizes, flavour changes or change in production facilities. No matter how regularly you buy a product, *always* read the label.

continued

2. If you are ever in doubt as to whether a product is safe for your child, don't give it to them without first checking with the manufacturer or your doctor or dietitian. If this is not possible, then avoid that food.

3. Always have your child's EpiPen and Action Plan on hand. If you are out and about and realise you have forgotten the EpiPen, then your child should not eat anything. No EpiPen, no eating.

Reading food labels for food-allergen information

While there is a legal responsibility for every food manufacturer and importer to ensure packaged foods contain accurate information about the presence of major allergens, the ultimate responsibility of keeping allergic children safe falls onto the shoulders of parents and carers of food-allergic children, who need to carefully read and interpret label information. (As children mature, they need to learn to take on this responsibility, too.)

Research conducted by FSANZ in 2003[3] found that consumers who belonged to an allergen support group (in this case Anaphylaxis Australia and Allergy New Zealand) were able to better identify foods that were not suitable for their food-allergic children than those who were not members of support groups, implying that increased education and awareness in regard to food labelling occurs through support groups.

This research is in line with the findings of a US study in 2002,[4] which reported that parents who had met with a dietitian or had contact with the Food Allergy and Anaphylaxis Network (a US support group) were better able to understand and interpret food labels. Both research findings indicate that further education about understanding food labels is imperative for families who need to avoid specific allergens in food.

Interpreting a food label

Below is an example of a food label with simple explanations of how to interpret each component of the label in regard to identifying food allergens. If you are interested in reading more about how to understand food labels (not only from a food-allergy perspective), visit the website of Food Standards Australia New Zealand at **www.foodstandards.gov.au** Paediatric dietitians are also highly skilled in educating parents on what to look for on food labels.

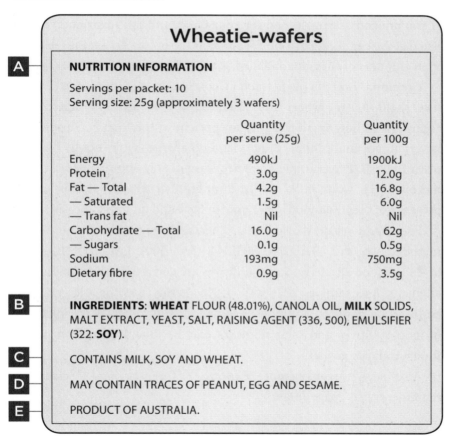

Wheatie-wafers

A

NUTRITION INFORMATION

Servings per packet: 10
Serving size: 25g (approximately 3 wafers)

	Quantity per serve (25g)	Quantity per 100g
Energy	490kJ	1900kJ
Protein	3.0g	12.0g
Fat — Total	4.2g	16.8g
— Saturated	1.5g	6.0g
— Trans fat	Nil	Nil
Carbohydrate — Total	16.0g	62g
— Sugars	0.1g	0.5g
Sodium	193mg	750mg
Dietary fibre	0.9g	3.5g

B

INGREDIENTS: WHEAT FLOUR (48.01%), CANOLA OIL, **MILK** SOLIDS, MALT EXTRACT, YEAST, SALT, RAISING AGENT (336, 500), EMULSIFIER (322: **SOY**).

C

CONTAINS MILK, SOY AND WHEAT.

D

MAY CONTAIN TRACES OF PEANUT, EGG AND SESAME.

E

PRODUCT OF AUSTRALIA.

A NUTRITION INFORMATION

In Australia, most packaged food products are required to have a nutrition information panel. The nutrition panel includes important details about the nutrients contained in a product as well as the amount of energy, protein, fat, saturated fat, carbohydrates, sugar and salt (sodium). The information must be presented in a standard format so consumers can see the amounts present per serve of the product and per 100g (or 100ml if it is a liquid product).

B INGREDIENTS

The ingredients of a product must be listed from largest to smallest by weight. So the ingredient that forms the largest component of the product is listed first and the ingredient that forms the smallest component of the product is listed last. This is very helpful information for parents to know. If you are considering a food for your child, and fat, sugar and salt are listed at the beginning of a label, you know the product contains relatively high amounts of these ingredients.

Common food allergens (such as cow's milk, egg, peanut, tree nuts, fish, shellfish, soy, wheat and sesame) *must* be listed as ingredients, regardless of how small the amount present in the food is. However, it is very important to understand that food allergens may not be listed in plain English. For example, the term 'casein' may appear instead of the more familiar word 'milk'. (A list of unfamiliar terms that indicate the presence of common food allergens can be found on pages 166–79.)

Food additives must also be listed, usually by a number. For example, in the above label 'RAISING AGENT (336, 500), EMULSIFIER (322: SOY)' are food additives. Some additives are derived from common food allergens, for example, '322: SOY'. If this is the case, the allergen must be listed by name in addition to the additive number. A complete list of food additives and their numbers may be downloaded from **www. foodstandards.gov.au**

Also see 'A word about "Flavours", "Colours" and "Spices" in ingredients lists', page 158.

C ALLERGY INFORMATION

Common food allergens must be included in the ingredients list (B), whether they are present as an individual ingredient or as a component of an ingredient. Some food manufacturers, as in this example, also highlight the presence of allergens in the product by mentioning them in their own entry, beneath the ingredients list. This is not mandatory under the *Food Standards Code*, however.

D VOLUNTARY ALLERGY ADVISORY STATEMENTS

In addition to specific allergens being present as ingredients in a food, there is also the possibility of very small amounts of an allergen being present in a food due to cross-contamination, which can occur at any point in the food's journey from 'paddock to plate'. This warning is a voluntary allergy advisory statement from manufacturers, and there is currently no regulation around the use or wording of these statements. However, a working party has developed a standardised allergen risk assessment tool for food producers to enable them to assess the risk of cross-contamination and provide appropriate and consistent warning statements for consumers. (See, VITAL: Voluntary Incidental Trace Allergen Labelling, below.)

E COUNTRY OF ORIGIN

The country of origin of a packaged food must be labelled as a separate statement. A country of origin label will be worded as either 'Product of X' or 'Made in X'. There are guidelines governing which statement should be used.

For a packaged food to qualify to be labelled as 'Product of Australia', for example, all of the major ingredients/components of the product must be from Australia.

For a packaged food to qualify to be labelled as 'Made in Australia', according to the *Food Standards Code*, it must be 'substantially transformed in that country for which the claim is made, and more than 50% of the cost of production or manufacture must be incurred in that country'.[5]

In simple terms, this means only products labelled 'Product of Australia' are made from purely Australian ingredients and 'Made in Australia' indicates that it is a composite product, with not all ingredients being Australian.

VITAL: Voluntary Incidental Trace Allergen Labelling

As you have read earlier in this chapter, when specific food allergens (as listed on pages 147–48) are intentionally added as an ingredient to a food, they must be labelled on the packaging of the food under the *Food Standards Code*.

However, food allergens may also be present in a product due to inadvertent contamination, which can occur at any point in the food's journey from 'paddock to plate'. The presence of an unintentional allergen in a food product is often referred to as cross-contact, or 'trace' allergens, hence the voluntary allergy advisory statements you see on food packaging: 'May contain traces of …' The labelling of cross-contact allergens is *not* mandatory under the *Food Standards Code*.

Ask any parent of a food-allergic child what they find most frustrating about reading food labels and most will tell you it is the glut of inconsistent voluntary allergy advisory statements, such as 'This product may contain traces of …', 'Produced on the same line as …', 'Produced in a facility …', that seem to be included as a generic disclaimer on a broad range of products.

The abundant use of voluntary allergy advisory statements often leads to one of two scenarios:

1) The food choices of food-allergic individuals who heed such warnings become even more limited.
2) Food-allergic individuals decide to ignore such statements and take an unknown risk every time they consume these products.

In an effort to improve this situation, the Australian Food and Grocery Council Allergen Forum facilitated a working group involving a broad range of contributors, including regulators, manufacturers, consumers and food scientists. The group developed VITAL (Voluntary Incidental Trace Allergen Labelling), which was launched in mid 2007. VITAL is designed to provide a consistent risk-assessment process for manufacturers to determine the requirement for allergen advisory statements on the labelling of processed foods.

VITAL is a 'methodology' (or, more simply, 'a tool') that enables food manufacturers to consistently assess the risk that allergen cross-contact poses to allergen-sensitive consumers.

If, after assessing a food using the VITAL methodology, a manufacturer determines that the cross-contact allergen concentration is present at a level deemed to be below the specified action level then it is not required to be declared on the label. If the cross-contact allergen is found to be at a higher level, then it will be labelled with the statement, 'May be present: [name of allergen] …'. This is the only voluntary allergy advisory statement to be used in conjunction with VITAL, and is only to be used when the cross-contamination is:[6]

- documented using the VITAL system
- unavoidable; and
- sporadic

In summary, the 'May be present: …' voluntary allergy advisory statement will communicate to food-allergic consumers that the food should be avoided. An outcome of VITAL should be to promote the removal of unnecessary precautionary labelling, and this will give allergic consumers more safe food choices.

Adoption of the VITAL system is voluntary, so at the time of going to press a myriad of voluntary allergy advisory statements are still commonly encountered at the supermarket, but there is hope on the horizon that the uniform adoption of VITAL by the food industry will lead to meaningful and consistent labelling information about cross-contact allergens in packaged foods.

The Allergen Bureau

In 2005, the Allergen Bureau was established by the Australian Food and Grocery Council. The role of the Allergen Bureau is to provide information and answer questions about the management of food-allergen risks in ingredients and manufactured foods in Australia and New Zealand. It is a central point where food manufacturers, retailers, suppliers, importers, exporters and others, including consumers, can go for accurate advice and help. It is another example of the food industry working collaboratively to improve education on managing the risks associated with food allergens within its own ranks. As a consumer, it is still hard work to find safe foods for food-allergic children, but it is encouraging to know that the industry is moving in the right direction. For more information, visit **www.allergenbureau.net**

A word about 'flavours', 'colours' and 'spices' in ingredients lists

While labelling of the most common food allergens added to a product in any amount is compulsory under the *Food Standards Code*, if your child is allergic to a more unusual food (that is, any food other than those listed on pages 147–148), you will need to be wary of generic terms such as 'flavours', 'natural flavours', 'colours' and 'spices' on ingredients lists.

Consider the following fictional scenario. Two mothers are at the supermarket reading the label on a packet of fruit biscuits. One mother has a child with peanut allergy and the other has a child with banana allergy. Peanut is one of the most common allergens, so if peanut is present as an ingredient in any amount in a product, it must be labelled. Banana is not one of the most common allergens, so it does not necessarily have to be disclosed as an ingredient if it is present in a small amount.

One of the ingredients listed on the packet of biscuits is 'flavours [contains peanuts]'. The mother of the peanut-allergic child immediately knows this product is not safe to feed her child; however, the mother of the banana-allergic child will have to do further research to ensure the product does not contain banana flavour: she will need to call the manufacturer and directly ask if the product contains any banana flavour.

Consuming products with 'May contain' statements?

Q My son is allergic to peanut and had a severe reaction as a toddler. He is now 8, and we are becoming increasingly frustrated by the number of products with 'May contain traces of peanut' statements. His diet seems so restricted, and if we could introduce some products with 'May contain traces', our lives would be so much easier. Is it safe for him to consume foods containing 'May contain peanut' statements?

A Often when parents of food-allergic children get together they ask, 'Do you do traces at your house?' It is a much-debated topic between parents, doctors, support groups and dietitians.

If your question was, 'Is it possible for a child to have a severe allergic reaction to a product containing a trace amount of their allergen?', then the answer would be yes. There are cases of children experiencing anaphylaxis after consuming products which didn't contain their allergen as an ingredient but carried a voluntary allergy advisory statement such as 'May contain [the allergen]'.

As mentioned earlier in this chapter, the *Food Standards Code* does not require a food company to list on the label the presence of trace amounts of an allergen due to cross-contamination. So, on the one hand, there are products on supermarket shelves that may contain traces of allergens but which do not include any voluntary allergy advisory statement at all. And, on the other hand, when a voluntary allergy advisory statement does appear on a product, it can be difficult to verify how real the risk of contamination may be. Clear as mud, right?

The position of Anaphylaxis Australia Inc. is that foods with 'May contain' warnings should not be given to children at risk of a severe allergic reaction — which is prudent, as the risk may be present. However, it needs to be acknowledged that some allergy specialists and dietitians disagree with this approach, especially if a child has never had a severe reaction to a food before. On a case-by-case basis, some might advocate that certain products may be okay to introduce into your child's diet — after talking to the manufacturer about the possible risks — but it must be stressed that the authors and publisher of this book are not suggesting you try this with your child. Any thoughts about giving your child products with 'May contain [your child's allergen]' statements must be discussed with your allergy specialist.

What many people do agree on, however, is that there are particular packaged foods that should always be avoided by peanut- and tree-nut-allergic children if they carry a 'May contain nuts' advisory statement, because the risk of cross-contamination is considered very high. These include: cereals, cereal products such as health bars, chocolate, ice-cream and bakery goods.

In summary, it is obviously safest *never* to offer to your child foods labelled with 'May contain' statements, especially as your child has a history of severe reactions. However, you really need to discuss this issue directly with your allergy specialist before making any decisions, as they need to take into account your child's clinical history and dietary needs.

Hopefully, the food industry will continue to move towards adopting a system of consistent and meaningful labelling of trace allergens (see the section on VITAL, pages 155–157), making it easier for consumers to really understand which products are safe for food-allergy sufferers to consume and which aren't.

Food allergens in non-food products

Carefully checking labels for allergens doesn't only apply to packaged foods. A wide range of products can contain food allergens as an ingredient, especially cosmetics, skin- and hair-care products, sunscreen, soaps, baby bath and moisturising products, cleaning products, pet food, medicines (prescribed, over-the-counter and complementary) and children's craft materials.

Many cosmetics and skin products are labelled as 'all natural' or 'hypoallergenic', but these terms bear no relevance to whether or not your child will be allergic to them. Many 'natural' products contain nut oils, and the last 'hypoallergenic' shower wash I purchased listed 'milk protein' in the ingredients.

Whenever your child is coming into contact with a product, especially one that is applied to the skin or, in the case of medication, is ingested, always check the ingredients carefully and be on the lookout for unfamiliar terms. If you are in doubt as to whether or not a product is safe, check with the manufacturer; if you are still unsure then check with your doctor before using it.

Making a complaint about a food you suspect contains an undeclared allergen

If anyone in your family has an allergic reaction from a food product that you believe has been mislabelled, or from an unlabelled product where you made it clear you were allergic to a food and were told the product did not contain your allergen (for example, a meal in a café or restaurant), there are certain steps you can take to lodge a formal complaint.

- Contact the relevant health authority in the state or territory in which the product was made or distributed from. For example, if you live in Victoria but the product you want to make a complaint about was made in New South Wales, you need to contact the New South Wales authority. (The name and address of a food manufacturer or importer must be present on a food label.) The contact details for state and territory authorities do change from time to time, so refer to the following link on the FSANZ website for up-to-date contact telephone numbers: **www.foodstandards.gov.au/thecode/assistanceforindustry/ contactslist/industrycontacts.cfm**
- When you call the authority, have the packaging of the food in question in front of you to help you answer questions. Your health authority may ask you for the following information:[7]
  —Your personal contact details
  —The brand name, product name and manufacturer of the food in question
  —The size and type of package of the food
  —Package codes and dates
  —Name and location of the store or restaurant where you purchased the food
  —Date you purchased the food
- Save (freeze if perishable) the remainder of the suspect food. Be sure to wrap it securely so it does not contaminate any other foods in your freezer and label it in a way that makes it clear the product is not safe for your child to consume. Do not leave the food anywhere it may be mistakenly eaten by (or offered to) your child. Also save the original container or packaging the food came in, especially the ingredients label.

In addition:

- Contact the manufacturer or distributor of the food in question and advise them of the allergic reaction that has occurred to the food. If the reaction took place in a café or restaurant, contact the manager or owner.

● Contact Anaphylaxis Australia Inc. and report the food that you suspect caused your child to have an allergic reaction. Telephone: 1300 728 000.

Remember, if you suspect a food contains an undeclared allergen, you are playing an important role in reporting this information to your local health authority.

Food recalls: what they are and how you can keep informed

A food recall is when formal action is taken to remove from sale, distribution and consumption a food which may pose a health and safety risk to consumers.[8]

If an undeclared allergen is found to be present in a packaged food, FSANZ will coordinate an immediate recall of the product to protect consumers.

For example, if a particular brand of soy cheese was found to contain undeclared cow's milk in the ingredients, it would be immediately recalled. Working with the company that manufactures, imports or distributes the soy cheese, FSANZ would coordinate the recall process, arranging for the product to be removed from sale, and assisting in how consumers are informed.

As a consumer, the best way to keep up to date with news of foods being recalled is to:

● Subscribe to the food recall email alert from FSANZ, at: **www. foodstandards.gov.au/newsroom/subscriptionservice.cfm**

● Regularly visit the food recall information page of the Anaphylaxis Australia website, at: **www.allergyfacts.org.au/foodalerts.asp**

● Keep an eye out for food recall notices in major daily newspapers (they are usually near the front of the newspaper and feature a black-and-white diagonally striped border).

If you have a food in your pantry that has been formally recalled, you should take it back to the place of purchase for a cash refund. Food recalls are taken very seriously by food companies and health authorities.

Finding safe foods to feed your child: helpful resources to get you started

What food is or isn't safe for your child depends entirely on their allergies. However, the following references are provided to help you in your *research* to find safe foods for your child. Not all of the products from the companies mentioned below will be suitable for your child: always read the label of every food you buy for your child *every* time you buy it — ingredients can (and do) change on a regular basis. If you are unsure if a food is safe for your child, always call the manufacturer to check the ingredients and check with your child's doctor or dietitian. If you have a child who is newly diagnosed with food allergies and you are struggling to find safe foods for them, ask your doctor to refer you to a paediatric dietitian with experience in food allergies. (See Chapter 7, Feeding your food-allergic child, page 122.)

Food company links

www.freedomfoods.com.au

An Australian-owned company specialising in healthy foods. They make a range of products that are free from many of the most common allergens. For each product in the range their website displays the ingredients list and any 'May contain' warnings.

www.kinnerton.com.au

An Australian subsidiary of UK company Kinnerton Confectionery. Makers of a character-based (for example, Thomas the Tank Engine, the Simpsons) range of nut-free chocolate products. They also make a range of chocolate products that are dairy-free, egg-free, gluten-free and nut-free.

www.orgran.com

Orgran is an Australian company specialising in producing gluten-free, wheat-free, dairy-free, egg-free, yeast-free, GMO-free vegan foods. Orgran products are available in most supermarkets and health food stores.

www.sweetwilliam.com.au

An Australian chocolate company producing a range of dairy-free, tree-nut- and peanut-free chocolates.

Shopping links

www.allergease.com.au

An online store selling allergy-friendly products. For each product featured on the website, the ingredients list is displayed.

www.allergyblock.com

A Melbourne-based store that specialises in sourcing foods from allergy-aware companies. You can also order goods online and have them posted to you. The website enables you to search for products based on ingredients you need to avoid.

www.glutenfreeshop.com.au

An online store specialising in gluten-free products which also stocks nut-free, egg-free, dairy-free and soy-free products. The website enables you to search for products by ingredients you need to avoid.

Understanding food labelling: a summary of important things to remember

- Read every label on every food package every time you shop for your food-allergic child. This is where complacency can really slip in and many parents I have spoken to (and I must include myself in this) admit they are guilty of not checking the labels on products they buy for their child every week.
- If you are out and you forget your child's EpiPen, do not let them eat any food, even if the label indicates it is safe. No EpiPen, no eating is a rule that should never be broken.
- Know what ingredients your child must avoid. Learn the unfamiliar terms on a food label that can indicate the presence of your child's allergen (see pages 166–179).
- Remember that the legislation around identifying allergens does not specify how and where an allergen needs to be

identified on a label. Take the time to read all information on a packaged food before offering it to your child.

- It is safest to stick to foods labelled 'Product of Australia'. Even though the same label regulations apply to imported foods, there is a greater risk of inaccuracy due to errors in translation or communication between the overseas manufacturer and importer.

- If you are ever in doubt about the safety of a food you would like to offer your child, don't give it to them. Call the manufacturer or distributor of the product and check with them first.

- Be wary of boutique products and ask questions before buying. For example, I was excited to find a nut-free muesli in a health food store but noticed the same muesli also came in a sesame variety. My son is allergic to nuts and sesame, so I asked the store owner about the risk of cross-contamination with sesame. He said the muesli products were hand-made locally in a mum's kitchen, and cross-contamination of sesame could definitely be an issue; I was advised not to buy the product, despite its seemingly 'safe' label.

- Trust your instincts: if a label looks unprofessional or something doesn't feel right (for example, a home-made label at a stall at a school fete), don't take the risk.

Decoding unfamiliar food terms

Food allergens do not always appear in 'plain English' on food labels. Sometimes scientific or more technical terms are used; for example, 'ovalbumin' to indicate the presence of egg. In this section we list a broad range of lesser-known terms that may be used on a food label to indicate the presence of a common food allergen. We also list products that often contain common food allergens: these lists are presented allergen by allergen.

It is really important to become familiar with the various terms in use that indicate the presence of your child's allergen in a food, remembering that there is no legal requirement for food producers to label allergens in 'plain English'.

While the following lists are helpful, allergens may be presented as an unfamiliar term not included here. If you see a term on a food label and you do not know what it means, check with the manufacturer, your allergy specialist or dietitian before offering it to your child. These lists are intended as a useful aid for living with specific food allergies. They are not meant to replace medical advice given by your child's doctor.

The following information is © Copyright Anaphylaxis Australia Inc. 2007 and is reprinted here with kind permission by Anaphylaxis Australia Inc. Handy wallet-sized allergen information cards that are ideal to keep in your shopping bag can be downloaded from **www.allergyfacts.org.au**

Cow's milk

Ingredients to avoid if you are allergic to cow's milk:
All dairy products
Ammonium caseinate
Butter/butter fat
Calcium caseinate
Casein
Casein hydrolysate
Caseinates
Cheese
Cream
Cultured buttermilk
Curds
Delactosed whey
Ghee
Hydrolysed casein
Hydrolysed whey
Imitation milk
Lactalbumin
Lactalbumin phosphate
Lacto acidophilus
Magnesium caseinate

Malted milk

Milk[+]

Nougat

Skim milk

Potassium caseinate

Rennet casein

Sodium caseinate

Sweet whey

Whey protein

Whey solids

Whey/whey powder

Yoghurt

Products which might contain cow's milk include:

Baked goods (for example, cake)

Battered fried goods

Canned products

Caramel lollies

Cheese

Cheese powder

Chocolate

Coated/seasoned foods

Custards and puddings

Deli meats

Dips

Egg replacers

Fat substitutes

Flavouring (natural or artificial)

Flavoured coffees and drinks

Frozen desserts

Fruit juice

Gravy

High-protein flour

Lactic acid starter culture

Margarine spreads

Meat pies

Non-dairy cheeses
Non-dairy whiteners
Pastries
Poultry/turkey (basted)
Protein hydrolysate
Salad dressings
Sauces and spreads
Sausages
Soups/soup mixes
Stock
Vegetable stock
Whitener

Lactose does not normally contain the protein that causes reactions, but there may be a risk of contamination with milk protein. Lactose found in medicine is generally safe, but check with your doctor.
+Any product containing the word milk from an animal source must be avoided, for example, 'goat's milk'.

Egg

Ingredients to avoid if you are allergic to egg:
Albumin
Apovitellin
Avidin
Binder
Dried eggs
Egg
Egg solids
Egg substitutes (some)
Egg white
Egg white solids
Egg yolk
Flovoproteins
Glaze (on baked goods)
Globulin

Imitation egg product

Livetin

Lysozyme

Meringue mix

Ovalbumin

Ovglycoprotein

Ovomucoid

Ovomuxiod

Powdered egg

Products which might contain egg include:

Baked products

Battered foods

Biscuits

Cakes (for example, sponge, angel)

Chocolate (some)

Confectionery

Crumbed foods

Custards

Doughnuts

Drink mixes

Frittatas

Fritters

Frozen desserts

Glazed foods

Icing on cakes

Macaroons

Malted drinks

Marshmallow

Marzipan

Mayonnaise

Meatloaf/hamburgers

Meringue

Mousse

Naan bread

Noodles

Nougat

Omelettes

Pancakes

Pasta

Pastries

Pavlovas

Pizza

Quiche

Quick breads

Rissoles

Salad dressings

Sauces (for example, Hollandaise)

Soufflés

Soups

Sushi

Sweets/lollies

Vegetarian meat substitutes, for example, vegetarian sausage

Waffles

Peanut

Ingredients to avoid if you are allergic to peanut:

Arachis oil

Beer nuts

Goober nuts

Ground nuts

Mandelonas

Mixed nuts

Monkey nuts

Nu-nuts

Nut pieces

Nutmeat

Peanut

Peanut butter

Peanut oil (cold-pressed, expelled or extruded)

Peanut sprouts

Products which might contain peanut include:

African dishes

Asian/Indian dishes

Biscuits

Breakfast cereals

Chocolates

Dried fruit mixes

Gravy

Health food bars

Ice-creams

Lollies

Marzipan

Mexican dishes

Nougat

Praline

Pesto

Salad/salad dressing

Sauces

Snack foods

Soup

Any products containing peanut or peanut derivatives must be avoided (for example, peanut flour, sodium peanutate, peanutamide).

Allergy specialists often advise peanut-allergic individuals to also avoid tree nuts.

Those allergic to peanuts are not often allergic to other legumes; however, peanut-allergic individuals may also react to lupin (for example, lupin flour and lupini beans).

Tree nuts

Ingredients to avoid if you are allergic to tree nuts include:

Almonds

Artificial nuts

Brazil nuts

Carponata

Cashews

Gianduja (a nut mix)

Hazelnuts/filberts

Hickory nuts

Indian nuts

Macadamia nuts

Marzipan/almond paste

Non-gai nuts

Natural nut extract

Pecans/mashuga nuts

Pine nuts+

Pistachios

Pralines

Shea nuts

Walnuts

Products which may contain tree nuts include:

African dishes

Asian/Indian dishes

Baked goods

Biscuits

Breakfast cereals

Cereals

Chocolate

Chocolate spreads

Dried fruit mixes

Flavouring (natural or artificial)

Flavoured coffees, drinks

Frozen desserts

Health food bars

Ice-cream

Lollies

Marzipan

Mexican dishes

Nougat

Pastries

Pesto

Salads

Snack foods

Vegan dishes

Any food containing nut or nut derivatives must be avoided (for example, nut butters, nut meal, nut oil).

Allergy specialists often advise those with tree-nut allergy to also avoid peanuts.

+Pine nuts are also known as: pinyon, pignoli, pignollia, pinon and pignon.

Fish

Ingredients to avoid if you are allergic to fish include:

Anchovy

Bass

Bluefish

Bream

Carp

Catfish

Caviar

Char

Chub

Cisco

Cod

Eel

Flounder

Grouper

Haddock

Hake

Halibut

Herring

Imitation crab

Mackerel

Mahi-mahi

Marlin

Monkfish

Orange roughy

Perch

Pickerel

Pike

Plaice

Pollock

Pompano

Porgy

Rockfish

Salmon

Sardine

Shark

Smelt

Snapper

Sashimi

Surimi

Tilapia

Trout

Tuna

White fish

Whiting

Products which might contain fish include:

Antipasto

Asian dishes

Canned spreads

Caesar salad

Dips

Gelatin

Greek dishes

Marshmallow

Pizza topping

Salad dressings
Sauces (for example, Worcestershire)
Soups
Sushi

Food served in a seafood or other restaurant may be cross-contaminated with fish or shellfish during storage, preparation and cooking.

Please note that it is possible for an allergic reaction to occur from cooking odours or handling of fish.

Shellfish

Avoid all foods containing any shellfish to which you are allergic:
Abalone
Clams
Cockle
Crab
Crawfish
Lobster
Molluscs
Mussels
Octopus
Oysters
Prawns
Scallops
Shrimp (crevette)
Sea snails
Squid (calamari)

Products which may contain shellfish include:
Bouillabaisse
Cuttlefish ink
Fish stock
Flavouring (artificial or natural)
Sauces (for example, fish sauce)
Seafood flavouring (for example, clam)

Squid ink
Surimi

Food served in a seafood or other restaurant may be cross-contaminated with fish or shellfish during storage, preparation and cooking.

Please note that it is possible for an allergic reaction to occur from cooking odours or handling of shellfish.

Soy

Ingredients to avoid if you are allergic to soy:
Bean curd
Edamame (or endamame)
Hydrolysed plant protein
Hydrolysed soy protein
Hydrolysed vegetable protein
Miso
Natto
Okara
Soja
Soy
Soya
Soyabean
Soybean
Tamari
Tempeh
Textured vegetable protein
Tofu
Yuba

Products which might contain soy include:
Vegetable stock
Vegetable broth
Vegetable gum
Vegetable starch
Flavouring (natural or artificial)

Any food containing soy or soy derivatives must be avoided, for example, soy drink (often marketed as soy milk), soy sauce, soy flour.

Research studies indicate that most individuals who are allergic to soy can safely eat soy lecithin and soyabean oil, but check with your specialist.

Wheat

Ingredients to avoid if you are allergic to wheat:
Bran

Breadcrumbs

Bulgar

Couscous

Cracker meal

Farina

Flour*

Gluten

Kamut

Matzoh

Pasta

Seitan

Semolina

Soy sauce

Spelt

Tabouleh

Triticale

Wheat+

Whole wheat berries

*all-purpose, bread, durum, cake, enriched, high-gluten, high-protein instant, multigrain, pastry, plain, self-raising, soft-wheat, steel ground, stone-ground, wholemeal, whole-wheat
+bran, germ, flakes, sprouts, cornflour

Products which might contain wheat include:
Baked goods (for example, bread, cakes, doughnuts, muffins)
Biscuits

Breakfast cereals

Flavouring (natural or artificial)

Hydrolysed protein

Baking mixes/powders

Battered fried foods

Canned soups/stocks

Chips

Chocolate

Corn chips

Crisps

Crumbed foods

Ice-cream

Icing sugar

Ice-cream cones

Lollies

Malted milk

Marshmallow

Mayonnaise

Noodles

Pancakes

Pastry

Pizza

Processed meats

Sauces/gravy mixes

Snack foods

Soy sauce

Starch (for example, modified vegetable, gelatinised)

Surimi

Vegetable gum/starch

Wraps

Sesame

Ingredients to avoid if you are allergic to sesame:

Benne

Benniseed

Gingelly seeds

Sesame

Sesame seed

Sesarmol

Sesomolina

Sim sim

Tahina

Tahini

Til

Products which might contain sesame include:

Asian foods

Bakery goods

Crackers

Dips

Dressings

Halvah

Herbs

Marinades

Middle Eastern foods

Nutritional snacks

Pâtés

Pretzels

Salads

Spices

Spreads

Any food containing sesame or sesame derivatives must be avoided (for example, sesame flour, sesame seed paste).

9

Eating out with food allergy

Eating out is one of the great social pleasures in life, but for those with food allergy, it also poses a risk: you are relying on chefs and service staff to vet the safety of your food, meals often contain hidden ingredients and there is always the risk of cross-contamination in the preparation of meals in busy kitchens.

However, if you are prepared to plan ahead, ask questions and work with restaurant staff in educating them about food allergies, then you may find eating out with your food-allergic child can become an enjoyable option — enabling your child to enjoy normal social experiences, and giving you some welcome time-out from the kitchen.

In this chapter, we look at how to safely plan a meal out, including communication and preparation tips, as well as explaining the risk of cross-contamination in a restaurant environment. We also explain what to do when things don't go to plan and suggest ideas for working with your teenager to help them make eating out with their friends as safe as possible.

A joint effort

It would be lovely to live in a world where we could tell a restaurant or takeaway outlet about our children's allergies and sit back and relax while we wait for them to prepare a delicious and safe meal. But as parents of food-allergic children, we know just how much knowledge and effort it takes to prepare safe meals for our children in our own home, so we need to acknowledge it is also a big (but not impossible) ask for restaurants to do the same. You can never eliminate all risks — eating out *always* involves some degree of risk — however, the following 10 pointers are designed to help you work together with a café or restaurant to plan an enjoyable and as-safe-as-possible dining experience.

1. Choose an appropriate restaurant

Carefully consider your choice of restaurant. For example, if your child has a peanut allergy, it is not a good idea to choose a Thai restaurant; if your child has a shellfish allergy then a seafood restaurant should be crossed off the list. Restaurants that offer buffet meals are a no-go zone for anyone with a serious food allergy due to the high risk of cross-contamination through serving utensils and food display. Cafés that specialise in desserts are also high-risk, as desserts and cakes are often made 'off-premises' so staff can't always accurately verify the ingredients or risk of cross-contamination; desserts also often contain 'hidden' allergens, for example, almond meal in the bases of cakes, nuts as decorations, egg in glazes.

If you are unsure if a restaurant has suitable meal options, pop in and view their menu in advance or search online; many restaurants have their own websites featuring their menu.

The Coeliac Society websites (state-based) can be a useful research tool in finding places to eat: visit **www.coeliacsociety.com.au** then click on the link 'Your State Society'. If a restaurant is listed as having gluten-free options available it *might* indicate that the restaurant is allergy-aware — a good starting point to consider when researching restaurant options.

> 'We eat out regularly, but we no longer go to Thai or Chinese restaurants, because the risk of cross-contamination is too high. On one occasion, we went to a Chinese restaurant and ordered a roast duck and chicken dish. Despite explaining Hugh's peanut allergy, when the meal arrived, we discovered a pile of peanuts beneath the chicken and duck. When we explained that Hugh could not eat this, they just removed the peanuts and served the same dish again, with one peanut remaining! Of course, he could not eat the meal.'
>
> —Tinmimi Maung (Vic), mother of Hugh (10), allergic to peanut

2. Contact the restaurant in advance

The best way to ensure a positive dining experience is to work with your chosen restaurant in advance of your visit. If you can, visit the restaurant in person at a quiet time of day, when staff will have time to communicate with you. If you can't visit the restaurant in person, then be sure to call at a quiet time of day.

Ask to speak directly to the chef and explain you would like to eat at the restaurant and your child has food allergies. Be polite and direct, and respect that chefs are really busy with preparation and planning, even during slow periods. It may be helpful to bring along written information about your child's food allergy; for example, an allergen information card that lists all the names used on food labels to indicate it contains your child's allergen (see page 166).

Ask the chef about menu items that might be safe for your child. Some chefs are willing to make a plain meal not offered on the menu to accommodate those with allergies. If the chef suggests a meal that might be safe, ask follow-up questions. For example, if the suggested dish is fried, ask what other foods are cooked in the same fryer. If the dish comes with a sauce, ask if it can be served without the sauce to reduce the chance of hidden allergens creeping in. Ask exactly what is in a dish and how it is prepared. It can help if you are willing to choose plain meals, for example, grilled meat and steamed vegetables (no sauce, no marinade), to minimise the chance of hidden allergens being present.

Importantly, find out which chef will actually be on duty when you intend to eat at the restaurant. You also need to have the discussion with whoever will be cooking your child's meal on the day.

While it isn't always possible to speak with a restaurant in advance, always do so if you can. Chefs do a lot of food preparation before you order a meal — for example, basting meats, baking desserts, preparing soups, sauces and so on — so putting your request in early can mean more options may be available, and they will appreciate the fact that you are not making last-minute demands when they are flat out in the kitchen.

If your child is attending a function, for example, a wedding, you should always call the restaurant or caterers in advance, as components of a meal for large crowds are often pre-prepared, and it may not be possible for them to whip up something safe for your child at the last minute. You also need to be aware of what other meals they will be offering on the day. For example, if they will be serving a dish with satay sauce and your child has peanut allergy, you may want to ask the restaurant if you can bring your child's meal to the function to avoid the risk of cross-contamination.

Finally, if after speaking to the restaurant you find staff are unhelpful, don't force the issue: simply choose another restaurant. Or, if the staff are helpful and cooperative but really can't cater for your child's needs, ask them if they mind you bringing along a safe meal for your child, or consider taking along your own dry food, for example, a safe pasta, that can then be cooked by the restaurant.

3. Consider the best time of day to eat out

Take into consideration your child's specific allergens when deciding what time of day to eat out. For example, if your child is allergic to egg, choosing to order a cooked breakfast at a time when eggs are flying around the kitchen — scrambled, in pancakes, omelettes, French toast and so on — is not a great idea.

If you are new to dining out with food allergy, try eating dinner early, for example 6pm, while you are gaining confidence and getting to know a restaurant. You may feel more relaxed being able to communicate with service and kitchen staff when they are not rushed off their feet and will have more time to listen carefully to your needs and check labels or talk to the chef.

If you are ordering takeaway from a restaurant, no matter how confident you are that the food will be safe, don't put your child to bed immediately after they have eaten. I confess this is exactly what we did when Noah recently ate some hot chips from a fish and chip restaurant that also does takeaway. Ten minutes after eating five chips he went to bed and was well. A couple of minutes later he was distressed and calling out to us — and when we went in to check on him he had welts near his mouth and swelling of the face. He is not allergic to potato or the oil in which they were fried, so we can only assume cross-contamination with one of his allergens occurred. After a dose of antihistamine he was fine, but we certainly learned from the experience.

4. Communicate clearly with staff

When you arrive at the restaurant of your choice ideally ask to speak with the manager or head chef — the most informed staff member. If you have spoken to the head chef in advance, check with the manager that the same chef is on duty now.

If you haven't reviewed the menu in advance, tell the manager or head chef what your child cannot eat and ask what items are safe to order for your child. Ask exactly what is in a dish you want to order for your child and how it is prepared.

When your child's meal arrives, be sure to check with the staff member again that the meal does not contain your child's allergen. Keep in mind that not all restaurants work the same way. In some establishments the person who takes the order is not the same person who delivers the order, so never hesitate to politely double-check before your child eats the food — often there are a lot of links in the food preparation chain before a meal lands on your table.

If you find a café or restaurant that serves some meals that are safe for your child, you still need to check with staff every time you order the meal for your child. Staff change, ingredients and recipes can change, and a meal that you have previously ordered for your child may no longer be safe.

5. Be nice — and tell the truth

Anyone who has ever worked in service or hospitality (myself included) will tell you that rude and demanding customers are hands-down the worst part of the job. The majority of staff in hospitality aim to please, but when special requests are delivered as curt commands, rightly or wrongly staff can become resentful and less helpful than you need them to be.

Remember, you need to work *with* restaurant staff, to educate them and help them understand your needs. This doesn't mean you should be apologetic or meek, and if a staff member isn't taking your concerns seriously you should ask to speak with the owner or manager. Be mindful, though, that your request is one of many being fired at staff in a busy and often stressful environment. Treat staff with courtesy and respect, and acknowledge that you are asking the restaurant for special attention.

In addition to being nice, you also need to be absolutely honest about what your child can and can't eat and how serious their allergy is — *never* fib about any other food preferences. It is galling for staff who bend over backwards to make a meal safe by eliminating an allergen — cow's milk, for example — only to have a patron do a backflip — for instance, then order a babyccino and say, 'Oh, they can have a little bit.'

6. Know when to leave

If you are in a restaurant and you don't feel your concerns are being taken seriously by staff or management, leave or, at the very least, do not order a meal for your child. If a restaurant is not prepared to take food allergy seriously, then it is not safe for your child to eat there. It is pointless trying to battle with staff who really aren't interested in becoming educated. It might not be fair, but do you really want to eat somewhere that doesn't welcome your child as a customer?

7. Remember that your child is listening

It is easy to forget that your child is listening to how you communicate their allergies to others. If you seem overly anxious or demanding in dealing with staff, your children will pick up on this and may become afraid to eat out or self-conscious about their allergies. Lead by example: show that politely asking questions about food safety and preparation is a normal and acceptable thing to do, and that their allergy is a part of life, not something to be embarrassed by.

> *'Don't be afraid to speak out about your child's food allergy. It's not an embarrassing thing and if you are positive about it, you are being a role model for your child. When I take Kate to a café, for example, I won't speak softly and make it a hidden thing. I will say this is my daughter Kate, and she would like to have this off the menu but she is allergic to peanuts, so I'd like to see the packaging please.'*
>
> —Jodie Bellchambers (WA), mother of Kate (9), allergic to peanut (and previously egg)

8. Carry a backup option in your bag

Despite your best efforts — and often the restaurant's — ordering a safe meal may not be possible, or may not eventuate. For example, if your child orders a meal and it comes out with a sauce it wasn't supposed to have, even if the chef offers to remake the meal, your child may no longer be willing to eat it or trust that it is safe.

Always carry some backup options with you in case this happens. It can also be a good idea to give your child a light meal before you eat out, so they aren't ravenous when you arrive and will therefore be less likely to tuck into a huge serving of a new food (or be upset if there is some delay, and consequently make what should be an enjoyable outing an ordeal for all concerned).

> *'We went to Canberra and we were staying in a hotel for a function. I rang them ahead of time and I said, we're coming, my daughter has allergies, what's going to be on the menu? I asked if it would be safe for us to bring her, and we organised a plate of boiled durum wheat pasta, with nothing else on it. Then when we got there, I said the same things. When they brought the pasta out, it looked yellow and glossy and had herbs on top. So I said to the staff, there is something on this, butter or oil. They took it away and brought another plate. Jess had a mouthful, spat it out and said, "No, no, no." I spoke to the manager and they said they had just run the pasta under hot water to wash the butter off. They got it right third time round but by that time she wasn't hungry any more.'*
>
> —Merryn Gibbons (NSW), mother of Jessica (9), allergic to cow's milk, egg and peanut

9. Be prepared

Anyone with a food allergy knows that eating out poses risks; the key is to be prepared, which means always carrying your child's EpiPen and Action Plan. If you have forgotten your child's EpiPen, you'll have to either postpone your plans to eat out or go home and get the EpiPen. No EpiPen, no eating.

If your child is old enough to be eating out on their own with friends, make sure they have friends with them who know what to do in an emergency — in other words, they know how and when to use an EpiPen, and where your child keeps their EpiPen and Action Plan.

> *'Eating out and eating good-quality food is a part of our life, and the children's too. It prepares Thomas so that when he approaches the teen years, if he goes out for dinner with friends, he will be confident. He will know the kind of restaurants that he will be able to visit, and be confident to say to his mates, "Hey, I can't eat there. Do you mind if we go here instead for a grill?" It gives him skills for when he is older and encourages that eating is a pleasurable experience, not one to be feared.'*

—Claire Bent (Tas), mother of Thomas (8),
allergic to egg, peanut, tree nuts and sesame

10. Say thank you

When a café or restaurant makes you feel welcome and accommodates the needs of your child with food allergies, remember to say thank you. Let them know how much you appreciate the extra effort they went to in order to prepare a safe meal for your child, or their flexibility in letting you bring safe food for your child.

Highchair hygiene

If you are eating out with infants and young children, you will need to give some thought to seating arrangements. If a highchair tray is contaminated with an allergen and pieces of food are placed directly onto the tray, the food may also become contaminated — meaning there is a definite risk of an allergic reaction. Tray tables need to be wiped with a clean cloth. Carrying wipes with your medical kit is a good idea: always be prepared.

When Noah was a baby, several times he experienced skin reactions from seemingly 'clean' highchairs that were wiped down in front of our eyes. In each case, staff had wiped with a cloth that had been contaminated with milk, and on one occasion peanut butter. We soon started to pack our own wipes

continued

to clean highchairs and, when Noah was a toddler, we invested in a collapsible booster seat that fitted onto most restaurant chairs. When folded, the seat fitted in our suitcase perfectly and could also fit in the storage tray beneath our pram when we were out and about.

Teens and fast-food chains

If you have a teenager who is keen to eat out at fast-food chains with their friends, you might be pleasantly surprised to find that safe options can often be found (depending on your child's allergy, of course). Many of the major fast-food chains list menu items on their website along with helpful allergen information. While the menu options aren't always healthy, food preparation in large chains is usually standardised, with strictly enforced cleaning procedures and other safeguards that can help to lower (but not eliminate) the risk of cross-contamination.

The 'standardisation' in the preparation of menu items also usually means that menu items contain the same ingredients at every store and are prepared in the same way. Spend some time with your teen researching safe menu options, but also educate your teen that they still have to alert staff to their allergy and every time they eat out check the meal they order does not contain their allergen. And, of course, they must always carry their EpiPen and Action Plan.

'Cross-contamination' in a restaurant environment?

Q I am new to the world of food allergy, with my teenage son recently diagnosed with shellfish allergy, having experienced anaphylaxis after eating prawn. Our family has always enjoyed eating out and I know he needs to avoid all shellfish, but I don't really understand cross-contamination. What cross-contamination risks do we need to be aware of in a restaurant environment?

A Cross-contamination in a restaurant environment refers to a safe food somehow being 'contaminated' by an allergen. In food preparation, this can happen in a variety of ways, including:

- Food-to-equipment contamination. For example, the same tongs may be used to pick up shellfish and then to serve plain pasta, or a grill plate may be used to cook shellfish and then a steak.
- Food-to-food contamination. For example, a container of yoghurt might leak onto other food items in the cool room, or fresh fish purchased from a market may have been displayed in such a way that it was touching shellfish.
- Food-to-hand contamination. For example, staff might handle shellfish wearing a pair of gloves, then handle a piece of fish while wearing the same pair of gloves.

With shellfish allergy, you need to avoid seafood restaurants, where the risk of cross-contamination is very high. When you are selecting a restaurant, in addition to trying to find a safe meal option, also take note of the dishes that contain your son's allergen. If the majority of meals on the menu contain seafood, or a prawn dish is the house specialty, then you might want to reconsider your restaurant selection. Do your research before choosing a restaurant.

When you or your son are communicating with staff about his allergy, ask very specific questions about the dish you want to order: what are the ingredients and how is it prepared? If he is ordering a steak, check what other foods are cooked on the grill. If he is ordering chips, check what other foods are prepared in the same fryer. Make sure you feel confident that the restaurant staff and chef understand the serious nature of your son's allergy before his meal is ordered. When the meal arrives, he should check again with staff that the meal does not contain his allergen.

Be aware that in addition to cross-contamination, shellfish can often be a hidden ingredient — for example, it can be found in fish stock, which may be used as a component of a seemingly safe soup or curry. He needs to become familiar with the names of all the ingredients he must avoid and products which commonly contain shellfish (see pages 175–176).

Importantly, as your son is a teen and only recently diagnosed, spend time educating him about what he has to know to keep himself safe. He needs to understand what foods to avoid and that he has to carry his EpiPen and Action Plan at all times. He should also educate some of the friends he socialises with frequently, in case he has a reaction and is not well enough to self-inject his EpiPen. On this topic, some doctors suggest that a child chooses one or two close friends to act as 'buddies'.

Because your son has not grown up with his allergy, he has a lot to learn and he may be feeling anxious after his recent severe reaction. Open up the lines of communication. If he requires help understanding his allergy, you might need to enlist the assistance of your allergy specialist, GP or dietitian — sometimes teens are more responsive when information comes from an outside source.

Also, while it is not common, some people who are allergic to shellfish can also react to cooking odours and handling shellfish, which is something your son should be aware of if he is socialising in an environment where shellfish is being prepared close by, for example, a Japanese teppanyaki bar.

In summary, your son always needs to make his allergy known to any supplier or server of food; ask questions about cross-contamination; and, above all else, always carry his Action Plan and emergency medications in case of inadvertent exposure. No EpiPen, no eating.

What happens when things don't go to plan?

Despite careful planning and usually the best efforts of restaurant staff, sometimes things do go wrong when you are eating out.

If you think your child is having an allergic reaction in a restaurant, get them to stop eating the food immediately and remove the food from their reach. Monitor your child's symptoms and treat them according to their personalised Action Plan. If they have any symptoms of anaphylaxis (listed on their Action Plan) do not hesitate to use your child's EpiPen and call an ambulance immediately.

When your child has recovered from the reaction, follow up with the restaurant and try to determine what went wrong. Was the meal contaminated or has your child developed a new allergy? Work with the restaurant to try to establish what triggered your child's reaction. In some cases, your allergy specialist might request a sample meal from a restaurant to try to identify the allergen.

If you specifically asked the restaurant if a meal contained your child's allergen, and you believe they served the allergen to your child, then you should report the incident to health authorities. The process for lodging a formal complaint is outlined on pages 160–162, in Chapter 8, Understanding food labelling.

Make a point of talking about the allergic reaction with your child. Try to focus on the positives: ask them what they think they did well in the situation, for example, remembering to tell you they weren't feeling well, keeping calm and listening. Acknowledge that things did go wrong but, importantly, let them know they handled the situation with strength and you think they coped admirably. Remind your child that there was a plan in place, you had their medication on hand, and that by following the plan and using the medication, everything was okay. Anxiety can snowball, so it is important to talk through how your child feels after an allergic reaction and use it as a learning experience. (See more on the emotional wellbeing of children with food allergies in Chapter 17, Anxiety in children, page 331.)

Be realistic in what you can and can't do

Sometimes, ordering a meal for your food-allergic child at a restaurant just isn't an option, so you have to come up with other ideas to let your child experience normal social situations while also keeping them safe.

For our family, ordering Noah a safe meal in a restaurant hasn't worked. Despite our best efforts, and restaurants trying hard, on three occasions Noah has experienced hives and facial swelling as well as other widespread skin reactions when eating out. At this stage, we interpret these reactions as a warning sign that it simply isn't worth the risk as he has so many allergens — especially milk, which, in our experience, has been the hardest to avoid and the allergen Noah reacts to in the tiniest of amounts. We also reason that it's not too big an issue for him socially while he is only 4 years of age and doesn't yet crave to order a restaurant meal.

We still eat out regularly with Noah, but we stick to our favourite local café, where they know about Noah's allergies and do not mind us bringing safe food for him. In addition, the café owner took it upon himself to specially order Noah's favourite bottled juice: he keeps a box of it out the back so Noah can still order something special when he comes in. (Thank you, George.)

We have also found a local café that only sells 'allergy-friendly' foods and provides a written ingredients list for every product they sell. We take Noah there to buy a special takeaway cookie (he has a choice of three!). He doesn't even particularly love the cookies but he thoroughly enjoys the fact that we can walk into a shop and he can choose something for himself and watch it being popped into a brown paper bag.

When Noah is older and hopefully outgrows his milk and egg allergy, at the very least, we will try ordering him a meal in a restaurant again. But for now, it just doesn't make sense to take the risk when he has reacted to unseen cross-contamination on a few occasions. You have to make decisions based on what is appropriate for your own child's safety.

> *'When eating out, we take safe chocolate and use it to crumble over frothy "babyccinos" instead of the powdered chocolate. Emily loves it even better.'*
>
> —Angela Batten (Vic), mother of Emily (10), allergic to peanut and tree nuts

Chef cards

Q I have a friend in the US, and her child — like mine — has peanut allergy. They seem to eat out regularly, and she mentioned to me that she uses a 'chef's card' that outlines her child's allergy. Are these used in Australia and where can I get one?

A A chef's card briefly explains a person's allergies and lists the names of foods they cannot consume, as well as a reminder about using clean utensils. These cards are then handed to restaurant staff to communicate food allergies to the chef. If you search online you will find various versions, most of which are free.

However, while chef's cards appear to be popular in the US and other countries, they aren't commonly used in Australia. Chef's cards can be a helpful *additional* communication tool, but nothing replaces the value of face-to-face communication about food allergies with restaurant staff. Handing over an information card does not guarantee it will be read, whereas a conversation with staff gives you the opportunity to assess how seriously they are taking your concerns, provides the chance for you to ask very specific questions and also answer any questions staff may have about your child's allergies. It also gives you the chance to build a relationship with a restaurant where you might be able to eat regularly, if they can accommodate your needs.

It can be helpful to hand over an allergen information card — listing a large variety of names that may be used to identify your child's allergen, as well as common foods where the allergen is usually found (available at **www.allergyfacts.org.au**) — after you have had a conversation with the chef or restaurant staff.

Important things to remember when eating out with food allergy

- Plan ahead.
- Communicate clearly with staff — ideally, the manager or head chef — and ask direct questions.
- Be polite.
- Order plain foods to minimise the risk of hidden allergens.
- Always carry your child's EpiPen and Action Plan. No EpiPen, no eating.
- Teens need to educate friends on how and when to use their EpiPen and understand how to follow their Action Plan.

10

Travelling with food allergy

Travelling anywhere with children can, even at the best of times, be challenging. Travelling with a child who has food allergy is even more so. Home is usually where parents of food-allergic children feel the most at ease: where they have control over what their child is eating and have safeguards and routines in place that enable the family to relax. The very thought of leaving the sanctuary of not only your own home but your own state or country can be a daunting prospect, but it can be done and, what's more, it can be a lot of fun.

Travel, whether it is an overnight stay or an overseas adventure, should be a wonderful and exciting experience. Food allergy will certainly influence travel plans to some extent, but it doesn't have to be the ruling force. No matter how far or wide you intend to roam, preparation and planning are the keys to a successful and safe trip the whole family will enjoy.

In this chapter we will provide some general tips on preparing to travel with food allergy. We will then look specifically at flying and cruising with food allergy, and preparing to eat out in a foreign land.

Preparing to travel ... anywhere

The steps you need to take in preparing to travel will vary depending on where you are going, the mode of transport, how long you intend to travel for and, of course, your child's age, allergies and any other related medical conditions they may have.

Below is a list of 20 things you might like to consider when preparing to travel. This list is not exhaustive, and not all measures will be appropriate for all families, but it is designed to illustrate a range of issues that may crop up when travelling. Keep in mind that there is no one-size-fits-all approach to preparing to travel with food allergies. Use the list below as a springboard for ideas on how you might individually plan for your own family adventure.

1. Check in with your GP or allergy specialist. Discuss your travel plans with your doctor so you can receive information specific to your child's allergies and your destination. If you are travelling for a long time or to a remote location, your doctor may prescribe additional medications for you to carry for your child. If you are travelling interstate, overseas or to a remote location it is advisable to carry a minimum of two EpiPens with you; discuss this with your doctor. If your child has asthma that is worse in winter and you are travelling to a colder destination, you may want to discuss increasing your child's preventer medication.

2. If you are travelling overseas, check if your family requires immunisations and always remind your doctor of your child's food allergies before an immunisation is scheduled. Some immunisations may not be safe for your child. For example, yellow fever immunisation is not recommended for children who have previously experienced severe reactions to egg.

3. Check the expiry dates on all medications. If you are planning a long trip, ensure the medications will be in date for the duration of your trip, with time to spare in case you are delayed.

4. Pack a medical kit, including your child's emergency medications and Action Plan. As well as any extra prescription medications your doctor has given you to take, think about any extra over-the-counter medications you might want to pack. For example, I recently dropped — and smashed — a bottle of antihistamine while giving Noah a dose. We now carry a spare, as it can be hard to replace after-hours when you are away from home.

5. Think about how you are going to carry your medication in your holiday destination. For example, if you are going camping somewhere hot, you might want to invest in an insulated wallet to store your EpiPen.

6. Think about any other health conditions that might affect your child in another destination and plan for these as well; for example, asthma, dustmite allergy, hayfever or eczema. These days our son Noah experiences only mild eczema in Melbourne; however, if we travel to a warm destination, his eczema flares. I always have a script filled for his various eczema creams prior to travelling and also pack his bath oil, moisturising creams and sunscreen, because the brands we use can be hard to find in other locations.

7. Pack scripts for medication replacement in case any medication gets lost or damaged somewhere along your travels.

8. If your child is at risk of a severe allergic reaction, consider purchasing a medical alert tag that indicates what your child is allergic to in case you are involved in an accident or your child gets lost in a new destination. Visit **www.medicalert.org.au** for more information on MedicAlert emblems, or call into your local pharmacy where other brands of medical alert tags can also be purchased.

9. If you are travelling with a group, be sure to educate those people about your child's allergies. Let them know what they can do to help keep your child safe and included in holiday activities; for example, not offering your child any food without checking with the parent first.

10. No matter where you are travelling, check you will have mobile phone reception at your intended destination. Do not assume you will have mobile coverage at your destination; check with your provider before you go. If you are camping or visiting somewhere remote without mobile phone reception, you may need to consider an emergency satellite beacon,[1] satellite phone or walkie-talkie. In summary, no matter where you are, ensure you have some means by which you can call for help.

11. If you are going camping or bushwalking, always let others know where you are going, your intended travel route and when you will be coming home. If you are visiting a national park, you might like to check in with the local ranger about what to do in an emergency situation. Make sure you know the most direct route to the nearest hospital or medical facility, and that you know your exact location if you need to call for medical help to come to you.

12. If you are travelling overseas, be sure you know what number to dial for an ambulance if you are in an emergency. If you are travelling to a country where English is not spoken, pack a translated script you can use to call an ambulance. There are numerous translation service companies, or you may know someone who speaks the language. Which service you use will depend on which language you need translated. Do your research and check the company you choose is reputable and that your script is accurate and appropriate for the specific region in which you intend to travel. (Also see page 212, for information about **www. foodallergyalliance.org** and **www.travelwithallergy.com.au**)

13. Think about your accommodation options when booking. Ideally, you should look for accommodation that is self-contained with kitchen facilities to ensure you can always prepare safe meals and snacks for your child along the way. If you are taking a long car trip and are staying in motels along the way, many have mini fridges and microwaves. (For more on self-contained accommodation, see page 209.)

14. Think about the kind of meals you will want to prepare at your destination: what ingredients might be hard to find? If you are visiting one location for a week or more, you might like to consider ordering some safe grocery items online and having them sent to your holiday address to save having to go on a hunt when you arrive (and also decrease the amount of foods you might otherwise be trying to squeeze into your suitcase or car boot). Stick to foods your child has already safely eaten before and, as always, read the labels on every packet. Ensure you pack or order more food than you think you might need.

15. If you plan on eating out, research cafés or restaurants before you go. Call and ask to speak to the owner or manager, or email them. Find out what meal options they have on offer and talk to them about your child's allergies. If you know others who have travelled to your intended destination (with or without food allergies), ask them if they can recommend any restaurants that were helpful and friendly: a good indication that they *may* be willing to cater to your child's needs. (For more information, see page 210, 'Eating out in a foreign land', and Chapter 9, Eating out with food allergy, page 180.)

16. If you plan on booking a hire car, it is worth mentioning to the hire car company that your child has food allergy and request that the car you are hiring (and any child safety seats) have been adequately cleaned. Although there is no guarantee this will happen, a formal request can help.

17. When travelling in a foreign country, don't expect the same standard of food labelling that you are used to at home. For a start, the label may not be written in English and, if it is, it may not reveal the whole truth about hidden allergens. Sticking to a diet of fresh fruit and vegetables and meats (being aware of cross-contamination from wherever you purchase fresh foods) is the safest option.

18. Always leave a copy of your itinerary and travel documents with close relatives in case you need help while travelling.

19. Make sure you carry with you the contact details of your allergy specialist or GP in case you need to contact them while you are away.

20. While a lot of planning is needed to ensure a safe and enjoyable travel experience, try not to burden your child with too much detail about all the effort you are going to. Certainly don't hide the fact that you are putting measures in place to keep them safe, but try not to make a huge fuss so that your child is worried that their food allergy might ruin the holiday. Keep the focus on the *pleasure* of travel, with food allergy being only one component of the planning involved. You want your children to relax and have fun on holidays.

> 'When we went to Fiji, the reason we chose the island we went to was that it had a store on it, so we could buy food, and we chose a self-catering accommodation option, with a kitchenette, so we could boil pasta and make simple things. The whole holiday really was directed around the allergies. And we met another couple by the pool that had chosen the same island for the very same reasons.
>
> 'It was a really well-stocked shop, because the island had a marina with boats coming in every day with stock. We were a 45-minute boat ride from the mainland, so we had to take that into consideration, but there was an airstrip on the island, so we would never be too far away.

*There was also mobile phone reception on this island and
I switched my mobile phone provider so I knew we would
have coverage while we were there. The allergies were a
prime consideration in planning the holiday, but then we
could relax when we were there. It gave us the confidence
to think, "We could do this again, as long as we self-cater."'*

—Anne Frisby and Phil Solomon (Vic), parents of Amelia (6),
allergic to cow's milk, egg and peanut,
and Hugh (4), allergic to egg and peanut

Ask yourself, 'What would you do if …?'

When you are preparing a trip away, it can be helpful to ask
yourself a few 'What would you do if …?' questions. For example,
we recently visited friends on a farm in regional Victoria. Before
going, I asked myself, 'What would I do if Noah experienced
anaphylaxis on the farm?' From there I knew I had to locate the
nearest hospital and work out how long it would take to get
to the hospital (I Googled the exact location of the farm); from
there I knew I had to pack an extra EpiPen, safe foods and have
a chat to our friends about Noah's allergies. I also had to check
that our mobile phone would still be in range in case we needed
to call for help. We packed safe non-perishable foods for Noah
and stopped at the closest town to pick up meat and fresh fruit
and vegetables. We packed all of Noah's medications and Action
Plan in a kit and placed it in a safe location in the house as soon
as we arrived and did not move it unless we were going out;
we carried the kit in a bag when we went on walks on the farm.
With the right preparation in place, we had a very relaxing
weekend away.

Flying with food allergy

Having moved from Sydney to Melbourne five years ago, our family is used to taking interstate flights to visit relatives — all of whom live in NSW and Queensland. Noah is a well-seasoned flyer and we are much better at it now than when we first started.

Most of our issues with flying have been related to inconsistent information from staff (being given certain information when booking with call centre staff then receiving conflicting information at check-in) and the cleanliness of the plane itself.

As mentioned previously, Noah is allergic to cow's milk, egg, peanut, tree nuts and sesame. Over the past few years we have collected several loose cashews from beneath Noah's seat, he has had a couple of skin-only reactions to dirty seats and, on our most recent flight, he pulled down his tray table to find it covered in powdered milk chocolate — all pretty minor stuff because we were prepared to deal with it when it happened. We find that if we do everything we can to prevent an allergic reaction and ensure we are prepared for the unlikely — that Noah might suffer a severe allergic reaction while flying — then we are, nowadays, very relaxed when we fly.

Below is a list of general information which may be helpful for your family when preparing to fly with a child who has food allergy. What your family needs to do to prepare for flying will vary depending on how far you are flying and your intended destination, as well as your child's allergies and clinical history (including any associated medical conditions). You should always discuss your child's individual needs with your doctor before flying.

Before booking your ticket

- Research the airline. When you have chosen the airline you want to fly with, call and ask them if they have a specific policy on food allergy (some do). Request a copy of the policy and ask questions if anything in the policy is unclear.
- Check with the airline what its policy is on carrying medication on board, and what kind of documentation you may need to provide to ensure you are allowed to bring your child's medication into the cabin.

- Ask the airline what kind of meals and snacks they serve. For example, do you serve packaged peanuts during the flight?
- Check with the airline that you are allowed to carry meals and snacks on board for your child. If you are going on a long flight, ask if they can assist with the heating of meals for your child — some might; many won't. If your airline is happy to heat your child's meal, be aware that airlines do not usually have microwaves on board, so you will need to pack your child's meal in an ovenproof container. Supplying your child's meal in an appropriate container also reduces the risk of cross-contamination during heating and serving.
- Check what liquids you are allowed to carry on board. There are security restrictions when travelling to and from Australia, which you need to know if you intend on packing safe liquid options for your child; for example, juices, milks, formula. It is a good idea to carry any liquids in their original packaging rather than containers so security can verify what you intend on taking on board (although you may need to 'decant' some of the packaged fluid into a bottle to comply with the maximum capacity allowed). In short, it can be complicated carrying liquids on a flight, so check with the airline *before* travelling about how much liquid you can carry and in what kind of container or packaging it must be stored.
- If you are taking out travel insurance, carefully read the policy document to ensure persons at risk of anaphylaxis are covered under the policy. If not, specifically request coverage in your policy (which will usually be at an additional cost) or find another insurer.

When booking your ticket

- Consider the time of day you are flying. For example, on a short domestic flight you may be better suited to flying at a time when only a light snack is served rather than a two-course main meal.
- If you are flying overseas, if possible, consider booking a direct flight so you do not need to change aircraft or airlines along the way.
- Book your ticket over the phone (as opposed to online or through a travel agent) direct with the airline. Alert the airline that your child has a severe food allergy and confirm your understanding of the airline's food-allergy policy with the staff member. Be sure what they

tell you when you book your ticket is consistent with what you were told on your initial research inquiry. Write down the name of the staff member in case you are told any conflicting information by another staff member further down the track.

- You won't necessarily be price-penalised for making a booking over the phone. Booking online is usually the best way to secure a discount fare, but some airlines (in my experience) will still give you the online rate if you need to book over the phone because your child has food allergies, so always check with your airline. You might be pleasantly surprised.

- If possible, request a seat where your young child won't be exposed to other passengers eating allergenic food; for example, a window seat.

Preparing to fly

- Visit your GP or allergy specialist in advance and ask them to provide you with a signed Travel Plan, which will outline your child's allergies, medications, and the fact that your child may need to carry safe food and drinks on board. (See page 204 for information on the ASCIA Travel Plan.)

- Ask your GP or allergy specialist for any scripts you may need to have on hand; for example, in case you lose any medication while travelling.

- Consider your child's health. If your child is generally unwell close to your departure date, be sure to visit your GP for a check-up before you depart.

- Check the expiry dates on your child's medication and ensure they are in date for the duration of your trip. Check with your doctor if you need to carry additional EpiPens and any other medicines for your child when travelling.

- Ensure all of your child's medications are pharmacy-labelled with your child's name. For example, often pharmacies only label the box the EpiPen comes in and some airlines specify that the EpiPen itself must be pharmacy-labelled.

- Pack all of your child's medication, their Action Plan and Travel Plan (both signed by your doctor) in a kit you can carry on board and stow beneath your seat for easy in-flight access.

- Pack some wipes/travel towels.
- Pack plenty of games and activities to keep your child busy during the flight. Often the desire to eat while flying stems from boredom rather than hunger.
- Depending on the age of your child, talk to them about how they are feeling about the flight. Ask them if they have any questions and, if they are worried, reassure them by explaining the steps you have taken to keep them safe during the flight. While it is important to talk to your child about any concerns they may have, try to keep it in perspective. Be organised and have one conversation about their allergies and then focus on the fun things about the trip.

The day you fly

- Double-check you have packed your child's medical kit and documentation in your carry-on luggage. If you are packing spare EpiPens to have on hand at your destination, they should still be packed in your carry-on luggage in the event you need them in-flight and in case luggage is lost. Also, there is no guarantee the EpiPen is being stored at the appropriate temperature in the cargo hold area.
- Call the airline and confirm your child's allergies have been listed with your booking.
- Ensure you have an abundance of safe foods for your child to eat on the flight (allowing for spillage and wastage if you have toddlers!). Some airlines might offer to prepare a safe meal for your child, but it is safer to bring your own food from home. Even when you fly domestically you can experience long flight delays. Expect the unexpected and pack accordingly.
- Arrive at the check-in counter in plenty of time so you and your family are relaxed and you have time to reconfirm your requests and show necessary documentation.
- When you board your plane, check that your child's seat, tray table and the carpet beneath their feet is clean. This may sound extreme but in my experience it is necessary. There is a risk of your child's 'safe' food becoming contaminated if consumed from a dirty surface, and even though skin contact with an allergen is extremely unlikely to cause a severe reaction, it can cause a local reaction. While local reactions

such as hives are not life-threatening, they are uncomfortable and can require a dose of antihistamine, so it is not being paranoid to check your child's seating area. A dose of hives is sometimes enough to cause a food-allergic child to be unnecessarily nervous about the flight ahead, which nobody wants.

- Alert your flight attendant that your child has food allergies.
- If you are on a particularly long flight, you may like to introduce yourself to your neighbouring passengers and tell them your young child has a food allergy.

'We have got into a mode of operating where day to day it's not that stressful. We stock the cupboards with stuff we know they can eat. We don't do takeaways or go out to eat with them, so we stay within our comfort zone. The real stress is when we have to go outside of our routine, which is usually on holidays.'

—Justine Sayers (Vic), mother of Esme (5),
allergic to cow's milk, egg, peanut and tree nut,
and Fred (2), allergic to cow's milk,
fish and sesame

ASCIA Travel Plan

The Australasian Society of Clinical Immunology and Allergy has developed and published a Travel Plan to make life easier for those at risk of anaphylaxis. The plan has been developed so individuals at risk of anaphylaxis can carry standardised formal documentation outlining that they:

- are at risk of anaphylaxis
- need to carry adrenaline in an autoinjector accessible at all times
- need to carry safe food and liquids

The plan has space for you to fill in your child's name and allergens and needs to be signed by your child's doctor and carried in conjunction with their Action Plan. To download copies of the travel plan go to **www.allergy.org.au** (then click on the Anaphylaxis Resources link).

Airborne exposure to allergen on airlines

Q Our 5-year-old son is allergic to peanut and has experienced anaphylaxis after eating a very small amount of peanut butter. We are travelling overseas soon and the airline we are flying with serves peanuts on board. I plan on packing meals and snacks for my son, but should we be worried about other people on board the aircraft consuming peanuts around us? Could the smell of peanuts trigger anaphylaxis?

A In a 1999 American study into peanut-allergic reactions on commercial airlines,[2] it was concluded that allergic reactions to both peanut and tree nuts do occur on commercial flights, with reactions caused by: accidental ingestion, skin contact or inhalation — but in most cases anaphylaxis was due to ingestion. In the study, most of the allergic reactions which resulted from airborne exposure to peanuts were *not* life-threatening, and the study found that the symptoms occurred when a large number (25 or more) of passengers were eating peanuts. (Passengers eating food containing nuts, for example, muffins, pose no risk to your child, as long as he doesn't eat it.)

There are several published studies of severe allergic reactions to airborne food particles, but these reactions are usually associated with fumes from cooking,[3] especially seafood,[4, 5] or airborne exposure in a workplace,[6] for example, a factory or agricultural research centre.

Remember that people with food allergies fly safely every day, but do check with your son's allergy specialist before you fly to see if they have any advice specific to your son's condition. Depending on the length of your trip and medical facilities available at your destination, your doctor may prescribe extra EpiPens and other medications for you to carry. Your allergy specialist or GP will also be able to help you with any documentation your airline might require you to carry in regard to your son's allergies and his emergency medications. Be sure to phone your airline in advance to advise them of your son's allergy and ask them about any documentation you may need to provide.

The most important thing to focus on is being prepared for your flight. Careful planning is imperative, including: packing safe meal and snack options, medications and your son's Action Plan and Travel Plan in your carry-on luggage, as well as effectively communicating to airline staff your son's allergy.

Cruising with food allergy

Taking a cruise on a ship with a child who has food allergy can be done; however — as always — you'll need to do your homework to ensure the cruise line you choose is educated about food allergies, willing to help make your family welcome and safe, and equipped to cope with an emergency situation should it arise.

Following are some tips to help you plan an enjoyable and safe cruise with food allergies.

- Before booking any cruise and paying a deposit, alert the company that your child has a severe food allergy and ask questions to gauge whether they are willing and able to accommodate your needs. You might ask, for example: Is the kitchen able to prepare safe meals for my child? Do you have a medical clinic and doctor on board? Does your company require me to provide any documentation about my child's allergies and medication in advance? Will our cabin have a bar fridge? Can we bring some safe snacks on board for our child? Write down a list of questions before you call. Record the date and the name of the person who is answering your questions.

- When you decide to make a booking, ensure you include reference to your child's food allergies on the booking form and mention that you have previously spoken to a staff member about the cruise line accommodating your child's needs.

- Before you leave for your cruise, be sure to check in with your child's allergy specialist, who may prescribe additional medications for you to carry on board. You should also ask your specialist to provide you with a signed Travel Plan (see page 204) outlining your child's allergies and any other important medical information that medical staff on board the ship may need to know. Written permission to carry EpiPens may also be required: check with your cruise line.

- Ensure you have travel insurance and that food allergy and anaphylaxis is covered under the policy.
- Wearing a medical alert necklace or bracelet (see page 196) can also be a good idea, especially if children are going to participate in kids' club activities.
- Pack a full medical kit, as well as a few photocopies of your child's Action Plan, Travel Plan and the contact details of your child's allergy specialist and GP. Always pack your medical kit in carry-on luggage and think about how you will carry the EpiPen, Action Plan and Travel Plan on board; you might need to invest in a bum bag.
- You might like to pack a bag of non-perishable safe snack options. Check with your cruise line about what you are allowed to bring, as quarantine regulations will vary depending on your cruise destinations.
- When you board the ship, introduce yourself to the Maitre d' and discuss your child's food allergies. Confirm with the Maitre d' your understanding of how your child's food allergies will be managed on board, including the ordering of meals, the hours of operation of the medical clinic and how you can access help immediately in the event of anaphylaxis.
- It is a good idea to introduce your child to medical staff on board and know exactly where the medical clinic is. You may also like to give the medical staff a copy of your child's Action Plan and Travel Plan so they are aware of your child's medical history in the event of an emergency.
- Avoid buffet meals while on cruise ships, as the risk of cross-contamination is always high. Keep to the dining room, where you can order your child's meals and remind staff of your child's allergies. Consider always sitting in the same area so you are likely to have the same informed staff serving you each day. Some cruise ships have chefs dedicated to preparing meals

continued

for passengers with special dietary needs. Sometimes special meals need to be ordered a day in advance.

- If you leave the ship on a day trip, ensure you take your medical kit with you and that you know how to call for help in the location you are visiting. If finding safe food on land is going to be a problem, talk to staff on board the ship about packing some safe food — that quarantine staff will allow — for your child for the day.

- If there is a kids' club on board, check with staff about their knowledge of food allergies. Make sure carers know how to recognise the signs and symptoms of an allergic reaction and administer your child's EpiPen in the event of anaphylaxis. Clarify whether they can or cannot offer your child any food while you are not with them. On some cruise ships, parents who leave children in a kids' club can be given a pager in case they are needed. Once the pager alarm is activated, the parent can ring the kids' club staff from one of the many phones around the ship.

- Be aware that if you need to see medical staff outside of clinic hours you may have to pay an 'after hours' fee for a consultation, so pack your credit card.

'We recently took a cruise where there were over 2,000 passengers and 700 staff. They were overall very well informed about food allergies and, in the areas where they needed further education, they were willing to listen. My son had to order his meals the day before but a dedicated chef then prepared his meals and they always arrived at the same time as everyone else's; there was no delay, so he always felt included. They took food allergies very seriously. We checked in with our son's allergy specialist before leaving and were well prepared with a medical kit containing an extra EpiPen and other medications. He

*carried his medical kit (in a bum bag) everywhere, both on
and off the ship. We were very impressed, had a wonderful
time and are definitely going to go on a cruise with the
same company again. I think it would be more of a
challenge if your child has multiple food allergies but I still
think that, with forward planning, it can be done.'*

—Maria Said (NSW), President of Anaphylaxis Australia
Incorporated and mother of Alex (18),
allergic to peanut

Self-contained accommodation

When travelling and managing food allergies, self-contained
accommodation is ideal, because it gives you the freedom to prepare safe
meals. If you are staying in one spot for a while, it also gives you the
chance to freeze some meals so you don't have to spend every night in the
kitchen while you are on holidays.

The one thing you do need to be careful of, though, is the cleanliness
of the kitchen and utensils. It's a good idea to wash utensils, bread boards,
cooking pots and other kitchen equipment before preparing meals for
your child. There is no guarantee that whoever stayed in the apartment
or house before you has taken the time to wash up appropriately. (We
recently stayed in an apartment and found cheese residue stuck to most
of the cutlery, and the pots and pans were dirty, too.) If you are going to
use the barbeque, consider buying foil or a barbeque liner to prevent the
chance of cross-contamination from recently cooked items.

Also think about food storage. I usually buy some cheap disposable
food containers so I can pack snacks for Noah when we go to the
beach or on day trips — that way we don't have to lug whole packets of
snacks around with us. If at your accommodation there are Tupperware
containers for guests to use, run them through the dishwasher to ensure
they are clean before using them, as you have no way of knowing what
previous guests have stored in them.

Eating out in a foreign land

Eating out in an overseas country poses additional risks as you will be dealing with unfamiliar cuisine. The risk compounds where there is also a language barrier.

As always, careful preparation is the key to staying safe. If you are travelling to a country where English is not the first language, consider purchasing a travel translation card that outlines your child's allergies and makes it clear what your child cannot eat, and explains that if they do eat the food in question they may experience a severe reaction. Pack several copies of the translation card. Have the translation card with you when you attempt to communicate. Do restaurant staff seem to comprehend what you are telling them?

When you are travelling, ideally, you would try to visit the restaurant where you want to eat before making a booking. Do this at a time of day when the restaurant is not busy, so you can make your needs known, review the menu and show the owner, manager or chef your child's allergy translation card. If you do not think the restaurant can safely cater for your child, ask them if you can bring your child's meal to the restaurant. If language is a barrier in the country in which you are travelling, you might consider eating out at a restaurant inside a hotel, where English may be spoken.

When you are looking at the menu, don't assume a dish your child safely eats at home will necessarily be prepared in the same way. Always check the ingredients and ask specific questions of the owner and/or chef; for example, 'Does this meal contain peanut in any form?'

Always consider the risk of cross-contamination. Obviously, a little common sense also goes a long way. For example, if your child has a severe shellfish allergy, avoid seafood restaurants.

If you do decide it is safe for your child to eat at the restaurant, remind staff of your child's allergy when you arrive for your meal. Again, show the translation card to staff and ensure that not only the waiter but the chef understands your needs. If your child wears some form of medical alert tag, it may be helpful to point this out to staff in addition to handing them the translation card. While a translation card can certainly help communicate your needs to a restaurant, in no way does it guarantee your child's meal will be safe.

Many parents I interviewed for this book who had travelled abroad (and whose children are not allergic to potato) worship the humble hot chip: choosing to feed their child at home or take their child's meal to the restaurant and then order their child a bowl of hot chips at the restaurant, so they can still participate in 'eating out' in a small way with limited risk. Of course, you always need to check the ingredients of hot chips and what other foods are prepared in the same fryer which can still pose a risk, depending on your child's allergies. But the point is that sometimes you can find a middle ground with ordering options; it doesn't have to be all or nothing. Another tip parents have passed on is that it can be helpful to look out for a restaurant that offers 'gluten-free' meals. While there is no guarantee, it *might* mean that the restaurant will be willing to engage in a sensible conversation with you about your child's needs.

No matter how confident you are that a restaurant can cater for your child's needs, always carry your child's emergency medication and Action Plan and ensure you know how to call an ambulance in the country in which you are travelling. (See Chapter 9, Eating out with food allergy, page 180, for more tips on eating out.)

'There was some apprehension the first time that we travelled because of the unknown. When the children were younger I felt that I would never be able to travel overseas because it was too "risky". As they grew older I realised that I didn't want them to miss out on the wonderful opportunities of exploring foreign countries and went about planning the trip [to Germany and England] to make it as safe as I possibly could.

'The children coped well with the limitations of travelling with food allergies. It is obviously easier having the two affected in that they don't feel alone. There were so many new and exciting things to discover while travelling, we tried to not make food a focus. Being at an age where they can rationalise things, they understood

that they couldn't take unnecessary risks with food while we were travelling and were happy to "play it safe". They still had the opportunity to occasionally eat out.'

—Sally Voukelatos (Vic), mother of Kosta (10), allergic to peanut, tree nuts, fish, shellfish and latex, and Sophia (8), allergic to cow's milk, egg, peanut, tree nuts, fish, shellfish, lentils and sesame

www.foodallergyalliance.org

The Food Allergy and Anaphylaxis Alliance was established in 1999 to unite organisations from around the world working in food allergy and anaphylaxis. Current members of the alliance include organisations from Australia, Canada, Germany, Italy, Japan, The Netherlands, New Zealand, Sweden, the United Kingdom and the USA.

The Food Allergy and Anaphylaxis Alliance publishes helpful information on topics including food labelling and how to access emergency care and treatment in each of the above-mentioned countries. Essential reading if you are planning a holiday to any of these locations.

www.travelwithallergy.com.au

Dr Preeti Joshi has registered this web address and will soon be launching a website aimed at helping those with food allergy access translated information to use while travelling with food allergy. The service will offer information cards for ordering meals in restaurants, as well as cards about how to call an ambulance.

Learn as you go ... then go again

Most parents of children with food allergy will tell you that, initially, travelling with food allergy is hard work, but each time they do it they become more proficient, picking up new tips and determining what works best for their family.

If your child has been recently diagnosed with food allergy, it can be helpful to 'start small' while you are building your confidence. For example, consider a weekend away where you can drive and pack safe foods, or visit a holiday destination where you know it will be easy to locate safe foods in major stores. Start with a short flight interstate before taking on a long-haul overseas journey.

The point is, the more you travel, the easier it will become — although the challenges will always vary depending on your child's allergies and your destination.

11

Childcare and pre-school*

For many parents, when the time comes to send their child to childcare, or pre-school, it is their first experience of entrusting the care of their child to someone other than family. It is a big transition for both the parents and the child.

In these early years, infants and young children are learning to explore the world around them — often putting anything and everything in their mouths, eating messily, dribbling, sharing toys — with very little (depending on their age) understanding of what they can and can't eat. Parents are entirely dependent on childcare workers and teachers to provide a safe environment in which their children can learn and enjoy normal childhood experiences.

These days, owing to the increasing number of Australian children with food allergy, many childcare centres and pre-schools do have experience in caring for children with food allergy, but no matter how experienced or well-informed a centre or pre-school appears to be, the only way to ensure a positive and safe environment for your child is to invest time and effort in working together with the staff who care for your child. A team approach is always the best approach.

In this chapter we will look at different ideas to help you find the right childcare centre or pre-school for your child, how to prepare you and your child for their first day of care and what to pack in your child's all-important medical kit. We also include suggestions on how to communicate and work with staff and what to do if you are having

---

* 'Pre-school' is used in this book as a term to describe the years of early childhood education undertaken before commencing the full-time years of school. Different states and territories in Australia use different terminology for early childhood education, as do private and public schools. Other terms include kindergarten and pre-prep.

problems with your childcare centre or pre-school. Finally, we outline information about family day care as a childcare option for children with food allergy and discuss the widely debated subject of banning foods.

A special note needs to be included here: this chapter has been written to help parents work together with their child's childcare centre or pre-school in managing food allergy and the risk of an allergic reaction. There is no universal formula for creating an ideal safe environment for a food-allergic child. The particular strategies your childcare centre or school implements will vary depending on a number of factors, including the age of your child, their allergens, whether or not they are at risk of anaphylaxis, staffing levels and whether staff have had adequate training in anaphylaxis management, the location of your centre or school, and its size. It is really important that you work in partnership with staff at your child's childcare centre or pre-school to establish an individual management plan suitable for your child and their environment.

We are grateful to early childhood professionals Naomi Harris, Ann-Maree Fisher, Loata Mataitoga and Kylie Sanderson for reviewing the content of this chapter and providing helpful feedback. We also thank Monique Webber, General Manager of Family Day Care Australia, and directors for their valuable contribution.

Finding the right fit for your child

The best way to discover if a childcare centre or pre-school is suitable for your child and is willing to work with you in managing your child's food allergy is to do your homework. Arrange to visit a selection of centres or pre-schools to meet with the manager or director well in advance of when you need care for your child. Many centres and pre-schools schedule open days so prospective parents can visit, tour the premises and speak with staff. With limited availability of care options in some areas, you need to consider a range of options and make sure you place your child's name on a number of waiting lists — the earlier you do so the better.

Prepare a list of questions and think about how you are going to communicate your child's allergies to staff. Preparation really is key: the more you prepare, the more likely you are to feel relaxed about the conversation, and you may then find it easier to talk in a positive manner about managing your child's allergies, rather than coming across as anxious or demanding (which can happen, even when it is not intentional).

Below are some ideas to help you put together your own list of questions, but when you do meet with staff, remember to approach any conversations about food allergy with an encouraging and cooperative attitude. Make it clear to staff that you are willing to help or support them in any way. Successful partnerships are always two-way.

- Does the centre have a food-allergy policy document you can review?
- Establish what experience staff have in managing food allergy.
- Can they run you through a typical day at the centre or school? (There may be practical implications: for example, if your child is allergic to milk and the day starts with the serving of breakfast at 7.30am, you may not want to drop your child off until after the breakfast clean-up; at some childcare centres, all children are cared for together in a communal room for the first hour or so, until more staff arrive, so you might like to find out what time children are taken to their own room with their regular teacher.)
- How many staff have been formally trained in managing anaphylaxis and administering an EpiPen? How recent was the training and who provided the training?
- How often do casual staff work there typically, and how does management communicate allergies to casual staff?
- Are there established practices for celebrating special occasions, such as birthdays? How is food managed at these times?
- Can you pack meals for your own child? (This may or may not be necessary.)
- If meals are prepared on the premises, ask if you can also speak directly with the cook.
- Does the cook have some kind of system for keeping track of foods served to children with allergies? (For example, some pre-schools and childcare centres have a system of always preparing foods for allergic children first and using colour-coded serving ware: cups, bowls, plates.)
- How are eating times managed and supervised?

- Ask if there is an orientation process. Some childcare centres and pre-schools encourage parents to stay with their child on the first few days while they adjust, which can be great for you to get a feel for the kind of situations that might arise during your child's day and also give staff the chance to ask you questions while you are on site.
- Don't forget to also ask questions about the centre or pre-school in general, not just food allergies.

Guidelines for managing anaphylaxis in childcare centres and schools

In Australia, there are currently no national guidelines around the management of anaphylaxis in childcare, pre-school and schools: different guidelines apply depending on the state or territory in which you live. The latest anaphylaxis guidelines for each state and territory are posted on the Anaphylaxis Australia website: **www.allergyfacts.org.au** (then click on the 'Schools and Childcare' link).

In July 2008, Victoria became the first Australian state to legally require anaphylaxis management, policies and training. All children's services and schools with a student enrolled at risk of anaphylaxis must have an anaphylaxis management policy in place; all children at risk must have individual management plans in place; and there is compulsory specialist medical training for all staff in early childhood services and the majority of staff in schools where there is an 'at-risk' student enrolled. It is hoped that other states and territories will follow suit.

The Australasian Society of Clinical Immunology and Allergy (ASCIA) has also published guidelines for the prevention of food-induced anaphylaxis in schools, pre-schools and childcare settings. The guidelines can be accessed at: **www.allergy.org.au** (then click on the link for 'Position Papers/Guidelines').

Before your child's first day

- If your child's centre or pre-school has a food-allergy policy, ensure you read it. In addition to outlining the responsibilities of the centre or pre-school, many policies also outline the responsibilities of parents. If you have any questions, raise them with staff before your child's first day.

- Check in with your GP or allergy specialist and ensure you have an up-to-date Action Plan signed by your doctor (ensuring the photograph of your child is recent), as well as all the necessary medications and appropriate dosages, which are often based on weight, so your child may need to hit the scales. (Also see 'The all-important medical kit', page 225.)

- Book an appointment with your child's teacher, ideally on a pupil-free day, when the teacher can schedule time to talk with you without being interrupted. Talk to your child's teacher about your child's specific allergies and any other medical conditions. Discuss any specific concerns: for example, you may be worried about how your child's milk allergy will be managed in an environment where babies are being fed milk in bottles.

- Ask who will be responsible for administering medication to your child in an emergency and who will be responsible if this person is away or on a break. An emergency response plan must be in place, and all staff need to be aware of it.

- Take your EpiPen trainer pen with you to the meeting to demonstrate how to use an EpiPen. A recent study in New South Wales[1] found that simply asking whether staff have been trained in how to use an EpiPen does not guarantee that they can correctly administer an EpiPen.

- Ask the teacher what strategies will be put into place to minimise the risk of your child being exposed to an allergen. (See 'Minimising the risk of allergic reactions in the classroom' page 221.)

- If your child's meals are going to be prepared by staff, ensure you have spoken with kitchen staff about the risks of cross-contamination and that they understand what your child can and cannot eat. Check there is a formal communication procedure in place for casual kitchen staff for the days when regular kitchen staff are sick or on leave.
- If you are packing food for your child, consider asking the cook for advance copies of their weekly menu plan so you can prepare the same or similar meals for your child.
- Be sure kitchen staff also understand that it can be an issue if they are hand-washing a food-allergic child's plates and cups in the same water as plates and cups that have had contact with their allergen. (For example, washing a milk-allergic child's plate in the same water as the yoghurt bowls.)
- Reinforce the message to your child's teacher that if they are ever in doubt about using your child's EpiPen, not to hesitate.

On the day your child starts childcare or pre-school

- Ensure the medical kit is stored in your child's room in an easily accessible location with clear and conspicuous signage.
- Check that your child's Action Plan is located in a prominent position and securely fixed to the wall or other surface.
- Pack your child's meals in a clearly labelled container and see if it can be stored in a location out of reach of other children; or check in with kitchen staff who are preparing meals to see if they have any further questions about your child's allergies.
- Pack your child's own clearly labelled water bottle.
- Pack a change of clothes in your child's bag in case there are any spills of allergens during the day.

continued

- Remember to focus on your child's other needs for their first day, too. For example, pack your child's teddy or favourite toy for them to sleep with at rest time, as well as sunhats, suncream and anything else the centre or pre-school suggests.
- Ensure you are contactable by phone in case staff have any questions during the day — or at any other time. Make sure staff feel welcome and encouraged to call you.
- Even though you may be feeling anxious, try to put on a brave and happy face for your child. If they see you are anxious, they may also become anxious. Not an easy task, but try! (I confess, despite my best efforts, I couldn't hide my tears on Noah's first day — yet I doubt it would have been any different even if he didn't have food allergies.)

'When our son started kindergarten, I made up a small laminated card which read: "Anaphylaxis Emergency Telephone Card". On the card we included a photo of our son — using the same photo we used on his Action Plan and medical kit — as well as his name and age, and then listed step-by-step instructions:

1. Call '000'.

2. Tell the operator that the child is having an anaphylactic reaction.

'At step 3 I inserted the phone number and address of our kindergarten, including the nearest cross street.

'This card was then placed on the wall beside the phone for easy reference. The staff felt this was a useful tool, because if a staff member (or perhaps a parent on duty in a kindergarten) had to phone for help, they would need to give the correct information to the emergency workers and may not perhaps be in the most alert frame of mind at

*that particular time. We decided this could work really well
as an easy reference for those then having to make that
difficult call.'*

—Kylie Sanderson (Vic), kindergarten teacher and mother of
Will (5), allergic to egg, peanut, tree nuts and sesame

Minimising the risk of allergic reactions in the classroom

No childcare centre or pre-school can give you an iron-clad guarantee that
your child won't experience an allergic reaction on their watch; however,
there are many strategies that can be put in place to help minimise the
risk. Different systems work for different centres and pre-schools, and
you should always discuss your child's specific allergies with staff to come
up with practical safety measures appropriate for your situation. Below is
a list of commonly used strategies that will hopefully provide a helpful
starting point for you and your childcare centre or pre-school to start
working together.

- Ideally the centre or pre-school will have an allergen-minimisation
  policy. (See 'Banning foods: a good idea ... or not?', page 231.)
- Children with food allergy should be educated not to share food with
  their friends.
- Other children need to be encouraged and reminded not to share their
  food with a food-allergic child.
- Parents of other children in the centre need to be informed and
  educated about what foods not to bring into the centre. For example,
  not to use nuts as decorations on birthday cakes, no peanut butter
  or hazelnut spread sandwiches in lunchboxes. A letter might be sent
  home at the beginning of the year followed by friendly reminders
  in newsletters.
- All staff need to be aware of the risks associated with cross-
  contamination when serving food, as non-kitchen staff can also be
  involved in serving food to children.
- Encourage all children to wash their hands and faces before and after
  eating.

- Provide individual face washers/hand towels for children to wipe their hands and faces. Wash face washers/hand towels after each use. Some centres and pre-schools use a different coloured face washer for food-allergic children to prevent any mix-ups.

- Meal times need to be carefully supervised to prevent food-allergic children from being exposed to an allergen, but they should not be isolated from their friends.

- Ideally all foods and drinks should be served by permanent room staff only (rather than casual or relief staff). But if that is unavoidable, a written summary should be provided that sets out which children are food-allergic and what food-handling procedures to observe.

- If any food is usually stored in the actual classroom (for example, crackers are sometimes taken out of a large box and placed in Tupperware containers and left in classrooms), these foods should also be clearly labelled. If the food is unsafe, it should not be stored in the classroom of the allergic child.

- A communication system needs to be in place to ensure that casual or relief staff are immediately made aware of children with food allergies.

- All craft materials and activities need to be evaluated in regard to the needs of children with food allergy. For example, if a child has a wheat allergy, then playdough poses a risk. Some paints and glues contain wheat. Food containers used in craft activities also need to be checked: for example, no egg cartons are to be used if a child has egg allergy.

- Music activities also need to be considered. A food-allergic child may need to bring their own recorder or harmonica to school, or staff will need to thoroughly wash any shared mouth or wind instruments.

- Some childcare centres and pre-schools provide sunscreen for children; parents need to check that the ingredients are safe (some sunscreens contain nut oils).

- If your pre-school has a bubbler, it may be best for your child to avoid using it at such a young age. If they are using the bubbler, staff need to teach them to let the water run a little first, and not to let their mouth touch the bubbler, only the water.

- Visitors to the centre, for example, parents or relatives volunteering, tradespeople or music teachers, need to be aware of food allergies.
- If excursions are part of the education program of a childcare centre or pre-school, parents of food-allergic children need to be informed well in advance so potential risks can be discussed, as well as how the child needs to be supervised.
- Staff need to be especially aware of food allergies and any potential risks on any occasion where there is a break in the usual routine of the childcare centre or pre-school, such as on a 'grandparents and special friends' day, a sports day or a 'parents volunteer' day (when parents often bring with them younger children who may be eating allergenic foods).
- Parents of food-allergic children should supply safe treats for teachers to have on hand for special occasions, especially cup cakes for when other children are celebrating their birthday. Cup cakes that can be kept in the freezer and thawed out quickly as needed are ideal. When any food is supplied to a childcare centre or pre-school, the container should be clearly labelled with a list of the ingredients. (A parent might be sending in a cake that is safe for their child, but may not be safe for other classmates. For example, a cake might be nut-free, but other children in the room might be allergic to egg and milk, and staff need to know.)

> 'In the childcare centre Esme used to attend, there were four or five other kids with similar allergies and they used to discuss their allergies: well I can't eat this and I can't eat that. Not that there is kudos exactly, but one of Esme's friends said to me, "I can't eat Vegemite, I'm allergic to it," and I asked her mum, "Is that right?" And she said, "Oh no, she's just saying that because you get extra attention at school." So I think the other kids are building awareness.'
>
> —Justine Sayers (Vic), mother of Esme (5), allergic to cow's milk, egg, peanut and tree nuts, and Fred (2), allergic to cow's milk, fish and sesame

Give staff the chance to work with you and your child

It cannot be over-emphasised how important it is to approach managing your child's food allergies in a cooperative manner: very few people will respond positively to being handed a list of demands. Teamwork is the mantra.

Remember that while keeping your child safe is imperative, when implementing any new strategies, staff always have to keep in mind what is practical and what is appropriate for *all* children in their care. For example, if you request that a certain food is removed from a classroom and replaced with something you suggest is safe for your child to eat, a teacher also has to consider what other children in their care can and can't eat; they also have to deal with all of the other parents who may strongly object to some measure you would like to see put in place. A childcare centre or pre-school is a community environment where the needs of all children need to be considered.

Staff often come up with inspired ideas to keep food-allergic children safe — some that parents would never think of — simply because: they are in a great position to assess high-risk times of the day; some staff have extensive experience in managing food allergies; and they also have a unique way of understanding a lot about how children view the world around them.

My husband and I have been so impressed by the ideas the staff at our son's pre-school have come up with to keep him safe, including: placing a sign on the wall of Noah's classroom that reads 'EpiPen' with a big red arrow pointing to the shelf where Noah's medical kit is stored. It is an instant reminder to all staff who come into the room that there is a child at risk of anaphylaxis in the class, and there can be no mistaking where the medication is stored. Only permanent room staff serve food to children with food allergies at Noah's pre-school, to ensure there is no chance of a casual or relief staff member making a mistake with their meals, and all meals served to children with food allergies have to be checked and signed off by two staff members.

When Noah moved classrooms this year, instead of eating morning tea on a mat, they eat morning tea on the tiles, so any spills can be cleaned up immediately, and they have initiated 'rolling meal times', where a small group of children eat and then the next group and then the next group. Noah always eats with the first group, when everything has just been cleaned, and still gets to enjoy socialising with his friends, but by not having all children eating and drinking at once, the risk of a reaction is further minimised.

The all-important medical kit

If your child has food allergies, you need to provide your child's childcare centre, pre-school or school with an appropriate medical kit before their first day.

If your child has been prescibed an EpiPen, your child's medical kit should include:

- An Action Plan for anaphylaxis (see page 371), signed by your doctor and featuring a close-up, recent photograph of your child's face (a passport photo is suitable).
- An EpiPen labelled clearly with your child's name.
- Any other medications your child needs, for example, antihistamine or asthma medications, labelled clearly with your child's name and correct dosage information.

If your child has not been prescibed an EpiPen, your child's medical kit should include:

- An Action Plan for allergic reactions (see page 372), signed by your doctor and featuring a close-up, recent photograph of your child's face (a passport photo is suitable).
- Any medications your child needs, for example, antihistamine or asthma medications, labelled clearly with your child's name and correct dosage information.

You might like to put your child's medications into some kind of easily accessible container (for example, a Tupperware food storage container) and affix a copy of your child's Action Plan to the lid. It is really important that an Action Plan is kept with your child's medication. Often an Action Plan is hung on a wall in a classroom but a reaction may take place elsewhere in the school — the playground, for example — so a copy of the Action Plan should always be kept with your child's emergency medication. Make sure you use the same photograph of your child on all copies of an Action Plan. Remember that there may be several other children in your child's class that also have medical kits, so it is particularly important to label all medications clearly to avoid confusion in an emergency.

Ensure that your child's medications are stored in an unlocked location, out of reach of children but easily accessible. They should also be stored away from any direct sources of heat (for example, not near a heating duct or in direct sunlight).

The medical kit needs to be at the school or centre whenever your child is present. Some parents choose to bring the medical kit to and from the premises every day, while others leave a permanent medical kit at the school. If you leave a permanent medical kit on the premises, be sure you have noted the expiry dates of all medications. It is also a good idea to check the contents of the kit from time to time to make sure nothing has gone astray and look at the viewing window of the EpiPen to ensure the solution is clear in appearance (if it is cloudy or appears dark in colour, the EpiPen needs to be replaced immediately).

Remember, if your school has EpiPen trainers, they need to be clearly labelled as training pens and stored in a location separate from the medical kit, so there is no risk of confusion in an emergency.

Personalise information about your child's allergies

In addition to staff knowing about the signs and symptoms of an allergic reaction and when and how to treat it, staff also need to know how their anaphylaxis training relates to your child.

When Noah started childcare, as well as providing a copy of his Action Plan, I put together personalised information about Noah's allergies. I presented the information about Noah as a series of questions and answers about his food allergies. For example:

- What is Noah allergic to?
- Can Noah consume any of his allergens in any form?
- What kind of allergic reactions has Noah experienced in the past?
- What kind of allergic reaction is Noah at risk of having?
- How much does Noah understand about his food allergies?
- What kind of measures can help to keep Noah safe?
- What medications does Noah need to have on hand at all times?

The feedback I received from staff was that this was really helpful and practical information. While all staff had undergone formal training in managing anaphylaxis, personal information about Noah's allergies helped staff to relate their professional training to his needs. They posted a photocopy of this information on the noticeboard, and attached a photo of Noah to the document. This, in addition to discussions at staff meetings, led to most of the staff in the centre being very familiar with Noah's allergy story, including relief staff.

Teaching staff understand children inside out, and personalising information about your child can really help them to understand more about managing their allergies. For example, telling staff that if Noah needs to take antihistamine and is resisting, a reminder that 'it's the special itchy medicine' helps

continued

him to cooperate, because he likes the taste of that particular medicine! Letting staff know that Noah has had a reaction from sharing a harmonica with his sister after she had eaten yoghurt (hours before), lets them know that sharing musical instruments with other children can pose a risk.

While a face-to-face meeting with staff is always needed, following up with some reader-friendly personal information about your child's allergies can reinforce what you chatted about, and also help staff come up with practical ideas to keep your child safe in their care. Writing information down can also ensure you are transferring information in a positive manner.

Family day care

Family day care is formal home-based childcare that caters for infants through to pre-teens. 'Home-based' means the care takes place in the home of a qualified carer, and 'formal' means that it is approved by the Australian Government

Family day care can be a good option for a food-allergic child, with the number of children in care at any one time being four or five under school-age, plus two school-aged children (it varies according to state and territory regulations). Fewer children means less food coming through the door and, in some cases, the carer is willing to plan all meals in advance and provide safe meals that all children in their care can enjoy together, so there is no risk of social isolation.

A family day care carer is in control of their own service, and has direct contact with you, ensuring continuity of communication, and you have the peace of mind of knowing that your child will always be cared for by the same person. Dealing with one carer also means you have a great opportunity to develop a meaningful and possibly long-term relationship, avoiding the need to have to educate a new carer at the start of every year — or possibly even more frequently if there is staff turnover.

Of course, there are also challenges specific to the family day care environment that you will need to consider. For example, if your child is allergic to peanuts, you will need to find out if your carer keeps peanut butter and other peanut-containing products in the house. If so, how is the carer going to ensure your child is not exposed to these products, and are you comfortable with the safety measures they are going to put in place? With only one carer present, what is their emergency response plan if your child has anaphylaxis? (Who would care for the other children?) Are the parents of other children happy to agree to no nut products being consumed in the home during the hours of care? As always, clear communication between parents and the carer can usually resolve these challenges.

If you are considering family day care as an option for your child, approach the carer in the same way you would a childcare centre: in the spirit of cooperation. Be honest and direct about your child's allergies. Ask questions: you'll soon know if the carer is willing and able to cater for your child's particular needs. Useful questions include:

- Do you have anaphylaxis training? How recent was the training?
- Do you have training in meal preparation for children with food allergies (including the risks of cross-contamination in food preparation, storage and serving)?
- Do you have any experience in caring for a child at risk of anaphylaxis?
- Do you keep my child's allergen in your house?
- If so, what safety measures would you put in place to ensure my child would not be exposed?
- Discuss how you will work with your carer to develop a risk management plan to minimise the chance of your child being exposed to their allergen, as well as an emergency response plan in the event of anaphylaxis.

continued

Just as you would when considering any childcare option for your child, ask yourself if you and the carer will make a 'good fit': you need to form a successful partnership in caring for your child.

For more information about family day care, visit **www.familydaycare.com.au**

Farmyard visits

Q My 3-year-old girl is allergic to egg and peanut and has experienced anaphylaxis. She attends childcare, and the director of our centre has just called to advise that a 'mobile farmyard' is going to be visiting next month. Baby chicks are part of the farmyard, and our director wants to know if it will be safe for my daughter to attend. I'm really pleased she thought to call me, but I'm unsure of what to tell her. Is it safe for my daughter to join in?

A Visits by farmyard animals are usually really fun and educational for young children and, with the appropriate safety measures in place, your daughter can certainly enjoy the experience.

It will be safe for your child to attend and watch, but whether she actually handles the chicks will depend on how old they are. It will not be safe for your child to handle a chick that has just hatched, as there may be residual egg protein on the chick. If the chick is more than a day old and has been washed, it is usually safe for the child to handle the chick, although all children should wash their hands after handling the chicks or exploring the incubator.

If possible, volunteer to attend the farmyard visit. This way you can check with the farmyard staff how old the chicks are and whether or not they have been washed. For added safety, make sure your daughter doesn't put her hands in her mouth after handling the chicks.

Because your daughter is allergic to egg and peanut, you should also ask the centre director to check with farmyard staff *before the visit* what is contained in all of the animal feeds they use during a visit. Some pet foods and animal feeds do contain egg and nuts, and ideally these should not be brought into the centre. (If they are, you need to be made aware and your child should not handle the feed; other children who do handle the feed will need to wash their hands thoroughly.)

Banning foods: a good idea ... or not?

Many schools and pre-schools advertise that they are 'nut-free' or that certain foods have been 'banned'; however, in reality, there is no way to ensure an allergen is not coming into a childcare centre or pre-school: you have to assume that it is. When children bring in their own food from home, while teachers do their best to be on the alert for allergens, most items in lunchboxes are unlabelled, and it can be difficult for teachers to know if an allergen is present as an ingredient of something. Is the mayonnaise on a child's sandwich egg-free? Does a health bar coated in yoghurt contain nuts? If a parent brings in a birthday cake, they may have purchased the cake from a bakery and have no idea there is almond meal in the base.

The Australasian Society of Clinical Immunology and Allergy (ASCIA), support group Anaphylaxis Australia Inc. and many doctors, do not recommend the blanket banning of allergens in school environments. Reasons why some of the experts do not recommend bans include:

- The practical challenges of enforcing any ban
- If you ban one allergen, such as nuts, what do you do about other common allergens, such as cow's milk or soy?
- The risk of complacency: if people believe an environment is 'nut-free' they may not be as vigilant in preparing for an emergency situation
- As food-allergic children mature, they need to be able to develop their own ways of avoiding exposure to an allergen in the real world; if they are never exposed to it, how will they learn?

Instead of promoting a school or childcare centre as being 'free' of an allergen, experts recommend a 'risk minimisation' approach is adopted (which usually means taking steps to reduce an allergen coming into a centre or pre-school but always assuming that the allergen is still coming in), combined with strategies to promote allergy awareness within a school environment.

While all of this makes sense, many parents I interviewed for this book still felt more comfortable sending very young children to a childcare centre or pre-school where an allergen was 'banned' or had a 'nut-free' policy; they felt it made other parents of children at the centre take food allergies seriously. It is a widely debated topic in food-allergy circles.

Regardless of what approach your childcare centre or school takes, or what your own personal beliefs might be, accept that there is never any way to guarantee that an environment can ever be made 'allergen-free' — it's an impossible ask. Always ensure that staff caring for your child have been formally trained to recognise the symptoms of anaphylaxis and that they know how to administer an EpiPen and follow your child's Action Plan in an emergency.

Talking to your child about their food allergies

Depending on the age of your child, it's helpful to teach them some basic concepts about their food allergies to prepare them for childcare or pre-school, but keep it simple. For example, remind toddlers not to share food, teach them by example at home to wash hands before and after a meal, buy them a special waterbottle and have them use it at home before pre-school starts so they learn to recognise it as their own (it may pay to purchase two or three identical bottles in case one goes astray), and encourage them to tell a teacher if they feel unwell or itchy.

Keep in mind that while gradual education of children about their food allergies is essential, it's just as important not to over-emphasise their allergies or give them information overload at a very young age, otherwise they may become anxious or fearful. Beginning childcare or pre-school is a big step for any little person, and they will have a lot of changes to cope with. Focus on helping them to feel safe and secure in their new environment, and work with childcare or pre-school staff on gradual and age-appropriate allergy education of your child and their classmates.

Supporting staff in caring for your child

When a teacher is initially charged with caring for a child at risk of anaphylaxis it can be daunting. Think back to when your child was initially diagnosed and how much there was for you to learn in order to keep your child safe. Your child's teacher has the same responsibility, along with a classroom full of other children, some of whom also have special needs.

Teaching staff will be grateful if you can acknowledge this and work with them to keep your child safe. Some of the ways you might be able to support your child's teachers include:

- Communicate clearly about your child's allergies at an appropriate time (don't turn up on the first day of care or school and announce your child has a food allergy).
- Be organised. Ensure you have supplied a full medical kit, labelled medications (checking expiry dates) and a current Action Plan prior to your child commencing.
- Tell the truth about your child's allergies: don't exaggerate or downplay your child's condition.
- If possible, make sure both parents are involved in communicating with the school about a child's allergies, so if the main carer does not answer their phone when a teacher has a question, the other parent or another nominated contact person also has a relationship with the teacher.
- If for some reason you are not going to be available by phone on a particular day, then make sure you tell staff who to contact in the event of an emergency so they don't have to try several numbers before someone picks up their phone.
- Consider ordering some form of medical identification bracelet or tag, to serve as a visual reminder for staff, and help casual staff identify your child at school.
- Become an active member of the school community, so you can build a relationship with staff members and give back to the community that supports your child and family. Remember, you have a role to play in a community environment as a regular parent, not just an allergy educator.

- Make practical suggestions to help the childcare centre or pre-school: for example, offer to provide your own safe snack options for your child, rather than have their cook always take that responsibility; offer to talk about food allergy at a staff meeting and demonstrate how to use an EpiPen.
- If you can afford to, offer to donate resources to the school, for example, an extra EpiPen trainer, an educational DVD, an age-appropriate storybook.
- Acknowledge when staff are doing a really great job. Let them know how happy your child is in their care, how much you appreciate their diligence or how pleased you are that they have come up with a new way of keeping your child safe. Give them feedback.
- If there is something you are not happy about, communicate directly and politely. Threatening or yelling at staff is never acceptable — or helpful.

Difficulties in working with a centre or pre-school

If you find that the childcare centre or pre-school you are dealing with is uncooperative or unsupportive, you should, ideally, consider alternative options. But that's easy advice to give out on paper: it's often just not possible.

When I was trying to find childcare options for my own son, I read a lot of advice about 'shopping around' for a centre that suits the needs of your child. I placed our son's name on 10 waiting lists the week after he was born and when the time came for me to return to work a year later, I had no offers at all! In theory, shopping around for suitable childcare or pre-school options is a great idea and exactly what parents want to do, but in practice, many parents simply do not have much choice at all. City parents often face extremely long waiting lists while some rural parents have few options (if any).

If you are in a situation where you have limited childcare or pre-school options available and you find that staff at the childcare centre or pre-school where you need to send your child are not being cooperative, or are not taking your child's food allergies seriously, consider asking your doctor to provide you with a letter outlining the seriousness of your child's allergies, especially if you have a request that is out of the ordinary for your particular centre or pre-school.

Joining education and support group Anaphylaxis Australia Inc. can also help. If you are having difficulties, a call or email from Anaphylaxis Australia Inc. to the centre or pre-school involved can enable teaching staff to access really helpful information and resources to start working with you.

It is also worth taking a step back and reviewing the approach you took with your child's centre or pre-school. Food allergy can evoke great anxiety in parents and affect the way we communicate with others. Did you plan in advance what you were going to say to your centre or pre-school or did you unload a huge amount of information and a long list of requests? Did you approach the conversation in a positive manner? Were all of your requests reasonable? Perhaps the staff you were communicating with responded negatively simply because they felt overwhelmed by how much information you were asking them to absorb at a time of year when they have a huge queue of parents wanting to talk to them about their child's special needs, too?

Sometimes, of course, this is not the case at all, and you do need to consider involving a third party such as your doctor or Anaphylaxis Australia Inc. But do keep in mind that a gentle and positive approach with staff is often the most effective. For example, consider pointing your child's carers in the direction of sources of information — such as the anaphylaxis guidelines for your state — rather than bombarding them with demands and expecting everything to be done your way. Ask yourself if it is worth scheduling another appointment and taking a different approach.

Childcare centres and schools are expected to provide a safe environment for all children and cater for individual needs, but in the real world this doesn't always happen. If, despite your best efforts, your relationship with a childcare centre or pre-school just isn't working out, then you might have to walk away. It might not be fair, but you can't leave your child in a centre or pre-school where they will not be in safe hands. Fortunately, this situation is becoming increasingly uncommon, thanks to the ever-growing awareness about food allergies and the adoption of anaphylaxis guidelines by many childcare centres and pre-schools.

Ongoing communication

Like any successful relationship, ongoing communication with your child's teaching staff is essential to keep things on track. While the beginning of every new school year is the perfect time to re-assess safety measures and update Action Plans, it's not a case of running through a checklist in January and thinking your job is done. The association you have with your child's childcare centre or pre-school is an evolving relationship, and you need to communicate with staff as new issues arise.

Keep staff up to date with any changes in your child's allergies or medications. For example, in our case, Noah's antihistamine dosage is based on weight and once or twice we have needed to advise the pre-school that the correct dosage — in the event that he has an allergic reaction — had increased. We let teachers know whenever Noah is going for his allergy test and what the results are. This is also of practical importance because following a skin prick test, hives seem to linger on Noah's back for a couple of days, and we want them to know why they are there, in case they think he is having an allergic reaction when they see him scratching.

If your child has outgrown an allergy, it is really important to tell staff. They go to great lengths to avoid an allergen coming into contact with your child, and if they no longer need to avoid a certain food in their classroom, they will want to join in your celebrations!

If your child suffers a severe allergic reaction at home or somewhere else, let the staff know. If your child has recently been diagnosed with a new food allergen or another medical problem — asthma, for example — staff need to know this, too.

Whenever you are communicating with teachers about your child's food allergies, try to avoid doing so in front of your child. Telephone staff or arrange to meet with staff without your child. Children need to learn about food allergies, certainly, but their exposure to it needs to be gradual. Yes, it is our role as parents to keep our children safe, but it is also our job to help them enjoy their childhood without feeling overly anxious or fearful.

Also remember to maintain an interest in all areas of your child's education, not just food allergies. Try not to let food allergies define your relationship with staff at your centre or pre-school.

12

The school years

It seems you have just mastered the art of managing food allergies in the pre-school environment and then it's time for the next leap: school. On the positive side, your child's level of understanding and education about their allergies will have improved, and they may have even outgrown some of their allergies. On the more challenging side, your child is now moving to a new and exciting world where class sizes will be larger, meal times are not as closely supervised, and children are often involved in a wide range of activities. Likewise, when your child jumps from primary school to high school, the challenges change again: into the mix come (usually) larger campuses, multiple teachers, peer pressure and a range of issues that accompany the teen years.

The recurring theme in managing food allergy in a school environment, regardless of the age of your child or their allergy, is to plan ahead, be prepared and communicate clearly. Parents need to develop a positive and successful relationship with staff at their child's school, and support them in caring for their child.

In this chapter we will look at different ideas in considering the right school for your child, how to prepare you and your child for their first day of school, and strategies for minimising the risk of an allergic reaction at school. We also look at ways of managing food allergy in school celebrations, at the canteen, during excursions and on camps. Importantly, bullying is also discussed, as well as ways to encourage your child to become increasingly responsible for managing their allergies. A list of resource materials available to help staff and school communities become 'allergy-aware' is listed at the end of the chapter.

A special note: this chapter has been written to help parents work together with their child's school in managing food allergy. Keep in mind that there is a wide range of factors to consider in how a school deals with the risk of anaphylaxis. What works for one family and their child's school may not work as well for another. Some of the strategies you implement in the early years of school may no longer be appropriate as your child becomes increasingly independent. Work closely with your school to establish an individualised management plan for your child that will keep them safe — and included.

We are grateful to Jane Danvers, Principal of the Wilderness School, South Australia; Karen King, Assistant Principal of Clifton Hill Primary School, Victoria; and Eric Patatoukos, Principal of Bradfordville Primary School, New South Wales, for their help with research for this chapter.

Finding the right fit for your child

For some parents, the management of food allergy is their primary concern in selecting a school for their child, while others simply choose a school based on whether it's a good fit for their child in general, and commit to working with the school to manage food allergy.

For any school, managing food allergy involves two main levels of responsibility: the first is to put allergen-minimisation strategies and education in place to reduce the chance of an allergic reaction taking place, and the second is to ensure staff and students are equipped to respond in the event of an allergic reaction, including anaphylaxis. Parents of food-allergic children must communicate clearly with staff to establish what strategies will be put in place to ensure these responsibilities can be met.

Whether you are considering a school for your child or have already chosen one, you will need to make an appointment with the principal, school nurse and whoever is responsible for managing food allergy at the school. Many parents have reported that taking a 'two-step' approach to communicating their child's food allergies to a school has been successful. This involves scheduling an initial meeting with the principal (and relevant staff members) to discuss your child's food allergies in general terms, followed by another meeting a couple of weeks later, where more specific details are discussed and agreed upon. When you are in planning mode, consider what you would like to say in your initial meeting and make a list of other points you might leave until your follow-up meeting. (See 'Approaching the principal', pages 241–242.) The better you prepare, the more likely you are to feel relaxed about each conversation. Consequently, you may find it easier to talk about managing your child's allergies in a positive manner, rather than coming across as anxious or demanding, which can happen, often unintentionally.

Below are some suggestions to help you prepare to meet with representatives from your school, but it is also a good idea to find out what safety measures your school already has in place. Turning up to a meeting with a list of specific requests for your child — especially if they involve placing restrictions on other children — probably won't go down well. Many schools have experience in managing food allergy and already comply with state- or territory-based guidelines.

When you do meet with staff, remember to approach any conversations about food allergy with an encouraging attitude and in the spirit of cooperation. While a school should always be willing to listen to your concerns, you also need to be willing to listen to theirs. Successful partnerships are always two-way.

- Does the school have an anaphylaxis policy? (If it doesn't, state- and territory-based guidelines are available. See 'Guidelines for managing anaphylaxis in childcare centres and schools', page 217, for more information.)
- Ask if the school has an orientation day or open day, when you can take a tour of the school and meet with staff. Taking a tour helps you to understand the size of the school, find out where the children play and eat, ask about staff to student ratios, enquire if there is a school nurse on staff and get a general feel for how willing staff are to engage with you about the needs of your child.
- Most schools will require you to fill in paperwork about your child's allergies and medications; ask if you can receive these forms before the meeting, so you can discuss any questions that might arise after reviewing the forms.
- Establish what experience the school has in managing food allergy. While a school with extensive experience in managing food allergy can be a great option, don't discount a school that doesn't have as

much experience if they have a positive attitude and are willing to listen, learn and work with your family.

- How many staff have been trained in managing anaphylaxis and administering an EpiPen?
- In addition to initial or annual anaphylaxis training, does the school conduct ongoing training and education with staff throughout the year? For example, do they run practice sessions with the EpiPen trainer at staff meetings?
- How does the school communicate about allergies to casual staff?
- Give staff the opportunity to ask you any questions about your child's allergies.
- Ask the school questions about issues other than food allergy. You are looking for a school where your child will be safe *and* happy.

Approaching the principal

When you are communicating about your child's food allergies to a school for the first time, it can feel as though there is a lot of territory to cover — and there is, but you don't have to communicate everything in one meeting. It is often more effective to schedule an initial meeting with your child's school principal where you have a general discussion about your child's food allergies and how the school currently manages food allergies. As appropriate, you might point the principal in the direction of reading materials, so they can do their own further research, or give them some examples of how other schools are managing food allergies. Then schedule a follow-up meeting for a couple of weeks later, when the principal has had time to do some research and consider how the school can manage your child's allergies. You can then have a more detailed discussion. Even if your child's school is already experienced in managing food allergy, ensure the principal understands your child's needs. For example, a school might be experienced in caring for a child with egg allergy, but perhaps that child can eat egg in baked

continued

goods and your child can't. Be sure that the school understands the needs of *your* child.

'It is a matter of reassuring parents and involving them in the discussion about what their child's management plan looks like. Communication is key to a successful relationship. You need to be very transparent in how you intend to deal with their child's food allergies, be prepared to listen to their concerns, and ensure that you then act.'

—Mrs Jane Danvers, Principal, Wilderness School (SA)

Before your child starts school

The list below is provided to help you prepare for your child's first day at school, but is by no means exhaustive. Work closely with your school to establish an individualised management plan suitable for your child.

- If your school has an anaphylaxis policy, ensure you read it. In addition to outlining the responsibilities of the school, many policies also outline the responsibilities of parents and students. If you have any questions or concerns about your school's policy, raise them with staff well in advance of your child's first day at school.
- Check in with your GP or allergy specialist and ensure you have an up-to-date Action Plan signed by your doctor, as well as all the necessary medications and appropriate dosages. (Also see 'The all-important medical kit', page 225.)
- The photograph of your child featured on the Action Plan needs to be recent; if your child wears a school uniform, take a photo of your child dressed in their uniform.
- After you have met with the school principal, schedule a time to meet with your child's teacher and other relevant staff

members (for example, the school nurse, if your school has one; if your child is going to attend before- or after-school care, ensure you can meet with these staff members, too). Make the appointment well in advance of when school starts, ideally on a pupil-free day, when staff members can speak to you without teaching commitments. Try to attend the appointment with your partner or another family member — you may feel more relaxed with support on hand.

- Prepare in advance so you can approach the meeting calmly and with confidence. Write down a list of questions and make sure you bring with you any necessary documentation to share with teachers, so they have the opportunity to read it before the first day of school, including: your child's Action Plan; a letter from your doctor outlining prescribed medications and any special requirements (if needed); and any personal information about your child's allergies you may have prepared. (See 'Personalise information about your child's allergies', pages 227–228.)

- Outline your child's allergens and be specific about what they can and cannot eat (for example, some children are allergic to egg but can safely eat it in baked goods).

- Check who will be responsible for your child in the event an allergic reaction occurs at school. What happens if that staff member is away or on a break? What happens if a reaction occurs in the playground? An emergency response plan must be in place and all staff need to be aware of it: an allergic reaction can happen anywhere.

- Agree upon where your child's Action Plan will be displayed and where their medical kit will be stored, and who will be responsible for carrying the medical kit when your child is off campus or a long way from where the medical kit is stored. (See more on page 225, 'The all important medical kit' on how a medical kit should be stored.)

continued

- For older children who might be carrying their own medical kit, has this practice already been put in place at home? Will your child need any support or reminders from staff in taking on this responsibility? Does there need to be a backup medical kit stored elsewhere in the school?
- Find out what strategies the school already has in place to reduce the risk of an allergic reaction and then discuss if any additional measures need to be incorporated for your child's situation. (Also see 'Minimising the risk of allergic reactions at school', pages 245–247.)
- If your child is going to use the school canteen, ask if you can schedule a time to meet with the canteen manager (see 'Canteen', page 253).
- Ask if there are any ways in which you can support staff in caring for your child. For example, would they like you to speak at a staff meeting? Would they like you to demonstrate how to use an EpiPen?
- You might like to reinforce the message to your child's teacher that if they are ever in doubt about using your child's EpiPen, not to hesitate.
- Remember to thank your teacher for their support, and let them know you are happy to be called at any time if they have questions, concerns or ideas they would like to discuss.

On the day your child starts school

- Ensure your child's medical kit is stored in a location that is easily accessible, unlocked and away from direct sunlight or sources of heat.
- Check that your child's Action Plan is located in a prominent position. If it is affixed to a wall, ensure it is secure — for example, use thumbtacks, not blu-tack or sticky tape (I once found my son's Action Plan behind a bookshelf — blu-tack does not hold on a hot day). An older child may not be comfortable with their Action Plan being on

display for all their peers to see. The location of a child's Action Plan needs to be easily accessible but also take into consideration the age of your child.

- If your child is carrying their own medical kit to and from school, check they have it packed in their bag.
- Pack your child's meals and snacks in a clearly labelled lunchbox. Pack plenty to eat so they aren't tempted to take food from others if they are still hungry.
- Pack your child's own clearly labelled drink bottle.
- For their first day of school for the year remember to focus on your child's other needs, too. Help your child to feel confident and happy about school.
- Make sure you are always contactable by phone, in case staff have any questions.
- Even though you may be feeling anxious about leaving your child at school, try to put on a happy face for your child. If they see you are anxious, they may also become anxious.

> *'I go in to meet the teacher, without Kate, before the first day of school. I take an expired EpiPen and an orange and I demonstrate how to use it. I give them an Action Plan — and the school nurse has a copy, too — and I make sure they are aware of what to do in the event of anaphylaxis. I try to educate the teacher as much as possible that if you are ever in doubt, just use the EpiPen. It is not going to harm her. They are really good with it.'*
>
> —Jodie Bellchambers (WA), mother of Kate (9), allergic to peanut (and previously egg)

Minimising the risk of allergic reactions at school

A school cannot guarantee that your child will never be exposed to their allergen, but there are many strategies that can be put in place to help minimise the risk. Different systems work for different schools, depending on the children involved, their allergies, their age, the size of the school, the layout of the school campus and other factors. Always discuss your child's specific allergies with staff to come up with practical safety measures appropriate for your situation. Below is a list of ideas that will hopefully provide a starting point for you and your school to work together.

- A system needs to be in place to ensure all staff can easily identify a child at risk of anaphylaxis. For example, photos of the child might be posted in key locations such as the staffroom, a child's home classroom and the canteen. Medical identification jewellery is also a good idea (see page 62 for more information).
- Children with food allergy need to be encouraged not to share food with their friends.
- Other children need to be encouraged and reminded not to share their food with a food-allergic child.
- Encourage hand washing before and after eating, especially in young children.
- A formal communication process needs to be in place to ensure casual and relief teaching staff are immediately made aware of children with food allergies.
- The wider school community should be educated about food allergy and the risk of anaphylaxis. A letter might be sent home to parents at the beginning of the year, with reminders prior to special events such as school excursions or class parties. Positive articles might be published in the school newsletter from time to time. The school might participate in Food Allergy Awareness Week or adopt the 'Be a M.A.T.E.' education program. (See page 255 for more information.)
- The school might ask parents of other children not to send certain products to school, for example, peanuts. (Also see 'Banning foods: a good idea … or not?', pages 231–232.)
- Staff members should be made aware that not all allergic reactions to food happen at meal times. Allergens can also be present in a range of activities, including: cooking, craft, science experiments and music activities. For example, egg-allergic children should not be handling egg cartons, and playdough contains wheat. Sharing mouth or wind musical instruments can also be an issue.

- 'Food rewards' in the classroom might be replaced with 'non-food rewards', when possible.
- Visitors to the school need to be aware of food allergy, for example, parents or relatives volunteering, music teachers.
- Children with food allergy should not be placed on 'rubbish duty', where they might be exposed to their allergen in food containers and wrappers.
- If any of the school's facilities are used for other purposes outside of school hours (for example, before- and after-school care, committee meetings, rehearsals for a school play), the same allergen-minimisation strategies that are in place during school hours need to be followed.

Celebrations at school

Food is an important part of most celebrations in life and many special occasions are celebrated during school hours. When a child has food allergies, they cannot always eat the same foods as their classmates, but they can still participate and enjoy the party. Below are some ideas to consider to keep your child safe and included.

- Ask your child's teacher to give you notice if there is a class party, birthday or other special celebration planned so you can check if the foods on offer will be safe for your child.
- If the foods will not be safe, then staff need to ensure your child does not share food at the celebration, and you can pack some special safe foods for your child to enjoy.
- If other children will be bringing in food from home on the day of the celebration, depending on the allergen and the age of the children involved, a letter might be sent home to parents reminding them not to send certain products to school (for example, no peanut butter or nut products), as part of the school's allergen-minimisation strategy.
- If it is your child's birthday, you might like to offer to provide all the food for the celebration, so your child can enjoy sharing food with their friends on their special day.
- As birthday celebrations are common, you might like to supply safe cakes for your child (in a clearly labelled sealed container) which can be kept in a freezer at school, ready to pull out at short notice as needed.

- Some teachers are happy to keep a safe 'treat box' (clearly labelled) in the classroom for food-allergic children.
- Check in with your child's teacher in advance of annual celebrations such as Easter and Christmas so you can come up with ways for your child to be kept safe and included in these celebrations.
- In the younger years, some parents choose to volunteer to help out at school during special occasions involving food.
- Parents of food-allergic children can feel worried that their child is missing out on eating the same foods as their classmates, but often the child is nowhere near as troubled by this as a parent — as long as they have a worthy substitute available.

Excursions

There is no reason for food-allergic children not to be included in school excursions; they are an important learning experience and integral to the school's curriculum. An excursion can mean a quick visit to a nearby location, a day trip or overnight stays. Planning and clear communication are essential to keep your child safe and enable them to get on with enjoying the experience with their friends. Below are some of the issues you might like to discuss with staff at your school in preparing for an excursion. (School camps require some additional preparation, and are discussed in detail on pages 250–253.)

- Ask your child's teacher to give you advance notice of any planned excursions.
- Consider the location. For example, if your child's class is visiting a food manufacturing plant, you might want to call the manufacturing plant, ask them what foods they produce and discuss the environment in light of your child's allergies. If your school group is visiting a dairy farm and your child is allergic to milk, it may or may not be a problem, but you will need time to make some calls and seek information in advance.
- If your child is still young, teachers appreciate parents volunteering to accompany their child and classmates on the excursion, if possible.

- Will staff be carrying mobile phones? Check there will be mobile phone reception at the excursion location.
- Work with staff to prepare an individual emergency response plan in the event of anaphylaxis. The plan must include which staff members will be involved in the event of anayphylaxis, and who will be responsible for carrying and administering the EpiPen in an emergency.
- The emergency response plan should include the exact location of sites being visited, and how to call an ambulance.
- Remind staff that your child's medical kit must not be left in direct sunlight or near any direct sources of heat.
- Are there any other parents or non-teaching staff volunteering to assist supervising children on the excursion? If so, have they been made aware about your child's allergies and the emergency response plan?
- Your child should be under the direct supervision of their usual teacher, not a parent volunteer or another staff member who does not have anaphylaxis training.
- Does the excursion involve any celebrations, sampling of food or games involving food? If so, check if the foods on offer will be safe for your child and, if not, supply safe alternatives.
- If possible, eating on transport should be avoided, especially with young children. Lunch and other meal breaks could be scheduled to take place in a specific location rather than allowing children to eat together on a bus or train.
- Pack plenty of safe food for your child so they won't be tempted to take food from others if they are still hungry.
- The school could remind parents of younger children not to pack specific allergens for their child: for example, no nut-containing products.
- If the excursion involves an overnight stay or meals being provided by others, refer to the tips given on page 250 under 'Camps'.

Camps

Parents of children with food allergy often feel uneasy about school camps. They commonly involve a combination of factors that increase the overall level of risk to your child, including: someone unfamiliar preparing foods; activities being supervised by staff members who don't usually teach your child; a location geographically isolated from a hospital; and participation by your child in activities where they are not under immediate supervision of a teacher, for example, orienteering.

There are definitely risks, but that doesn't mean they can't be managed or that your child has to miss out. Firstly, visit your child's doctor and let them know your child will soon be going on a camp. Specify the location of the camp and how long your child will be away and discuss the provision of adequate quantities of medications, for example, EpiPens. Also be sure you have an up-to-date signed Action Plan. Secondly, meet with your child's teacher well in advance of the camp to ensure safety measures can be put in place. Some of the issues you might like to discuss with your teacher include:

- What is the emergency response plan if a severe allergic reaction takes place on camp?
- Has it been confirmed that there is reliable mobile phone coverage at the camp site? If not, the school will need to consider another communication device, for example, an emergency satellite beacon,[1] satellite phone or walkie-talkie. (Staff may also need training in how to use unfamiliar communication devices.) No matter where your child is on camp, there must be some means by which staff can call for help in an emergency.
- The emergency response plan should include the exact location of the camp site and the number to call for an ambulance (staff may need to know you can call '112' from mobile phones where the service is out of range).
- Some emergency call operators accept GPS (Global Positioning System) positions, but you will have to check with the emergency services authority in your state or territory. If a GPS system is taken on camp, it should be seen as an additional safety measure and not as

a replacement of all other safety measures that need to be in place.

- Will staff carry on them at all times an emergency telephone card, including the name and age of the child at risk, their photograph, allergies, and instructions on how to call an ambulance?
- Which staff members attending the camp have been trained in anaphylaxis management and treatment? How recent was their training?
- Who will be responsible for administering the EpiPen in the event of anaphylaxis?
- Where will your child's Action Plan be displayed?
- Who will be responsible for carrying and storing your child's medications?
- Ensure staff understand that your child's medication needs to be easily accessible at all times and also stored away from direct sources of heat. It must not be left sitting inside a hot school bus or on a window sill in a kitchen that might be flooded by direct sunlight during the day.
- It is advisable to pack a second EpiPen for school camps; let staff know how many EpiPens you are providing for the camp.
- Parents should check the expiry date and condition of all medications before packing them for camp.
- Are there any parents or other non-staff members volunteering for the camp? If so, have they been made aware of your child's food allergies and have they been briefed on the emergency response plan?
- Can staff have an education revision session before leaving for camp, including practice with the EpiPen trainer? (Educational DVDs are also available from Anaphylaxis Australia.)
- Parents might like to call the ambulance station nearest to the camp site, explain that a child at risk of anaphylaxis will be camping in the area on a certain date, and check how long it would take an ambulance to reach the camp site.
- If teens are involved in activities such as bushwalking or orienteering, they should carry their medical kit with them at all times, and their friends should also be educated about what to do in an emergency.
- How are other children and their families going to be made aware that food allergies need to be considered on camp? For example, the

school may need to send home a note requesting that children not bring along snacks containing peanuts or tree nuts.

- What kind of activities will be taking place on camp? Do any involve food games? Cooking? Craft? All staff need to understand that exposure to an allergen can take place outside of meal times.
- Discuss with staff whether you need to send along all or some of your child's food or whether you can speak directly with the caterers to see if they can provide safe meals for your child.
- When you speak to caterers, ensure you are speaking with the staff member who will be in charge of food preparation while your child is at the camp. Send them a copy of your child's Action Plan or some form of documentation that clearly outlines the foods to which your child is allergic, to confirm your phone conversation.
- If you are packing meals for your child to take, discuss with staff how the meals will be stored and prepared. Make sure staff understand the risk of cross-contamination in storing, cooking and serving food.
- If your child is eating food supplied at the camp, encourage your child — in addition to teachers — to check their meal is safe before eating it.
- At the beginning of every school year, you might like to ask staff to let you know if any camps have been planned. If you intend to volunteer (which schools often appreciate, especially with younger children), knowing dates and locations in advance can help you plan ahead.

> *'If you are worried about anything on a school camp, don't be afraid to speak out. Ring up and speak to the caterers, speak to the teachers. Constantly make sure that people know. Don't let yourself go home thinking, "I wish I had told a particular person about their allergy." Always make sure that you keep people informed.'*
>
> —Jill Ahmed (SA), mother of Shana (15), allergic to peanut and tree nuts, and Alisa (13), allergic to peanut, tree nuts, honey and kiwi fruit

'We will sit down with the parent before camp and check that their child's Action Plan is in date, because information does change and a parent may have forgotten to tell us something; for example, their mobile phone number might have changed. It happens. Before the camp, we do a comprehensive risk assessment — physical risks, medical risks — and every staff member going on the camp is involved in the discussion. So we might, say, have three children with EpiPens: where are we going to store the EpiPens; who is going to be responsible for taking the EpiPens if we go for a walk on the beach; what is the plan if a reaction happens? We have very detailed conversations.'

—Karen King, Assistant Principal,
Clifton Hill Primary School (Vic)

Canteen

Children enjoy being able to buy food from the school canteen with their friends, and many schools work closely with families of food-allergic children to ensure safe options are available. Using the canteen also encourages children with food allergy to take increasing responsibility (while supervised) for choosing safe foods.

Meet with your school's canteen manager and discuss your child's allergies and how the risk of an allergic reaction from canteen products can be minimised. Ideally, the canteen manager will be the only staff member who serves your child (and will be responsible for checking the label every time your child purchases something). As your child matures, they can take on the responsibility of reading and checking food labels. The strategies put in place at your school will vary, depending on the age of your child, their allergies, the products available at your school's canteen and the level of education and training your canteen manager has. Following are some ideas you might like to consider when you are preparing to meet with your school's canteen manager.

- Take a copy of your child's Action Plan to give to the canteen manager. It is important to provide a written list of your child's allergens, and the Action Plan also serves as a great visual reminder for all canteen staff that they need to be aware of your child's food allergies. Staff will also learn how to recognise your child if they have a photo on hand.

- Ask what allergen-minimisation strategies your canteen already has in place. It is much easier to work out if any additional measures are needed for your child when you know what measures are already in place. For example, some canteens use a different-coloured lunch bag for children with food allergies, and these lunches are prepared before all other orders and only by the canteen manager.

- Ask if the canteen manager and any other canteen staff have taken part in food allergy and anaphylaxis training.

- Discuss the risk of cross-contamination during preparation, storage and serving of food. Benches need to be cleaned prior to food preparation, and clean or separate bread boards and utensils need to be used during food preparation. Ask if all staff in the canteen, including volunteers, have been educated about the risk of cross-contamination.

- Review the menu and product options on offer and identify some products that will be safe for your child to buy. Once you have done so, remind staff that food labels still need to be checked every time your child purchases the product, as ingredients can and do change.

- If your child has multiple food allergies and there are very few products available for your child, discuss with the canteen manager the possibility of sourcing some new menu items that are safe for your child.

- Consider introducing younger children to the canteen gradually. For instance, you might pack their lunch but they can buy a safely packaged drink, for example, a juice, or labelled treat.

- Discuss with your canteen manager if they are happy for you to donate education resources about food allergy and school canteens. (See 'Education resources', page 264.)

Be a M.A.T.E. program for schools

Many schools are now taking on the responsibility of creating an allergy-aware community, with teachers educating all children, staff and families about the seriousness of food allergy and its management. Educating the school community often involves sending a letter home to families and including awareness articles and positive reminders in newsletters. It can also include education in the classroom.

Anaphylaxis Australia runs a positive education program called 'Be a M.A.T.E.' (**M**ake **A**llergy **T**reatment **E**asier). The program is aimed at school-aged children and is designed to get them educated and involved in keeping their food-allergic friends safe.

It is hoped that if schools can '**M**ake **A**llergy **T**reatment **E**asier' during the early years of education, then by the time these children reach their teens, they will take fewer risks and feel more at ease about allergies by:

- Letting others know they have a serious food allergy
- Always reading food labels and making enquiries about foods before they eat
- Always carrying their emergency medication
- Letting others know if they suddenly feel unwell, especially after eating

Friends of children with food allergy can also be nominated for 'Be a M.A.T.E.' awards as part of the program, in recognition of special efforts made to keep their food-allergic mate safe.

For more information on the 'Be a M.A.T.E. program' or to order a resource kit for your school (containing posters and a discussion guide to help teachers with ideas for lesson plans) visit **www.allergyfacts.org.au**

Bullying

Bullying exists in varying degrees: at one end of the spectrum might be a one-off event of a child being teased; at the other end, it can involve a child feeling constantly unsafe or being physically threatened. How the child, parents and school handle bullying often depends on the nature of the bullying itself.

Bullying is a very complex issue and, regrettably, something many young people experience during school — it is not something that necessarily goes hand-in-hand with food allergy. Children will often pick on any point of difference in another child. In some cases, a particular child may be vulnerable to bullying and their allergy is the very thing the bully has singled out, because they know that child is already self-conscious about it. It's almost like a sixth sense with some children; they know exactly which buttons to push.

According to psychologist Olivia Keene, Clinic Director of Keene Insight Child and Adolescent Specialists, it's essential for parents to be willing to see the 'big picture', in order for them to be able to help their child.

'Children are bullied for all sorts of reasons; for example, for being too tall, too young, too fat, too thin, or even over scores on a test. It's important for parents to try to get a picture of exactly what is going on in a situation, rather than immediately linking bullying or teasing to a child's food allergy. They need to question how much of what is going on is based on the child's allergy itself, and to what extent is it a result of a child possibly having too much focus on their allergy, so that the child has become so self-conscious they are unwittingly drawing a lot of attention to it.

'Whatever the case, the child's social skills need to be encouraged through building self-esteem and resilience, because the more focus the child can take off the allergy and put onto their social skills, the better they will cope.'

In some cases, bullying occurs because there may be systemic issues going on with the culture of the school or your child's peer group, where food allergies are not being well handled. A school has an important role to play in 'normalising' allergies and educating others about keeping their food-allergic friends safe (see more information on the 'Be a M.A.T.E. program', page 255) while also maintaining a culture of inclusion — ensuring children with food allergies are not isolated during regular school activities.

A community approach to food allergy in a school can make a positive difference for food-allergic children. Some parents interviewed for this book reported that when their child's class was given a lesson focused on food allergy (not in relation to their child, just on food allergy in general), the class became very effective in monitoring the behaviour of their peers. While there will always be bullies, it's also lovely to remember that children can also be very protective of one another.

Most children don't really *like* bullies, and if your child's school encourages positive education around food allergies, as well as clear expectations in regard to bullying and unacceptable behaviour, then this will hopefully create an environment where students might want to come to the aid of a friend who is being bullied, or at least not join in by laughing, or cheering on the bully.

Unfortunately, there have been reported cases of food-allergic children being threatened with their allergen; for example, a child waving a peanut butter sandwich in the face of a peanut-allergic child. (Some of the parents interviewed for this book confirmed that their children had been subjected to this kind of bullying.)

Any form of bullying that involves a physical threat to your child needs to be dealt with immediately. In the case of your child being exposed to their allergen, it is a potentially life-threatening situation: the child needs to tell an adult, and parents need to contact the school directly. A child should not be expected to take responsibility for dealing with the bully in these circumstances.

However, when bullying is occurring at the lower end of the spectrum (for example, teasing), Olivia Keene says that
continued

a child needs to be empowered to deal with their bully.

'The reality is that a parent cannot be beside their child in the playground the whole time, and that's not going to develop resilience or the child's ability to deal with the situation.

'Kids need to have a few standard responses up their sleeves. It is important to encourage children to, as much as they can, not take bullying too personally — the bullies are relying upon getting a particular response; they rely upon the other children being "hurt" by their words or actions.'

As parents, we can tend to want to rush in and fix everything for our children, but often this doesn't help — in fact, it can magnify the issue and further ostracise your child from his or her peers. Olivia Keene says this can also create or perpetuate a victim mentality at a time when we need to be encouraging children to become increasingly responsible and confident to handle themselves in the world as young adults.

'Challenge your child to focus upon what is in their control (for example, their own behaviour and response), rather than other factors that are not in their control (for example, the behaviour of the bully, school or other families). An over-focus upon factors outside the child's control will often lead to a level of "learned helplessness" or a "victim" mentality — this acts to kick-start, and then maintain, the bullying cycle.'

If your child comes to you for advice about handling a bully (again emphasising that we are talking about teasing as opposed to physical threats), listen to their concerns and resist the urge to step in and take control. Instead, encourage your child to come up with solutions to deal with the situation. While there are numerous websites and brochures that list practical suggestions for dealing with bullies (two of which are mentioned below) and they are really useful resources, children shouldn't be expected to follow a prescriptive list. Different strategies will work for different children in different situations, and it is essential that children are involved in decision-making around how they handle a bully.

'A child needs to feel comfortable — as much as possible — with how they are going to handle a bully,' says Olivia Keene. 'If they are involved in coming up with solutions that feel right for them, they will be more confident in handling the situation.

'Whatever approach they do take, the message they need to give the bully is "I'm okay, regardless of you."'

Keep the lines of communication with your child open and encourage them to continue talking to you about the bullying. Also let your child know that if the bullying is escalating and they feel unsafe or they can no longer cope with the situation, they need to tell an adult at school immediately.

More information — for parents, teachers and children — on specific strategies for dealing with bullying is available at: **www.friendlyschools.com.au** and **www.bullyingnoway.com.au**

'Thomas copes very well with his allergies but lately, as he's becoming more aware, he does get a bit down. Now that he is in a school environment he says things like, "Wish I was like the girls [his sisters]" or "Why can't I be normal?" I tell him he is really special and that we love him, and anyone who holds your allergy against you is not worth having as a friend.'

—Claire Bent (Tas), mother of Thomas (8),
allergic to egg, peanut, tree nuts and sesame

'In my experience in a classroom where there was a child with severe allergies, the other children were actually really very caring. They were always asking their friend if he was sure he could eat a certain food, before he ate it.'

—Karen King, Assistant Principal,
Clifton Hill Primary School (Vic)

Your child's responsibilities: an evolving process

Encouraging your child to become increasingly responsible for managing their food allergy is an essential and evolving process. From a very young age children can be taught simple concepts to keep them safe, for example, not to share food, and what their allergens look like. This learning process can be gradually built upon as the child matures, preparing a child to take ownership of their allergies in their teenage years. When you are educating your child about their allergies, remember to emphasise that they can enjoy a normal life, as long as they have safeguards in place. Avoid trying to 'scare' your child into taking responsibility for their allergies. (If you are struggling with your teenager taking allergies seriously, read Chapter 13, The teenage years, page 265, for more information.)

Following is a list of ideas to help you think about some of the responsibilities your child may be ready to take on.

- Understanding the importance of not sharing food and drinks.
- Learning how to recognise their allergen as well as knowing about which foods are likely to contain their allergen as an ingredient.
- Learning how to read and interpret food labels.
- Recognising the symptoms of an allergic reaction.
- Telling a teacher if they think they are having an allergic reaction.
- Understanding that they should never go to a bathroom or any other location on their own if they think they are having an allergic reaction.
- If they are experiencing an allergic reaction in the playground or somewhere away from teaching staff, they should tell a friend who can find a teacher or call another child to run for help. They should never be left alone if they feel unwell.
- Tell a teacher if they think they have eaten something that might have contained their allergen — reassure your child that they will not be in trouble for eating the wrong food.
- Knowing where their medication is kept and who can access it for them (if they don't carry it themselves).
- If older children carry their medication, they need to educate their

friends about where they keep their medication in case they can't speak for themselves in an emergency.

- Teens carrying their own medication without adult supervision (for example, travelling to and from school) also need to educate their friends about what to do in an emergency.
- Learning to be confident in social situations and asking if a food is safe for them to eat.
- Understanding not to use bubblers or, if there is no alternative, to let the water run a little first and never place their mouth in direct contact with the bubbler.
- To understand that bullying or threatening behaviour towards them is unacceptable and they should tell an adult.

'The teacher assigned Jess two guardian angels, who have to try to remind her — if they go to the science room or the library or wherever — that she's got to take her EpiPen.'

—Merryn Gibbons (NSW), mother of Jessica (9),
allergic to cow's milk, egg and peanut

Growing independence: Children carrying their own medications

Q My son has egg allergy and needs to carry his EpiPen at all times. He is starting high school next year, and I am wondering if he is old enough to carry his own EpiPen, or if it should still be left in the care of teaching staff? Is there a recommended age when children are responsible enough to carry their own medication? So far we have taken total responsibility for all his medications, and I suspect we have been cocooning him for too long.

A This is a dilemma for many parents. On the one hand, we want to encourage our children to be independent and take ownership of their allergies; on the other, we worry if they are really ready for the extra responsibility, and is it actually putting their safety at risk?

There is no accepted age when children are ready to carry their own medication: it will depend on the maturity of your child and his personality.

Ideally, by the time they are going out on their own or with friends, for example, playing sport or travelling to and from school, they will be experienced and educated in carrying their own EpiPen and Action Plan.

You are right in wanting to encourage your son to take responsibility for his allergies — the school years are really important for preparing your child to become self-sufficient in managing their allergies in the real world.

As your child is starting a new school, is still young, and hasn't had to take any responsibility for his medications before, it is probably safest to still have his EpiPen in the care of teaching staff or the school nurse (or whatever system and location you and your school agree upon). However, you can encourage gradual independence by having your son take responsibility for his allergy in other ways. For example, consider having your son carry his medical kit to and from school each day and dropping it off in a designated location and remembering to bring it home (although you might want to leave a backup kit at school with the teacher). Outside of school, when you are going out as a family, make your son responsible for remembering to carry his EpiPen instead of carrying it for him. Teach your son how to read food labels and involve him in selecting safe foods when shopping. In social situations, allow your son to ask questions of others, for example, 'Does this meal contain any egg?' instead of doing the asking for him. Think about all the responsibilities you currently take care of and then decide which ones are appropriate to start handing over to your son.

While you are making your decision, talk to your son's school. In some schools, staff encourage self-responsibility in many ways but prefer the EpiPen to be located in a central position, so there is never any risk of staff being caught without one. Your child's personality may also need to be considered. Some children feel embarrassed about wearing an EpiPen in a bum bag or constantly carrying around a bag. Some kids are also really good at losing everything that comes their way. Is your child likely to leave his medication in his school bag on a hot day? If so, again encourage independence and responsibility, but do so gradually. Another consideration is the safety of your child's classmates: is your child likely to produce the EpiPen for other kids to look at and possibly hurt themselves?

(Inadvertent injection involves a trip to hospital.) If your child carries his own EpiPen in a school bag, the school needs to allow your child to bring his bag with him into the classroom — it cannot be left outside in the sun. In addition, in an emergency, no teacher has time to search through a sea of school bags looking for your son's EpiPen.

A very important point to think through when a child is carrying their own medication, is whether or not they are capable of self-injecting, and whether or not their friends know what to do in an emergency. It is one thing for a child to carry their own medication, but someone who is trained in using the EpiPen must be available to administer it in the event of anaphylaxis (during which he may not be able to communicate clearly or be capable of self-injecting), and know exactly where your child keeps his medication.

Talk to your school regularly about the need to encourage independence and responsibility in your son while keeping him safe. A gradual process is usually the most manageable and safest way to approach the situation.

> *'Students used to carry their own EpiPens, but we prefer them not to. Students have said they are uncomfortable with carrying their own pens, and we have full-time medical staff here. When the pen is in our health centre we always know where it is. And our campus isn't huge, so all staff know how to access them, and we have a clear process in place.'*
>
> —Mrs Jane Danvers, Principal, Wilderness School (SA)

Providing support and communicating with teaching staff

Being responsible for a child at risk of anaphylaxis can feel overwhelming for some staff members. While the majority of teaching staff accept the responsibility as a part of their duty of care, it doesn't mean that individuals don't feel anxious or fearful about effectively caring for your child in the event of anaphylaxis, no matter how much training they have undertaken. As any parent will remember, when you are new to managing food allergies, there is much to learn — and it takes time and support.

Establishing a positive personal relationship with teaching staff can really help, and ongoing communication is essential. Both of these topics have been covered in Chapter 11, Childcare and pre-school, and the points made there are relevant to all levels of education. (See 'Supporting staff in caring for your child', page 233, and 'Ongoing communication', page 236.)

Education resources available to help schools become 'allergy-aware'

The following resources are available from Anaphylaxis Australia to help schools create an 'allergy-aware' community:

- Food allergy awareness posters.
- EpiPen trainers.
- Educational DVDs, including 'Living with Severe Allergy'. Produced in association with Dr Preeti Joshi, this DVD also contains excellent resource materials for schools, including discussion documents and sample correspondence that schools can use and adapt to educate their own community about food allergy and anaphylaxis.
- Canteen checklists.
- Storybooks appropriate for varying age groups.
- Be a M.A.T.E. posters and discussion guide.
- Fundraising wrist bands and pencils.
- Information about becoming involved in Food Allergy Awareness Week (an annual event aimed at increasing awareness of severe food allergies and the risk of anaphylaxis).

To view the complete product catalogue, visit **www.allergyfacts.org.au**

13

The teenage years

Managing food allergy in the teen years presents families with an entirely new set of challenges. Parents have to adjust to no longer being in charge of managing their child's allergies and instead shift their focus to supporting their teen in the transferral of responsibilities. Teens have to learn how to avoid their allergen by making appropriate food choices, carry emergency medications at all times and know how to recognise and treat the symptoms of an allergic reaction. In addition, their close friends need to be educated about what to do in an emergency.

The period in which teens need to become self-reliant in managing their condition coincides with a time when they are exploring their independence, engaging in risk-taking behaviour, spending an increasing amount of time socialising without parental supervision and experiencing a strong desire to fit in with their friends. Tensions in families often arise as teens seek increased freedom from parental limitations at a time when parents are acutely aware of their teen's 'invincible' outlook and worry over their safety. The transition from childhood to adolescence and then adulthood is a learning process for both parents and their children. While the teen years will never be 'pain-free' for either party, they can be made a lot easier if parents and teens can work together to understand each other's needs.

In this chapter, we look at some of the research findings around risk-taking and coping with food allergy in the teen years and consider some of the factors that can affect how a teen manages their condition. We also provide practical suggestions for how parents can support their teen and include important additional information on controlling asthma, the risks associated with alcohol and food allergy, and kissing and food allergy. We also explain the process of transition from paediatric to adult specialist care.

We are grateful for the assistance and enthusiasm of Olivia Keene, psychologist and Clinic Director of Keene Insight Child and Adolescent Specialists, in preparing information for this chapter.

Research on increased risks in the teenage years

Although fatal food allergy reactions remain rare, adolescents and young adults are at the highest risk of death from food allergy,[1, 2, 3, 4] comprising more than half of deaths from food-related anaphylaxis.[5]

Media coverage of teen fatalities from food allergy brings home to parents just how real the risk of life-threatening reactions can be. Many parents interviewed for this book made the comment that while they are not overly anxious about their young child's food allergies, they do worry about the future, when they have to hand over the reins of management to their teens.

Significant research has been conducted into risk-taking and coping strategies of teens with food allergy, as well as studies on how teens perceive their allergies.[6, 7, 8, 9] While the focus of each of these studies has been different, overall, three main factors have been identified as placing adolescents and young people at greatest risk of fatal food-allergic reactions (especially those with asthma and those with allergy to peanut or tree nuts).

1. Increased risk-taking behaviour

Risk-taking is accepted as a common behaviour in the teen years, and research confirms that many teens with food allergy intentionally engage in risk-taking behaviour in relation to their food allergy. An important study conducted in the US in 2006[10] looking at risk-taking behaviours in teens found that more than half of the participants had *knowingly* eaten at least a small amount of a food known to contain (or possibly contain) their allergen. Reasons for doing so included: desire to eat the food, being undeterred by 'may contain' statements, reluctance to ask questions, curiosity and pressure from friends.

2. Lack of access to, or timely administration of, adrenaline

A significant percentage of teens at risk of anaphylaxis do not always carry self-injectable adrenaline (for example, an EpiPen). In the same study as mentioned above,[11] of the 71 per cent of adolescents participating in the study who had experienced anaphylaxis, 38 per cent were not carrying self-injectable adrenaline during their last anaphylaxis. Overall, 61 per cent of teens involved in the study reported that they did carry their emergency medication at all times (but their compliance in doing so was found to be influenced by social circumstances, convenience and their own perceptions of risk: see below).

3. Skewed perceptions of risk

The concerns of teens with food allergies are very different from those of their parents. In one research study, when parents and teens were asked to list the 'hardest/worst' aspect of the condition, teens listed social isolation while parents listed issues related to fear of their child dying.[12] Most teens are very 'now'-focused, meaning they are more concerned with how their food allergies affect their life right now rather than thinking through the risks and consequences of an allergic reaction.

Research also suggests that teens may have an incorrect perception of risk about certain social situations. In the 2006 US study,[13] teens were asked to rate 10 situations in terms of degree of risk for triggering an allergic reaction. Teens ranked 'kissing after an allergen' as the highest risk situation. While kissing can pose a risk (see page 281), the authors of the study expressed concern that teens ranked several high-risk situations much lower on the list, including restaurants, friends' houses and parties.

> 'They think they are invincible at this age. It is difficult: you don't want to frighten them but you do need to make them aware that they have to be responsible for their own safety … Eventually our children have to go out into the real world and they won't have a bubble around them, so at some stage they have to deal with it and create their own safety.'
>
> —Judy Browning (Vic), mother of Geoffrey (17), allergic to egg and peanut

What affects how a teen manages their food allergies?

While there has been important research into how teens manage and cope with their food allergies, it should be emphasised that many teens effectively manage their food allergies and are not rampant risk-takers. All of the parents of teens interviewed for this book indicated that their teens did not take risks in regard to their food allergy (although many were happy to take risks in other ways). A wide range of factors may affect how a teen manages and copes with their food allergies. Discussion of some of the main ones follows.

- **History of management of their allergies**
  If a child is taught to gradually take responsibility for managing their allergies from a young age then the transition to self-management in the teen years won't be as challenging for them. Children who have been empowered to self-manage their condition are less likely to take unnecessary risks.[14]

- **Education**
  A teen's level of education about their allergy will directly impact on their ability to self-manage the condition. For example, teens are taught to carry their medication and Action Plan at all times and to use it in the event of anaphylaxis, but research[15] indicates many teens are unclear about the symptoms that constitute anaphylaxis (and therefore *when* to administer adrenaline). The same research study also revealed that many teens did not believe they needed to read food labels every time they used a product and did not heed 'May contain' warnings.

- **Personality**
  Outgoing and confident teens are better equipped to manage their food allergies in social situations. Managing food allergies in social situations requires teens to communicate clearly and speak up about their needs; for example, questioning restaurant staff, talking to potential boyfriends or girlfriends about kissing or asking friends to learn how to help them in an emergency. Teens who are quiet, shy or introverted may find communicating about their allergies much more

difficult. One parent interviewed for this book reported that one of the main reasons her teenage son found his multiple food allergies difficult to cope with was his very shy personality. Even though he had been encouraged from a young age to become self-reliant, the practices needed to manage his allergy in social situations were highly challenging for him because, from his point of view, it meant attracting unwanted attention.

- **Attitudes of parents**
  As covered in detail in Chapter 17, Anxiety in children, page 331, anxiety and negative attitudes about food allergy in parents can be transferred to children of all ages, affecting their abilities and making them more fearful of their condition.[16] A positive attitude can also be contagious, and research studies have associated a positive outlook about food allergies with empowerment in regard to managing allergies.[17]

- **The allergen itself (and the number of allergens)**
  Some allergens are much more difficult to avoid than others. For example, a teen with an allergy to a particular fruit, for instance kiwi fruit, may find this much easier to avoid in social situations than a teen who has milk allergy. (Teens with milk allergy often find themselves in environments where pizza and ice-cream are consumed, where the risk of cross-contamination and contact skin reactions may be high.) Similarly, a teen with multiple allergies will probably find it more challenging to avoid their allergens as opposed to a teen who only has to worry about one.

- **Previous experiences of allergic reactions**
  One research study that examined the psychosocial impact of anaphylaxis on young people and their parents reported that adolescents described their condition as 'no big deal'.[18] However, the majority of adolescents in this study had very little memory of anaphylaxis. If the study participants had more recent and memorable experiences of anaphylaxis, their condition may have been viewed differently.

  Anecdotally, most of the teens whose parents were interviewed for this book had experienced either anaphylaxis or severe symptoms that they could remember. This may be an important contributing factor in these parents reporting no known problems with risk-taking in their teens in regard to food allergies.

● **Education and support of peers**

Peer pressure and embarrassment have been identified as contributing to risk-taking behaviour in teens with food allergy.[19] If teens are in an environment where food allergy has been 'normalised' through education, they may be less likely to be teased or bullied (for information on bullying, see page 256) about their condition and also less likely to be excluded from participating in activities.

> *'Most of the time, I leave the management up to Samantha, and she has always been exceptionally calm and level-headed, even as a young child. She is the one who controls it and is very independent and aware. She carries her EpiPen and antihistamine everywhere. It is more challenging when she is out at restaurants, but her friends have also become more aware and exceptionally accommodating.'*
>
> —Peta Mawson (Qld), mother of Samantha (17), allergic to peanut, tree nuts and avocado

The importance of controlling asthma

Having asthma combined with food allergy increases the risk of a severe allergic reaction. Asthma, especially when poorly controlled, has been identified as a significant contributing factor in fatalities from food-related anaphylaxis.[20, 21, 22, 23]

More research is needed into understanding the role of asthma in severe allergic reactions; however, it is thought that people with asthma have highly reactive airways, so their lungs are more likely to be involved in an allergic reaction to food (resulting in severe symptoms associated with anaphylaxis).

Ensuring your teen's asthma is well controlled may help to prevent a fatal outcome. A teen needs to be responsible for using their asthma medications as prescribed, especially preventers, and to be encouraged to take responsibility for their health, for example, by carrying their Asthma Plan and medications at all times.

Ensure your teen receives ongoing and regular care from a doctor (in some cases this may be the same doctor who manages their food allergy; in other cases it may be a specialist respiratory physician, paediatrician or GP). Having lung function measured regularly, annually in most cases, will provide helpful feedback in regard to how well the asthma is being controlled.

Overall, 'well-controlled' asthma usually means infrequent use of relievers, minimal disruption to daily living and minimal use of oral steroids. If your teen is experiencing more frequent symptoms or difficulties breathing during sport, these could be indicators that the asthma is not being well controlled.

If your teen ever suspects they have been exposed to a potential food allergen and they start to experience asthma symptoms, they should use their EpiPen. (This may be more obvious if they are experiencing other symptoms of an allergic reaction, for example, hives or swelling, but this will not always be the case.)

Make sure your teen understands that using an EpiPen for an asthma attack will not do any harm (and may even help), but using asthma reliever medications for anaphylaxis is dangerous, as a delay in the administration of adrenaline is associated with fatalities from anaphylaxis.

The golden rule applies: if in doubt, *always* use the EpiPen.

Supporting your teen to self-manage and cope with food allergies

It's tough being the parent of any teen: no matter how hard you try, you will no doubt experience at least some door-slamming, and at some point be on the receiving end of 'That's not fair!' But teens too often get a bad rap:

they are mostly very capable and willing to take on new responsibilities and may surprise you with their positive attitudes and abilities. Never underestimate a teen: your confidence in them and support can make a difference in how they handle any challenge, including food allergy. Below are 10 ideas to help you work together with your teen to help them effectively and confidently manage their food allergies.

If you have any concerns about how your son or daughter is managing their food allergies, always consult your allergy specialist for advice specific to your teen's diagnosis.

1. Open communication

Parents need to support teens in becoming responsible for self-managing their allergies. For this to happen, the lines of communication need to be wide open, and this involves hard work and patience on behalf of both parties.

According to psychologist Olivia Keene, parents need to make a conscious effort to make time for their teens and prioritise the relationship they have with them. 'The relationship between a young person and their parents is pivotal. Not having open communication in this relationship is probably one of the biggest risk factors for a young person becoming isolated in the family — and then they gradually stop talking about what's happening in their world.'

To keep the lines of communication open, parents sometimes have to step back from a situation and listen, rather than reacting with threats of punishment, or judgment. Olivia Keene offers a practical example. 'Often a teenager will not talk to Mum and Dad about a party because there was alcohol there, and they know Mum and Dad will "freak out". If parents can pull back on their responses, by not turning information into disciplining issues, then they are actually going to know what kind of risks their teens are being exposed to. Parents can then help teens to manage those risks much better than if they did not have access to that information.'

2. Negotiate boundaries

When it comes to parties and social invitations, parents and teens often have conflicting views. Teenagers want to join their friends and break away from parental authority while parents worry about their safety.

Wrapping teens with food allergy in cotton wool won't work, according to Olivia Keene. 'Preventing teens from going to parties is going to create resentment, and the rubber band will flick back in the other direction, with the teen potentially partaking in quite risky behaviour the tighter a parent hangs on.'

When parents refuse to allow teens to attend parties, the message they are conveying to their child is: 'I don't trust you to be able to make good decisions.'

'That's a catch-22 situation for the young person,' explains Olivia Keene, 'because they feel, "Well hang on, you've never allowed me to be in that situation, so what are you basing that view on?" They then become really angry and that then affects trust which, in turn, can start to break down the relationship between parents and the young person.'

This doesn't mean that you let your teen attend every party and do whatever they please. Instead, discuss and agree upon expectations around social situations. Boundaries still need to be in place but they need to be clearly negotiated between parents and their teen, rather than dictated by the parents. According to Olivia Keene, the process of negotiating boundaries with your teen acts to:

- give your teen a voice and input into decision-making
- give your teen less to rebel against
- decrease your teen's feelings of disempowerment (which can result in anger)
- model a process that is actively building your teen's skills in communication and negotiating, which are important skills for life

For example, you might agree with your teen that they can go to a party, but they will eat before they go and take snacks in their bag (along with their Action Plan and medical kit) so they aren't tempted to share food. Discuss with your teen who else is going to the party and make sure some of their friends know about their allergy and have been educated in what to do if your teen does have an allergic reaction.

Negotiate boundaries with your teen and, with the right education in place, help them to understand you do trust them to be responsible for their safety.

'Our son said to us when he was about 14 that his anaphylaxis will never stop him from doing anything, and that if we say no to something, a social event or whatever, "It had better not be about anaphylaxis, because that's never an acceptable reason for you to stop me from doing anything." And he was right.'

—Barbara (NSW), mother of a 19-year-old son
who is allergic to cow's milk

3. Take responsibility for your own anxiety

If you are feeling anxious about your teen managing their allergy in social situations, that's completely understandable, but it will help your teen if you can be honest about your anxiety.

Parents often expect children to carry out things based on their own anxiety. For example, a parent might say, 'You can only go to the party if you call me at 10pm and let me know what's going on.' In this example, the teen will feel as though you are checking up on them and you don't trust them to make the right decisions on their own.

However, if in the same scenario, parents can acknowledge their anxiety and take ownership of it, the outcome can be very different. If you instead said to your teen, 'I'd like you to give me a quick call halfway through the party, not because I don't trust you, but because then I'll be able to sleep,' this sends them a very different message. Your teen understands you are worried and asking them to call is about supporting you.

(See Chapter 16, Anxiety in parents, page 313, for more information.)

4. Prepare your teen to deal with an allergic reaction away from home

In studies examining fatalities from food-related anaphylaxis, the allergen is most commonly found in foods prepared outside of their own home.[24] While all aspects of allergy education are important — especially avoidance — it is essential that your teen is prepared to deal with an allergic reaction away from home.

Set aside some time to talk to your teen about how to recognise and manage an allergic reaction. Many parents think their teen knows what to do but, as mentioned earlier in this chapter, research indicates that teens often do not understand the symptoms of anaphylaxis. Education messages your teen needs to understand include:

- Allergic reactions can happen any time and anywhere: their EpiPen and Action Plan must be carried at all times.
- Anyone with food allergy must be able to recognise the specific symptoms of anaphylaxis and know when to use their EpiPen. Reinforce that symptoms of an allergic reaction can present in any order. Ask your teen if they have any questions about what certain symptoms might look or feel like.
- Symptoms of an allergic reaction can vary from one reaction to another. If your teen has previously experienced an allergic reaction, remind them that the symptoms may not be exactly the same the next time they have a reaction.
- Buy an EpiPen trainer and have your teen practise using it from time to time. Let them use expired EpiPens on an orange so they understand how much pressure needs to be applied. Do everything you can to ensure your teen is capable and prepared to self-inject in the event of anaphylaxis.
- If they think they are having an allergic reaction, they must tell someone immediately and never seek refuge in a toilet cubicle or anywhere else where they will be on their own.
- If in doubt, they should always err on the side of caution and use their EpiPen: never 'wait and see'.
- Reinforce the strengths your teen possesses to cope with an emergency. For example, talk about some situations that demonstrated how they are a great communicator or have the ability to stay calm. Let them know you have confidence in their ability to handle an emergency.

EpiPens at the beach

Q My 14-year-old son has peanut and milk allergy and needs to carry an EpiPen at all times. We live on the coast and my son is a keen surfer. He is refusing to take his EpiPen with him to the beach, claiming he doesn't eat at the beach, and it will only be left sitting on the sand in the sun while he is in the water. Should he be taking his EpiPen to the beach and, if so, how should it be stored?

A Yes, he should be carrying his EpiPen at *all* times (the exception being when he is actually surfing!). EpiPens contain adrenaline, which can be affected by extreme temperatures: it should never be refrigerated or exposed to direct heat, so how your son stores his medication at the beach is really important.

Your son should keep his EpiPen in its carry tube inside a padded and insulated pack (similar to a cooler pack you might take on a picnic) and this should then be placed inside another bag; for example, a backpack. He might also like to throw his towel over the top of the bag (preferably one that is light in colour).

An insulated pouch is available that has been specially designed to store EpiPens (visit **www.allergyfacts.org.au**). However, if your son has other medications, for example, antihistamine and asthma medication, consider a larger pack so all medications can be stored in the one bag. In addition, your son's Action Plan for anaphylaxis must always be kept *with* his medications. He should also carry his mobile phone in case he needs to call for help.

There are two main reasons why your son probably doesn't want to carry his EpiPen to the beach. The first is that he doesn't perceive any risk of an allergic reaction while at the beach. Help your son to understand that allergic reactions can happen anywhere at any time. He may not plan on eating, but if the opportunity arises, he might change his mind. For example, if he is surfing with a mate who brings food to the beach, he might be tempted to eat or he might share an unsafe drink.

The second is that he may feel self-conscious about carrying his medications. Allow your son to have some say in how the medication is stored. You might purchase an appropriate insulated bag or pouch but then let your son visit a surf shop to buy a backpack or bag he feels comfortable taking to the beach. Most of the large surf brands produce a range of backpacks and bags. Helping your son to feel less self-conscious about carrying his medications may make a difference to his attitude.

If your son regularly surfs with mates, he should also communicate his allergies to them and let them know what to do in an emergency situation. Also be sure to encourage your son to regularly check his EpiPen. The viewing window of the EpiPen should be clear: if it becomes discoloured or appears cloudy, the EpiPen will need to be replaced immediately.

5. Continue specialist medical care

Ongoing specialist medical care will ensure your teen has access to objective information about their condition. If your teen has not experienced an allergic reaction in a very long time, regular review by an allergy specialist will reinforce to them that their seemingly 'invisible'[25] condition is real. If your teen has experienced recent allergic reactions, seeing their doctor will be reassuring and offer them the chance to talk about any concerns they have and ask questions. If you and your son or daughter disagree on any issues related to managing their food allergy, your specialist may be able to act as a neutral party, providing the facts you and your teen need to come to an agreement.

Just as you are encouraging your teen to become responsible for managing their food allergies, also encourage them to take greater ownership of their relationship with their specialist. Before an appointment, ask your teen to make a list of any questions they have, or work on one together, and let your teen run through the list during the appointment.

At some point during the teen years, your specialist will discuss the need for your child to transition from paediatric to adult medical care (for more information see page 283). It is important that your teen is working towards becoming confident and capable of communicating with doctors.

> *'Our allergy specialist is excellent with the girls. He directs his questions to them and they answer him. He will ask them if they have any issues, and "When was the last time you had a reaction?" He has been really supportive and reminds them that they always need to have their EpiPen with them. It's important a doctor talks to teens.'*
>
> —Jill Ahmed (SA), mother of Shana (15), allergic to peanut and tree nuts, and Alisa (13), allergic to peanut, tree nuts, honey and kiwi fruit

6. View the process of education as a 'partnership'

As we have already mentioned, research indicates that a teen's perception of risk is often poor and they are very focused on what is happening 'now'. Parents need to provide teens with ongoing education in a way that *supports* them to be able to make the best possible decisions they can around their food allergies.

'Young people work much better when they're given information that they can then use in making their own decisions "in the moment", rather than being told, "You really need to think through the consequences of your actions" — that doesn't compute with them,' says Olivia Keene. 'Telling them what to do is not the answer, it's about working alongside them by providing information.'

Accept that you are no longer 'the boss' in regard to managing your child's food allergies, you are their partner.

7. Stick to your new role

Once you have gradually handed over responsibilities to your teen in managing their allergies, you need to stick to your new role as an encourager rather than an organiser. For example, if you expect your teen to speak up for themselves when eating out with friends, don't revert to talking to restaurant staff on their behalf when you eat as a family; if you are going on a family outing, don't throw the EpiPen in your bag: ensure your teen is responsible for both remembering and carrying it.

Teens need to understand that making consistent safe decisions is an important part of managing their condition. Allowing your teen to be consistently responsible creates good habits and reinforces the confidence and trust you have in them.

8. Plan ahead

Planning ahead goes hand-in-hand with almost every aspect of managing food allergies. Some challenges in the teen years are predictable (for example, dating and exposure to drugs and alcohol), so work with your teen ahead of time in helping them feel prepared to make informed decisions in potentially difficult and risky social situations.

Ask your teen how they think they would handle certain situations, for example, being offered food at a party or explaining their allergy to a boyfriend or girlfriend. Get them thinking about situations before they happen so they have time to access the information they need and may then feel more confident in handling those situations when they do arise. (See 'Alcohol and food allergy', page 282 and 'Kissing', page 281.)

Also, think ahead about any new practical education points you will need to share with your teens in new situations. For example, when your teen starts driving, make sure they understand that adrenaline can be affected by extreme temperatures, so leaving an EpiPen in the glovebox is not a good idea. Remind your teen that food allergens can be present in skin-care products and cosmetics.

Make time for these conversations with your teen so you can have an open and detailed discussion rather than constantly hounding them with reminders and rules.

9. Help your teen learn from mistakes

Any learning process usually involves mistakes. If your teen experiences an allergic reaction, try to work out with them what went wrong. Remain calm and be empathetic: don't jump to the conclusion that they have done something wrong.

When they talk you through the experience, remember to praise them for any aspects they handled well, for example, telling someone when they felt unwell, taking their antihistamine and remembering to have their EpiPen and Action Plan with them.

If your teen's reaction was the result of risk-taking or not taking responsibility for their allergies seriously, still resist the urge to reprimand or punish. Try to work out why their reaction occurred and/or why they weren't well equipped to cope with the reaction. For example, did they not carry their medication because they are being teased at school or perhaps feel embarrassed?

Parents need to make their teens feel confident that they can open up to them about mistakes without fearing the consequences. If you know when and why mistakes are happening, you are then well placed to provide your teen with the education and support they need to prevent the same mistakes from happening again.

10. Support your teen in creating their own support network

Teens who are surrounded by educated and supportive friends will feel more confident (and less embarrassed) about clearly communicating their needs around their allergies, and less likely to take risks in order to 'fit in' with their friends. They will also feel safer in social situations knowing that their friends are capable of taking care of them if they do have an allergic reaction.

Research indicates that teens believe having friends and teaching staff educated about food allergy would improve their life; however, they are not always able to easily provide this information themselves.[26]

Third-party education is one solution; for example, working with your teen's teachers to see if they can include a general education session on food allergy in the classroom may be helpful. Encourage your school to become involved in education and fundraising activities around Food Allergy Awareness Week (visit **www.allergyfacts.org.au** for more information). Ensuring your teen has a trusted and educated member of staff to turn to when they are feeling stressed or need help in making a decision around their safety can also provide reassurance.

Educating friends of a food-allergic teen is essential, but your teen won't want you to tell the world about their allergy: parents need to respect their teen's need for privacy. Talk to your son or daughter about identifying a small number of trusted friends to become educated about their allergy and ask them if they need your support in doing this, for example, by providing an EpiPen trainer, helping them to explain symptoms to friends or perhaps offering to pay for their friends to do an anaphylaxis training course or for an educational DVD for them to watch. Keep in mind that it is your job to support them in educating their friends, not take over.

The process of educating friends can have unexpected positive side effects, too, says Olivia Keene.

'It's important to remember that teens like being given responsibility. We have found with many young people who have chronic health issues, they nominate friends in their group to be educated, and a buddy system emerges, where the role of caretaker is rotated, and they sometimes fight over the role! It can make the young person with allergies feel special rather than being too embarrassed to talk about it. They feel cared for and nurtured without feeling like a victim. They feel like they belong, which is a protective factor that plays a key role in the development of resilience.' (See Chapter 15, Resilience in children, page 306.)

> *'My friends are supportive. I've taught a few of them how to use the EpiPen and I've told them not to be scared of using it on me if [anaphylaxis] happens, and they are okay with that ... Having friends around who know how to use it does give me peace of mind.'*
>
> —Geoffrey Browning (Vic; 17), allergic to egg and peanut

Kissing

If a food-allergic person kisses someone who has recently eaten their allergen, then they are at risk of an allergic reaction. Getting down to specifics, the nature of the kiss is likely to dictate the potential severity of a reaction. For example, a peck on the cheek is only likely to cause a local (minor) reaction, such as a hive at the site of the kiss. Passionate kissing, however, involving the transfer of saliva, can lead to a more general or even severe allergic reaction.

Research has not established with any certainty the amount of time or oral hygiene procedures (for example, brushing teeth and using mouthwash) needed after someone has consumed an allergen before it is safe for them to kiss an allergic partner.[27] Advice from one research study to reduce the risk of an allergic reaction from peanut includes waiting a few hours after eating peanut butter *and* consuming a peanut-free meal.[28] However, the safest way for anyone with a food allergy to avoid a reaction from kissing is for their partner to join them in not eating the allergen. *continued*

This is awkward territory for teens. While kissing is probably a topic many teens do not want to be chatting to their parents about, they do need to understand that they have to be upfront with anyone they want to kiss. There is no way around it: they have to communicate about their allergies to anyone they want to kiss, preferably before the kissing opportunity arrives. Reassure your teen that their friends are supportive about their allergy and any boyfriend or girlfriend worth having will be equally so. Having an allergic reaction would be far more embarrassing (and dangerous) than telling someone about their allergy.

Alcohol and food allergy

As everyone knows, in Australia teens under the age of 18 aren't supposed to be drinking alcohol, but parents need to acknowledge it is a possibility that their teens will be experimenting with alcohol well before the legal age.

Alcohol consumption in teens with food allergy poses some additional risks that your son or daughter needs to be made aware of. Below are some education points about food allergy and alcohol worth discussing with your teen.

- Alcohol impairs judgment: when teens consume alcohol they may make unsafe food choices and be incapable of self-managing an allergic reaction.
- Many alcoholic beverages contain food allergens. For example, many liqueurs contain nuts and/or milk; beer and some ciders contain barley, and some beers contain wheat. Cocktails often contain milk, egg, fruits, nuts and nut-containing chocolate: cocktails are an absolute no-go zone for anyone with a food allergy, because even if a cocktail doesn't contain an allergen as an ingredient, the likelihood of cross-contamination in a busy and usually poorly lit bar or nightclub is very high.
- All alcoholic drinks must contain warning notices to indicate if they contain any of the common allergens (covered under the *Australia*

New Zealand Food Standards Code). You may also notice that some wines or beers may say that wheat, eggs or fish have been used during production as a fining agent. The jury is still out as to whether food allergens used as fining agents can cause severe allergic reactions, but anyone with a food allergy needs to understand there may be a risk.

- It is thought that alcohol consumption may increase the absorption of food allergens in the stomach, which may result in a more significant allergic reaction if the allergen is consumed at the same time as alcohol.[29]

Transitioning from paediatric to adult medical care

Q My 15-year-old daughter is allergic to peanuts and pistachios and she has been seeing the same paediatric immunologist for more than 10 years. My daughter wholeheartedly trusts her immunologist and looks forward to her annual appointments for reassurance. During a recent consult, the doctor mentioned that my daughter will soon need to start the transition process to see an adult immunologist. My daughter is really upset and told me she is worried about having to see a new doctor. How should I help my daughter manage this transition?

A After such a long and happy relationship it is not surprising your daughter is upset by the prospect of changing doctors. Transitioning from paediatric to adult care can initially feel daunting. The process will be gradual, however, and the better it is managed, the better your daughter will start to feel about seeing her new specialist. You will need to support your daughter on both the emotional and practical fronts.

On the emotional front, firstly reassure your daughter that this transition won't be immediate. The issue of transition is usually discussed some time in the teenage years but doesn't take place until the age of approximately 17 (although the age will vary depending on the clinic your daughter attends). Your daughter needs to know that she will be seeing her doctor again and will have the opportunity to say goodbye.

Also help your daughter to understand the reasons why she will soon need to see an adult doctor. Make it clear that it is not because her doctor isn't interested in her any more. Explain that doctors have different areas of specialty and her current doctor specialises in treating children — and now that your daughter is close to becoming an adult (a fact most teens feel quite positive about!), she has almost outgrown the expertise of her current doctor. Also let your daughter know that her current specialist will recommend a new specialist and pass on her file notes. In other words, it is a coordinated handover.

On the practical front, planning ahead will make this transition run smoothly. At your daughter's next appointment, be sure to raise the issue of transition early in the appointment and ask your specialist to explain to you and your daughter how it will be handled. Also ask your specialist to explain how your daughter's care might change under an adult immunologist. If your daughter currently attends a clinic in a children's hospital, some hospitals have 'transition coordinators' who can support your teen through this process, so check with your specialist if this service is available.

Start encouraging your daughter to become independent in managing her relationship with her current specialist and GP. Ask your daughter to call and make medical appointments for herself, explain to her how Medicare works, ask her to prepare a list of questions in advance of any medical appointments and allow her to ask the questions during any consults. Your natural urge may be to do all of these things for your daughter but allowing her to do them, while she still has you for support, will make the transition much easier for her in the long run. Also ask your daughter if she has any suggestions about how she wants to handle the transition; be sure to involve your daughter in any decisions around the transition.

One of the most significant changes for you and your daughter when she changes doctors will probably be the style of care: there is a lot less 'hand holding' in an adult consultation, and the doctor will communicate with your daughter rather than you. If your daughter needs access to other support, such as a dietitian or psychologist, you may have to organise this independently (although obviously this will depend on your doctor). The first time your daughter visits an adult immunologist, by all means go along, but perhaps suggest you only stay for part of the consultation and wait in the sitting room for the remainder of the appointment, so she has the opportunity to establish her own relationship with her new specialist.

14

Enjoying celebrations and socialising

Any situation that involves eating food away from home, especially in a party atmosphere, means that the risk of an allergic reaction is increased. But celebration doesn't have to mean deprivation; you just need to plan ahead to minimise the risks, take appropriate safety precautions and, depending on your child's allergies, probably spend some extra time in the kitchen.

Celebrations should be pleasurable, and it's important for children with food allergies to understand they can enjoy living as close to a normal life as possible. If parents set the example for young children that it is possible for them to be included in all the fun things in life, hopefully they won't feel self-conscious or resentful about their allergies as they grow older.

This chapter offers some helpful suggestions in preparing for common special occasions, including: birthday parties, sleepovers, Easter and Christmas. We also look at the often tricky situation of visiting friends and family. Keep in mind that the precautions needed in any social situation will depend on your child's age, personality and their allergies, as well as the attitude of the friends and family attending the occasion. Not all of the ideas outlined in this chapter are necessary for every child with food allergies.

Birthday parties

There's nothing quite like the enthusiasm of a room full of children surrounded by balloons, cake, treats and presents. Celebrating birthdays with friends is a wonderful rite of passage for all children.

Birthday parties, however, are also a common cause of stress for parents of food-allergic children, especially those who are dealing with a recent diagnosis. The challenges of keeping a food-allergic child safe at birthday parties are varied. Toddlers often have multiple food allergies and parents are charged with the task of keeping their child safe in a roomful of very messy little friends — but on the up side, they are still at an age where they need and want their parents to be with them at a party. As your child matures, they may outgrow some of their allergies, will hopefully have a good understanding of their allergies and what they need to do to avoid a reaction, but will no longer want their mum or dad tagging along.

When Noah is invited to a birthday party, I don't think about whether or not he can go, but rather how I can minimise the risks and make it as safe as possible for him to enjoy himself. Whatever challenges you are facing, by preparing in advance and communicating clearly with the host — and your child — birthday parties will hopefully become manageable *and* enjoyable for your family. Below are some tips to help you on your way in planning for your child to attend birthday parties.

- When you RSVP to the hosting parents, let them know about your child's food allergies. Even if you already know the hosts, you still may need to remind them of the specifics.
- When you talk to the hosting parents, do so with a positive attitude and realistic expectations. If you are thinking about asking them to make their child's birthday party completely allergen-free for the benefit of your child, you will almost certainly get them offside. Asking a parent if any peanut or nut products will be served is an understandable request, but running through a list of your child's multiple allergens and expecting them to cater accordingly is not.
- Talk to the parents about what foods will be served to determine if it will be safe for your child to eat the same as everyone else. If the foods on offer won't be safe, tell your hosts you are happy to bring food for your child.
- If you are taking food for your child, make sure you offer them similar or worthy substitutes, so your child feels just as special as all the other partygoers.

- Teach your child not to eat anything in their party bag without first checking with you that it is safe. If the party bag contains unlabelled or unsafe treats, let your child know you will trade them for safe lollies: they won't miss out. (Some parents interviewed for this book have made deals with their kids that they will always receive double the amount of safe lollies in exchange for their unsafe lollies, which has proven to be a very effective incentive.)

- The same rule as above applies to lolly-filled piñatas, which are becoming increasingly popular at birthday parties.

- If your child is going to a party where none of the foods will be safe, feed your child before the party, so they are not overly hungry when they arrive. (But do still take along safe treats for your child to enjoy.)

- Parties are often held at special venues: for example, toddler parties are sometimes held in indoor play centres, young children might be invited to a party at a zoo, and teenagers might hold their party at a café or restaurant. Call the venue ahead of time and ask to speak to the food service manager to see if they can cater for your child's special needs. Ask the same questions you would if planning to eat out at a restaurant with your child. (See Chapter 9, Eating out with food allergy, page 180.) Also ask if they will be serving any products containing your child's particular allergens.

- If you have toddlers or young children and are attending a party as a family, make sure you and your partner are clear on who will be supervising your food-allergic child. My husband and I take turns so we both get a chance to relax and chat to other parents and children at a party, knowing that Noah is being watched.

- If the party involves a barbeque, ask the host to cook your child's meat on a piece of foil or offer to bring along a barbeque liner.

- Make sure you and your child understand cross-contamination risks in a party environment. For example, Noah is allergic to milk, so if there is a bowl of cheese Twisties on the table, we are mindful of little fingers covered in cheese powder dipping in and out of all the other bowls on the table, making those foods unsafe for Noah to eat. We put a selection of safe treats in a bowl for Noah before the other children start eating.

- If your child is at an age where parents are no longer staying at parties with their children, but you are still not confident your child is ready to make appropriate food choices, you will need to talk about this with your hosts. It is a lot to ask another parent to be responsible for looking out for the symptoms of an allergic reaction and being prepared to cope with an emergency on top of hosting a party. If the host wants you to attend, that's fair enough. Ask if you can be given a job — taking video footage or photos, or being the barbeque chef, for example — so your child understands you are helping out, not keeping them under surveillance.

- Over time, your child needs to become confident and knowledgeable about what they can and can't eat, how to recognise the symptoms of an allergic reaction and what to do in an emergency. However, while they are in the transition stage, gradually taking on these responsibilities but perhaps not quite there yet, you might agree to leave your child at the party and take the weekend newspaper to a nearby park or café and settle in for a couple of hours. (Some parents interviewed for this book have said they happily park their car in a nearby location and read a book.) The hosting parent will appreciate you being nearby, your child will appreciate being trusted and given their independence, and you will have peace of mind knowing that if something doesn't go to plan, you can get there quickly. (In this scenario, your child's medical kit and Action Plan must be left with your hosts and they must understand the signs and symptoms of an allergic reaction and know when and how to use an EpiPen.)

- If you have very young children, it might be encouraging to know that when your child starts childcare or school, other parents are often highly allergy-aware. Now that Noah is at kindergarten, we find that his friends tell their parents he can't eat certain foods or the parents have noticed his Action Plan on the classroom wall. Noah has never been invited to a party where nut products have been on the menu, and I think this is because most parents are already used to being asked not to send nut-containing products to school. Parents are becoming increasingly conscious that food allergies are a serious issue.

- Just before a party, remind your child of relevant safety measures, for example, not sharing foods, but keep this to a single conversation. Don't make food allergy the focus for your child; let them enjoy the anticipation and excitement of the party.
- Always pack your child's Action Plan and medical kit. If for any reason you forget the EpiPen, take your child with you and go home and get it. No EpiPen, no eating.

We are still at the stage where it is perfectly acceptable for parents to stay at a child's birthday party, so I haven't yet had to sit in a car or ask a parent to take responsibility for Noah in a party situation. However, I have been overwhelmed and touched by the lengths the parents of some of Noah's friends have gone to in order to make him feel included.

When Noah was invited to the birthday party of one of his best friends last year, his mother rang me in advance and said she wanted to make everything on the party table safe for Noah, and that she would not be serving the birthday cake (which would not be safe) until the end of the party. I told my friend it was a lovely but unnecessary gesture, but she insisted and was keen to learn more because another boy with food allergies was also coming to the party. We ran through a range of party foods that were safe for Noah, and my friend then checked these were safe for the other little boy. My friend kept the packaging of all the foods she bought for the party and asked me to check the labels when we arrived at the party. All the children enjoyed eating the same foods together and, after the cake was cut, Noah rummaged through my bag looking for his container of safe cake — he knows the drill. The birthday boy's cake was a racetrack featuring chocolate cars on top: one for every child to take home. Noah was thrilled when my friend produced a toy car for him so he wouldn't feel left out.

We would never expect the parents of Noah's friends and classmates to go to such lengths, but the fact that this mum did was so lovely. This is only one positive experience of many. It does take time, but as family and friends gradually learn more about food allergies, you may find that others approach you about your child's allergies, rather than the other way around.

Your own child's birthday party

At Noah's birthday parties, we enjoy all the same things that every parent does when watching their child celebrate with their own little buddies, but we also get to relax. All the food we serve — for children and adults — is milk-, egg-, nut- and sesame-free. There is no mention of food allergies (unless another child attending has an allergy, which we will happily cater for): the focus is on Noah and fun.

Planning ahead (as always) is essential. Prepare your menu and go shopping for safe treats well before the big day — some specialty products can be hard to find — and, if you aren't a great cook, schedule a trial baking session so you don't feel stressed on the day of the party. While a range of cookbooks specialising in allergy-free recipes is available (see Appendix 1, page 370), you might need to experiment to find out which recipes actually work, and which ones your child likes.

Don't discount regular birthday cookbooks for inspiration, either. My son always chooses his own birthday cake from a popular birthday cake cookbook. None of the cake recipes are safe for him, so I use my own recipe for the sponge, and then adapt decorations and icings without too much trouble.

If baking isn't your thing, beautifully decorated cup cakes can be easier than making large cakes (especially if you have to eliminate eggs), and the perfect serving size for toddlers. Also remember that with the help of icing and a hot knife you can usually decorate or carve a disaster of a cake into anything. Noah's third birthday cake — a lady bug — looked good, but was underdone in the centre, because I couldn't get the egg-free cake to cook all the way through in an enormous pudding basin. Noah blew out the candles on his beautifully iced but seriously inedible lady bug cake and then I whisked it back into the kitchen and served cup cakes instead.

If you have young children, choosing the right time of day can also make catering easier. We always hold Noah's parties at morning- or afternoon tea-time, so we don't have to provide lunch, which is more challenging (but not impossible) to keep allergen-free when you are dealing with multiple allergies.

'My aim, when I am planning a birthday party at our house, is for our children to be able to eat all the food at the party. It means that they do not have to ask what is in each food and I can relax and enjoy the party chaos. All our family parties are dairy-, egg- and peanut-free — even for our child who is allergy-free.

'Dairy-, egg- and peanut-free food can be delicious, attractive and look like any other child's party food. Other children are not even aware they are eating cakes without these three ingredients. Our children love planning their parties. We have a birthday cake recipe book, and many hours are spent deciding on the cake design (with a little guidance from me, taking into consideration my cake construction skills). I then spend time sourcing safe lollies to use as decorations and any other alternative ingredients needed. The icing and lollies seem to be the most important components!'

— Anne Frisby (Vic), mother of Amelia (6), allergic to cow's milk, egg and peanut, and Hugh (4), allergic to egg and peanut

Sleepover invitation

Q My 6-year-old son is allergic to milk and wheat and experienced anaphylaxis after ingesting a very small amount of milk last year. Generally, we manage his allergies very well, because I usually take food for him wherever we go. I have a friend with a son the same age, and the two boys are the best of friends. My son has been invited to his house for a sleepover and my friend has offered to prepare his meals, but I feel anxious about anyone other than me providing food for my son. How should I prepare for his first sleepover?

A It is only natural for any parent who has witnessed their child experience anaphylaxis to feel nervous about letting others take responsibility for caring for and feeding their child. A big positive here is that you already have a friendship with the person who is offering to care for your son. As this is the first time your child has been away from you, and you are feeling anxious, explain to your friend that you would feel more relaxed if you could send along your son's own meals and snacks. You might also like to pack a safe supply of staples, such as dairy-free margarine, a fresh jar of jam (or whatever safe spread your son likes), dairy- and wheat-free bread and cereal, as well as his milk-alternative for breakfast and any other things your child usually likes to eat. Clearly label all foods you pack for your son so that no one else in the family uses them.

Letting someone else cook for your child is always a tricky situation, even more so when you won't be in the same house while your son is eating. Preparing safe food isn't as straightforward as many people think — there is a lot to learn about interpreting food labels and cross-contamination — so it is probably a good idea to aim towards educating your friend gradually, until you reach a point where you are confident she understands the lengths she will have to go to in order to prevent an allergic reaction. Run her through the safety measures you take at home to avoid a reaction, including: using clean utensils, wiping down benches with a cloth that hasn't already been used to wipe milk or wheat products, checking food labels. Be specific about all the necessary precautions in food preparation. Also talk to your friend about the risks of cross-contamination in the storage, preparation and serving of food; use examples to help her understand. Explain that your son can't use their jar of jam if a knife that has come into contact with butter and toast has been dipped into the jar. The fact that your friend is offering to take on the responsibility is wonderful, and probably means she is very willing to be educated in what needs to be done to keep your son safe.

For this first sleepover, in addition to providing safe food for your child, you will also need to educate your friend in how to recognise the symptoms of an allergic reaction and what to do in the event of anaphylaxis, including the administration of an EpiPen. Consider purchasing an EpiPen trainer to demonstrate how to use it.

Also think about any other potential risks in her home. If your friend has other young children, do they usually wander around with cups of milk? Will the boys be playing with any craft materials that might contain wheat (for example, playdough and some glues)? Ensure your friend understands that allergic reactions can happen anywhere. Ask her to let everyone in the household know about your son's allergies, and to see that no one else offers him food while he is staying there.

You should also have a chat to your son before the sleepover. At 6, he probably has a good understanding of his food allergies — and no doubt remembers his trip to hospital last year. Explain you are packing safe foods for him as well as his medical kit, and that you have spoken to his friend's mum about everything that needs to be done to keep him safe so he can have a great time. Remind your son not to share food or drinks, and to tell an adult if he feels itchy or unwell (or whatever language you usually use around the symptoms of food allergy). Once you have had this chat, let your son focus on the excitement of hanging out with his friend and enjoying his first taste of independence.

It is really important to let children with food allergies enjoy normal childhood experiences, and letting go gradually, by providing his meals for the time being, can help in managing your own anxiety as well as minimising the risk of an allergic reaction. You might also like to arrange to call or message your friend after the boys have gone to bed, if it means you will then sleep soundly. I'm sure your friend will understand that you have been through a traumatic experience, and only recently, and will be happy to support your needs as well as those of your son.

Easter

Many children with food allergies are already used to checking the labels on any chocolate treats before eating, and Easter is no different — except, of course, that there is a *lot* more chocolate on offer.

We are lucky that Noah's group of friends have very allergy-aware parents. Last Easter Noah was one of three children with food allergies joining in an 'egg' hunt in the local park. The mothers who organised the hunt, one of whom has two children with food allergies, spent an evening hand painting and decorating a huge basket of foam eggs. When Noah was invited, the other mums told me they had already decorated safe eggs and were asking all parents to bring along their own bag of treats to trade for the foam eggs at the end of the hunt. Easter was weeks away and they had it all under control before I had even thought of anything so creative. On the day, the excitement for the children was definitely focused on the thrill of the 'hunt', and the fact they were collecting foam eggs instead of chocolate made no difference to their enjoyment.

Following are some tips to help you get ready for Easter:

- Craft stores and educational toy shops often stock Easter craft materials, such as foam, plastic or paper eggs that can be decorated for use in hunts or parades. Children also like to be involved in decorating them.

- If your child only needs to avoid tree-nuts and peanuts, there are now various brands of nut-free chocolate eggs available that taste great. You might like to provide all the eggs for a hunt, or other parents might be happy to agree to only supplying nut-free eggs.

- There are now quite a few food-allergy-aware companies that produce specialty Easter products that may be safe for your child, even if you are dealing with multiple allergens. Among these are: Kinnerton (**www.kinnerton.com.au**), available at department stores and many larger chain store retailers; Sweet William (**www.sweetwilliamcom. au**), available at supermarkets and specialty stores; and Alpha (no website available), often carried in large department stores. As always, you will need to read the labels of any product to ensure it is safe for your child. If you find a company that makes an egg which is safe for your child, don't assume all products made by this company will be safe: read the label of every product every time before allowing your child to eat it.

- You might want to offer a taste of your child's allergen-free chocolate to your child in advance of Easter, to find out if they actually like it. Last year I spent a lot of time sourcing some safe (and expensive!) Easter eggs for Noah, so he would feel the same as his friends. Noah took one bite and spat it out: not because he was allergic to it, he just didn't like the bitter taste of dark chocolate. Noah now asks the Easter bunny to bring him marshmallows, jelly snakes and dinosaurs.

- Chat to your child's school teacher or care provider in advance of any Easter activities and offer to provide safe chocolate for your child and the class. If your child is allergic to egg, check there will be no activities involving real eggs.

Christmas

While any special occasion requires forward planning, Christmas requires that little bit more. Christmas is universally recognised as a time of indulgence when it comes to food, and it can be tempting for anyone with a food allergy to sample a high-risk food in a party atmosphere. Christmas celebrations can involve back-to-back meals (lunch with parents, dinner with in-laws), and the hosts of Christmas meals can be tired and distracted while preparing food. A string of public holidays can also mean pharmacy and medical services are in short supply, especially outside of major cities.

The good news is that most of the challenges that go hand-in-hand with Christmas can be met with careful preparation and clear communication. As always, the precautions you need to take will depend on your individual situation, but below is a list of tips to get you thinking ahead.

- If Christmas meals are being hosted by friends or relatives, call the host well in advance and gently remind them of your child's allergies. Approach the conversation with a positive, as opposed to policing, attitude.
- Talk to the host about what foods will be served to determine if it will be safe for your child to enjoy the same menu as everyone else. If not, inform your host you are happy to bring or prepare food for your child. If there are foods on the menu that pose too great a risk for your child, for example, satay sticks on the barbeque when your child is allergic to peanut, you will need to explain that you are not comfortable with this level of risk. Most people do not set out to intentionally make a social situation unsafe for your child, they just don't realise the risks until they are explained.
- If particular foods that contain your child's allergen are commonly on offer at social events, then you might want to ask if these foods will be served at Christmas. For example, often people aren't aware that dips such as hummus pose a risk for a child with sesame allergy, or pesto may be a risk for a child with nut allergies.
- Be pragmatic in your expectations: while risks need to be minimised, it's unreasonable to expect the host to plan their entire menu around

your child, especially if you are talking about multiple allergens.

- Offer to help the host. For example, bring a dessert you know will be safe for your child to eat and that everyone else will also enjoy, a salad with a safe dressing or safe chocolates for the table.

- Remember to talk to your host about other aspects of Christmas preparations. Don't let food allergies define your relationship with family and friends.

- If a barbeque is planned, bring along foil on which your child's meat can be cooked, or a barbeque liner.

- Seafood has become a popular choice for Christmas meals, so if your child has a seafood allergy you should make your hosts aware well in advance of Christmas. While it is uncommon, some people with shellfish allergy can react to cooking odours. If your host *is* serving shellfish, and you are comfortable with the safety precautions in place, be *very* careful that there is no cross-contamination in the cooking, storing or serving of your child's meal.

- If you are taking food for your child, make sure you offer similar or worthy substitutes, so your child feels included. Make sure you pack a large supply, too. Sometimes other children enjoy your child's food better than their own, so you need to make sure there is always enough to go round.

- Freeze a lot of treats in advance of the Christmas period so you are prepared to say 'yes' to spontaneous social invitations.

- Be conscious of the role alcohol can play in any social situation. Alcohol can affect the thinking and judgment of people you usually trust to keep your child safe.

- If you don't know all of the guests attending a Christmas function, you might want to ask the host to let others know about your child's allergy, so they don't bring along any inappropriate foods.

- If you are hosting Christmas, most guests want to contribute to a meal. It can help to be organised and ring guests in advance with a plan of what you would like them to bring — for example, fresh fruits (which you can cut and serve at your house), or wine and soft drink — or at least be very specific about what you would like them *not* to bring.

- If you have guests staying at your house, be sure to label any foods that are only to be used by your child to avoid any confusion or cross-contamination. For example, we label one jar of Vegemite 'Noah only' and another jar 'Not for Noah', to ensure guests don't contaminate Noah's jar of Vegemite with their butter knife. If you have made a special meal for your child, label it clearly so a guest doesn't help themselves to a portion with a contaminated utensil. If guests are bringing food for a celebration, for example, a salad or dessert, label it as safe or unsafe for your child before it goes into the fridge, to avoid any mix-ups.

- Lollies and chocolate are popular stocking fillers for children and adults; ensure your child does not sample anything before checking it is safe.
- If you are travelling to be with friends or relatives, ensure you know the address of where you are staying in case you need to call an ambulance, and check that you will have mobile phone reception at your intended destination. (See Chapter 10, Travelling with food allergy, page 194.)
- No matter where you are celebrating Christmas, ensure you have your child's Action Plan and medical kit with you at all times, that all medications are in date and stored appropriately, and that you always read the label of every food before allowing your child to eat it (or an older food-allergic child can check for themself).
- Remember to thank family and friends for their help in keeping your child safe and included over Christmas. Letting others know what a difference they can make means they may feel both acknowledged and empowered — and willing to help again at the next family gathering.

For our family, Christmas usually involves travelling interstate and staying with relatives. When Noah was newly diagnosed, I found his first Christmas really stressful, mainly because I wasn't very confident in communicating his needs, he had recently had a reaction to a very small amount of milk, and had only just been prescribed his EpiPen. I still had a lot to learn and, because I felt anxious about his allergies, I have no doubt I transferred this anxiety onto others (sorry ...).

Since that first Christmas, things have improved immeasurably, and I no longer feel any added worry at Christmas time; I just know that I need to invest time in planning ahead and cooking. For Noah's second

Christmas, we travelled to my sister's family in country New South Wales. My sister called me in advance and ran through the planned menu. Pavlova is usually a dessert at their Christmas table and my sister assured me there would be 'no pav' and no nut products — at her insistence — while we were staying, and that she would buy sesame-free bread. Dairy was still a part of the main meal and dessert (she asked all guests to wash their hands after eating) so I knew to expect that and could plan accordingly. Having that one conversation in advance meant we both felt comfortable that we were minimising the risk of an allergic reaction, and my sister could get on with the task of preparing a meal for 14 guests (an entirely separate cause of anxiety).

This year we hosted our first Christmas at home in Melbourne, with a seafood banquet and marinated chicken, as well as salads. All of the main meal was safe for Noah except for the adult dessert, and the children enjoyed home-made chocolate cupcakes and gingerbread men that were Noah-friendly.

Now that Noah is older, it is so much easier; he knows to check with Mummy or Daddy before eating food offered by anyone else. It also helps that Noah isn't the only one at our family's Christmas table with special dietary needs. This year we had a gluten-free plum pudding to cater for Nana, no cucumber in the salads for an uncle, and one of Noah's aunties is a fish-eating vegetarian. Noah understands that there are lots of reasons why people can't eat certain foods.

Staying with friends and family

If you are intending to stay with friends or family, it can be helpful to plan in advance exactly how you are going to communicate your child's needs before you raise the issue with others. Take some time out and write down a list of points you would like to talk about with the friend or family member you are going to stay with.

Once you have decided on what you want to say, spend some time thinking about how you are going to say it. How

continued

you communicate your needs to others will usually dictate the outcome. If you approach another person with an expectation that they must follow orders from you and then proceed to rattle off a list of food rules, the response may not be what you are looking for. Most people do want to help others in need, they just don't know how and appreciate being asked in a positive way. It's also important not to try to 'scare' hosts into taking food allergy seriously — creating an environment of fear won't make the stay enjoyable for anyone — and to keep your assessments of risk in proportion.

Offer specific practical solutions for your host to help them understand exactly how they can help, but also make it clear you do not expect them to be directly responsible for keeping your child safe, and that you are not going to try to dictate the menu for a special event they are planning. For example, you might offer to bring a supply of safe snacks for your own child and let your host know you are happy to prepare your child's meals while you are staying in their house, but ask if it's okay that other children don't eat peanut butter while you are visiting and that no nut products be served while you are there. When we visit my husband's family in Sydney, my young nieces still eat, drink and enjoy dairy, but my lovely sister-in-law has them eat it at the table, supervised, and washes their hands and faces as soon as they have finished eating, and then cleans the table.

If there are other school-aged children in the house, you might be surprised by how educated they are about food allergies (especially if they attend an allergy-aware school). When we were staying with my sister a couple of years ago, my nephew, who was 7 at the time, saw me walking out of the kitchen with a plastic cup of soy drink in my hand. He came running towards me, calling out, 'Aunty Ali, didn't Mum tell you? Noah can't drink milk.' When I told him it was soy drink, he said, 'Oh, okay then, he can have that.' He has a friend at school with peanut allergy and was used to looking out for her.

It is also helpful to appreciate that unless someone is living with a food allergy, they will be unfamiliar with the lengths you often need to go to for making food safe for your child. Offer your friends and family small pieces of information at a time and build on that, teaching them more at each get-together. Something that you take for granted about keeping your child safe may not even occur to others, not because they are thoughtless but just because they genuinely don't realise it poses a risk.

Importantly, always let your hosts know that you appreciate the extra effort they are taking to keep your child safe and included. A thank you note or leaving behind a small gift lets others know you really noticed all they did for your family while you were staying with them.

'Before a family ski holiday, my brother asked me to write something down [about Jess's food allergies] so everyone could understand it a bit better before we went. We produced a little brochure, which has a little photo of Jess on it, and it tells people this is Jess and explains what she is allergic to, what the potential reactions are, including information about anaphylaxis and how dangerous it can be … a typical menu of what she might eat in a day, a list of foods she can eat as well as a list of symptoms. People still ask for the brochure.'

—Merryn Gibbons (NSW), mother of Jessica (9), allergic to cow's milk, egg and peanut

Babysitters

The topic of babysitting is included in this chapter because it is important that parents get to enjoy socialising, too. Many parents can rely on family and friends for babysitting duties, but not everyone is so lucky. The thought of leaving a food-allergic child with a new babysitter can evoke anxiety, but once you meet and educate the right one, you will hopefully soon feel at ease and begin to enjoy some 'time out' every now and then. Following are some pointers on how to find and work with a babysitter.

- There are many babysitters available who already have experience in caring for children with food allergy. Some childcare workers with anaphylaxis training advertise for casual babysitting on babysitting websites or register with babysitting agencies, as do registered nurses and students studying health-related courses.
- A babysitter doesn't have to be experienced in managing food allergies, as long as they are willing to learn and are mature enough to cope with an emergency.
- Once you have found a babysitter, pay them to come over to play with your children for a few hours while you are at home. This way your children can get to know the babysitter, and you can begin to educate your babysitter about managing your child's food allergies. We did this a couple of times before we left Noah with our babysitter, so by the time we actually left him alone with her, he felt like he was hanging out with a friend, and we felt confident that she had a very good understanding of how we needed her to care for him.
- Run through your child's Action Plan, including the symptoms of an allergic reaction, and how and when to administer an EpiPen and any other medications prescribed for your child. An EpiPen trainer is a great way for you to demonstrate how to use the EpiPen and your babysitter will probably feel more comfortable being able to practise. (You should run through this information again before you go out for the first time.) Make sure your babysitter understands if they are ever in doubt about using the EpiPen, not to hesitate.
- If you are looking for a long-term relationship with a babysitter, consider paying for them to do an anaphylaxis training course. If you live in an area where this is impossible, consider ordering an educational DVD for your babysitter to watch. (Visit **www.allergyfacts.org.au**)
- Show the babysitter where you keep your child's medications and Action Plan.
- Show your babysitter where the phone is and how to call an ambulance (including your address, telephone number and the nearest cross street).

- Ideally, feed your child before you go out. If the babysitter needs to feed your child, leave prepared meals and snacks. When our babysitter first started, I used to leave out a basket of food and ask our babysitter to only offer Noah these foods while we were out, but now that we have known each other for years (and she has completed a training course on anaphylaxis) we are happy for her to be responsible for preparing food for Noah.

- Agree with your babysitter upon any special requests specific to your situation. For example, some parents don't feel comfortable with babysitters bringing any food into their 'safe' zone, while others don't mind as long as the babysitter understands they need to wash their hands thoroughly after eating. Whatever the case, make sure you communicate clearly so there are no misunderstandings.

- Some babysitters are used to bringing 'treats' for the children they care for. Ensure your babysitter understands that any treats need to be vetted by you before being offered to your child.

- Be sure to tell your babysitter all the usual things a parent should tell a babysitter: what time you expect to be home, ways in which your child likes to be comforted, any particular fears or habits they have, favourite books and toys, their bed time. Focus on the overall wellbeing of your child, not only food allergies.

- Before you go out, make sure your mobile phone is charged and on, and that the sitter has all your contact details. Remind your babysitter you are happy to be called if they have any questions.

Part 3

The emotions of food allergy

15

Resilience in children

There is no denying that food allergies present significant challenges for children and adolescents. They have to cope with daily vigilance, carrying medication at all times, not being able to enjoy eating everything their friends can, feeling 'different' from their peers at times when they may be longing for 'sameness' and, in some cases, the knowledge that they are at risk of a potentially life-threatening reaction.

In many research studies on food allergy, as well as media stories, there is a lot of interest in the anxiety and fears that can and do develop around the condition. This is certainly warranted — and anxiety in parents and children will be covered in the following chapters — however, it is also important for parents to acknowledge that all children in life face challenges (health-related or otherwise) and times of hardship, and some children are able to cope with whatever comes their way better than others.

What is it that enables some children, when faced with adversity, to negotiate a pathway through their problems, learn from their experiences and maintain a positive outlook? Psychologists believe that resilience may be the answer.

Resilience can be a complex concept and there is a wide range of psychological literature and books published on the subject. In this chapter we offer a simple overview of resilience, explain why it is important to be fostered in all children and then look at how the concept of resilience can be applied to children with food allergies.

The authors are grateful to Olivia Keene, psychologist and Clinic Director of Keene Insight Child and Adolescent Specialists, for contributing her time and knowledge in preparing information and reviewing the following three chapters in this book. Her positive outlook and enthusiasm combined with clinical experience and professional expertise was invaluable.

Resilience: what is it?

When parents hear the term 'resilience', they often simplify it to mean the ability to bounce back. However, to appreciate the importance of resilience — especially in the context of children — it needs to be understood on a much deeper level.

A widely cited and accepted research-based definition of resilience is:

'the human capacity to face, overcome and be strengthened by or even transformed by the adversities of life.'[1]

Resilience is not just about recovering from a setback. It also encompasses using challenges in life as reference points for growth, and attaining self-knowledge and confidence through the experience of adversity.

Olivia Keene explains: 'A child's core life experience is small to begin with and, as they grow and are allowed to experience challenges, they realise, "Okay, well I can do that," and every time they do this, their world becomes larger, and their ability to cope with challenges also improves. Over a period of time, this process internalises, so young people end up feeling, "No matter what comes my way, even though it might be really hard, I'm going to be able to deal with it."'

The concept of resilience is not new. Resilience came to the attention of researchers in the 1970s while studies were being undertaken to identify factors that place young adults 'at risk' of negative outcomes, for example, mental health problems and drug abuse. In the process, researchers discovered that some of the young people exposed to 'risk factors' were able to cope better than others. Researchers then turned their attention to identifying 'protective factors' that help young people to not only cope in the face of adversity, but learn from their experiences and succeed in life.

While initially the concept of resilience was almost stumbled upon, it has been widely researched and analysed ever since. Many studies have focused on resilience in children facing major adversity (for example, abuse, neglect and poverty); however, resilience is now universally seen as a factor for all children facing everyday difficulties, stress and problems.

When children do experience adversity, it is their parents who directly influence how they respond, meaning parents play a central role in developing resilience in their children. While various studies have identified a range of 'protective factors' that can promote the development of resilience in children, Olivia Keene says parents can help their children by understanding and encouraging the following three attributes:

1. 'Connectedness': a sense of belonging and being valued and supported by family, friends, school and the wider community. Parents need to support and encourage children to seek and participate in friendships, school activities, and family and community life.

2. Social and emotional competence: a child's ability to recognise, acknowledge and manage their emotions; display empathy — being willing and capable of reaching out to others; solve problems and talk things through positively, with a sense of optimism. Parents need to foster all of these skills in their children and lead by example. The more skilled a parent is in managing their own emotions, the more skilled the child is likely to become.

3. The presence of a 'charismatic' adult in the life of a child: a charismatic adult is someone who a child identifies as taking an active and genuine interest in them, and who is concerned about the child's development as a person. It may be a teacher or sporting coach, a relative or extended family member, but parents shouldn't force this relationship or try to choose someone for their child — a child needs to identify their own mentor. Parents just need to allow and support their child to have the relationship.

A resilient child feels supported by others, is socially competent, a good problem-solver, possesses positive self-esteem and a positive outlook about his or her future. Resilient young people see difficulties as challenges to overcome and as being points for growth and learning, rather than the world conspiring against them. Importantly, resilient children usually become resilient adults.

> # Emphasising the importance of 'protective factors'
>
> In very simple terms a 'risk factor' is a negative influence that can inhibit resilience, while a 'protective factor' is a positive influence that can foster and support resilience and help combat 'risk factors'. The presence of protective factors is far stronger in predicting resilience than the presence of risk factors. This is good news for parents, because by focusing on building protective factors (such as optimism, problem-solving skills, social and emotional skills and self-esteem) in a child's life, you will make a significant difference to the long-term strength and wellbeing of your child.

The role of resilience in children with food allergies

Resilience can be developed around all sorts of challenges in life, including food allergies. Children are not born with resilience, but rather the capacity to develop it. The way in which parents manage their child's food allergies can have a direct impact on the development of resilience in their child. At one end of the spectrum, if parents adopt a lax approach, children may be unconcerned by their allergies but also at risk of allergic reactions, while at the other end, if parents veer towards extreme vigilance, it can result in over-protected and even helpless children. Olivia Keene says parents need to aim for an even-handed approach.

'If parents set boundaries too tight, in terms of what is okay and what is not okay for a child to experience, the child's world will become smaller, because there is no room for growth. But if parents set the boundaries too loose, the child may end up feeling — and actually being — unsafe. In terms of promoting resilience, it is much better to have a balanced approach, where you have agreed boundaries with your child, as well as a consistent implementation of consequences if the boundaries are overstepped.

'One of the things that can get in the way of promoting resilience in these children is overprotective, or "helicopter", parents: this is where a parent is constantly over-focusing on everything that the child is doing. When this happens, the message a parent is unconsciously delivering to their child is that they are not going to be able to cope if the parent isn't there. One of the key factors in developing resilience is the experiential nature of it; so a child has to experience adversity and learn to cope with it to realise they *can* do it over time, and their confidence increases with practice.'

A practical example to consider is a parent who demands that their child's multiple allergens are banned at their primary school. In doing so, the parent is trying to control their child's environment, rather than supporting their child in adapting to a new environment. While the intentions of the parent might be admirable — wanting to protect their child — it is not going to help their child develop resilience. Instead, the parent is creating the illusion that the 'problem' of food allergy at school has been 'fixed' for them.

'A "learned helplessness" cycle can be accidentally reinforced by parents,' says Olivia Keene. 'This can be remedied by identifying all the ways that the child can help themselves. It is the ability to take action that allows the child to adapt to difficult situations and this is an important factor in the development of resilience.'

To promote resilience in children with food allergies, parents have to balance the need for their children to be protected, depending on the age of the child, with the fact that the child has to be exposed to adversity in order to develop confidence in managing their condition. This doesn't mean parents should ever consider not putting risk-minimisation strategies in place to avoid allergic reactions or stop carrying emergency medication. Rather, the ideal is to support children to directly experience challenges *around* their food allergies.

Take the example of a school-age child with multiple food allergies being invited to a birthday party. In one scenario, the parents won't allow their child to attend the party unless their child's allergens are not going to be present in any form; they also insist on staying with the child at the party. By taking this approach, the parents are trying to control an environment (which isn't possible), the child is being prevented from learning to take responsibility for their allergy, and denied the opportunity to create a sense of belonging with friends. The child is also being given an underlying message that other friends and adults cannot be trusted to care for them.

In another scenario, the parents take an entirely different approach. While sharing in their child's excitement about the party they also remind their child the foods on offer won't be safe so they will need to take their own food, and remember not to share food with their friends. The parents would still put usual risk-minimisation strategies in place; for example, calling the hosting parents of the party and explaining their child's allergies and ensuring the host is prepared to be educated in taking responsibility for their child's emergency medication. The parents drop the child at the party, checking the host knows how to contact them, and then visit friends in the area to make sure they are nearby if a reaction happens. When the child attends the party under these circumstances, they are learning to experience social challenges around their allergy — that they can't eat the same foods as everyone else, that they can't enjoy a slice of the special birthday cake — but they also realise, through experience, that this is not the end of the world and they can still enjoy other aspects of the party, such as a sense of belonging. They also learn that other parents and other children can be trusted to take care of them, and that their own parents trust them to think for themselves. They learn to ask others questions: 'Does this food contain nuts?', for example, and speak for themselves, 'No thanks, I can't have that. I have my own treat bag.' The child is not only learning from birthday party experiences, but also growing in confidence, and at each social situation they attend they will learn that missing out on some foods is sometimes hard, but they can deal with that. They also understand they can have an allergic reaction at any time, but their medication and caring adults are there for them if they need help.

In working towards finding the right balance, aiming for your child to experience *gradual* exposure to challenging situations is often the most manageable pathway.

'With graduated exposure you are building the child and the family's ability to cope with different levels of stress and discomfort around the allergies,' says Olivia Keene. 'It is also helpful to look back afterwards and ask, "What did we do really well?", and reinforce the positive.'

Of course, with food allergy, mapping out how your child can be gradually exposed to challenges isn't always possible: sometimes adversity arrives in the form of a sudden and unexpected severe allergic reaction. If this happens, resilience can still be fostered from the experience itself.

For example, after a reaction, parents can talk to their child about what they did well during the reaction. Did your child tell you or another adult when they were feeling unwell? Did they communicate their symptoms clearly? Did they stay calm? Did they lie down when they were asked to do so? From a resilience point of view, reinforcing to your child the internal strength they displayed during an allergic reaction gives them the confidence to know that if it does happen again, even though they might feel frightened and it will be really difficult, they do have the ability to get through it.

'As a parent, it is helpful to reinforce the positives in regard to your child's ability to cope with a reaction, rather than living in fear of a reaction,' Olivia Keene explains. 'Anxiety in a child can stem from feeling as though an allergic reaction is going to be completely out of their control, so helping them understand that they do have control over their internal strength, can help.'

A resilient child is not immune from adversity and stress, but is well equipped with skills to adapt, cope and grow from their experiences. In regard to food allergy specifically, a resilient child is able to self-manage their condition and accept it with an educated and positive outlook — something all parents of food-allergic children hope for.

If you are interested in reading more on the subject of developing resilience in children, the following reference is recommended as an inspiring starting point:

A Guide to Promoting Resilience in Children: Strengthening the Human Spirit, Edith H. Grotberg, 1995. The International Resilience Project, from the Early Childhood Development: Practice and Reflections series, Bernard Van Leer Foundation.

This publication can be accessed at: **www.resilnet.uiuc.edu**, in the 'Virtual Library' section, along with other recommended publications related to resilience in children and families.

16

Anxiety in parents

Diagnosis of food allergy in a child can have a significant impact on the whole family — especially parents. It is very common for parents to experience a wide range of emotions about their child's food allergies, including: fear, anxiety, anger, grief and guilt, as well as hope and optimism. For many parents, however, anxiety is at the top of this list.

It is natural for parents of children with food allergy to experience anxiety, and anxiety levels will fluctuate over time. However, parents have to be aware of the extent of their anxiety and work towards ensuring they find a balance between reasonable levels of anxiety and a sense of normalcy in family life.

In this chapter, we look at why and when parents of children with food allergy may feel anxious, include an overview of common patterns of anxiety in association with the condition and refer to some research findings in relation to anxiety in parents of food-allergic children. We then offer some practical tips for parents to help manage their anxiety levels about food allergy.

In some cases, anxiety can become unmanageable, even debilitating, getting in the way of a family's everyday enjoyment of life. At the end of this chapter, we list some of the symptoms that may indicate professional help is needed and explain how parents can access professional help. We also describe post-traumatic stress disorder symptoms, which can occur in parents or children following anaphylaxis.

Why and when parents may feel anxious

If you consider the many ways in which managing food allergy impacts upon daily family life, it is little wonder that many parents report feeling anxious. Parents interviewed for this book were all asked to list the most significant ways in which their child's food allergy had affected their family's life. The most common responses included a range of both practical and emotional concerns:

- Fear of their child dying
- Guilt: many parents reported feeling as though they were somehow to blame for their child's food allergies
- Lack of understanding from friends and family members: many parents sense that they have been labelled 'neurotic' by others
- The time involved in food preparation, reading of labels and shopping
- Financial stress: the cost of specialist appointments, medications and specialty foods
- The constant struggle of trying to find a balance between keeping their child safe and still letting them enjoy normal childhood experiences
- Tension between parents over the management of their child's allergies
- Loss of spontaneity in family life
- Geographic isolation from specialist medical care
- The amount of time involved in preparing for social situations, for example, eating out, attending birthday parties
- Limitations on travel options
- The fact that it affects life *every* day; you can never let your guard down
- In some cases, ongoing trauma from having witnessed their child experience a life-threatening reaction

For anyone living with a food-allergic child, these responses won't come as a surprise. For others, however, it can be difficult to comprehend just how much goes on 'behind the scenes' to manage the condition, and the extent to which it can affect parents. To an outsider, a child with food allergies appears to be perfectly healthy and happy (which they are, for the most part); the condition, as described in a 2005 Canadian research study, is largely 'invisible'.[1] Children with food allergies are expected to function normally — and are capable of doing so. But if they are inadvertently exposed to their allergen, it can result in a medical emergency, where the child's life may be at risk. The *threat* of an allergic reaction is chronic, but the event of anaphylaxis is sudden and unpredictable.

A major cause of anxiety for many parents is the fact that medical science cannot yet determine with certainty which children with food allergies will or will not experience life-threatening reactions. The repercussions of labelling a child 'at risk' of anaphylaxis are significant. Statistically, there is only an extremely small chance a child with food allergy will suffer a fatal reaction but statistics offer little comfort to parents. A parent's fear of what *could* happen to their child is often what remains foremost in their mind. An article recently published on the uncertainty of childhood food anaphylaxis contains a pertinent observation: 'Threats to the safety of children activate deep-seated fears and intensify perceptions of risk.'[2, 3]

While fatalities from food-related anaphylaxis are rare, medical literature reports that 90 per cent of deaths from food-related anaphylaxis are preventable,[4] meaning parents are also weighed down by the responsibility of avoiding a preventable, but at the same time unpredictable, life-threatening reaction.

To Oliva Keene, a parent experiencing fear about the potential severity of their child's allergic reactions fits with the definition of anxiety. 'Anxiety is about the brain going forward in time in a negative way. So parents can project a possible situation forward in time, for example, an allergic reaction, but experience it emotionally as if it is real and happening now.'

Anxiety levels in parents vary significantly. Some already have a predisposition to anxiety (courtesy of genetics or life experiences), or are perhaps worriers or perfectionists by nature, and a diagnosis of food allergy in their child will add another layer to their existing anxiety levels. Other parents are quite 'laid back', taking a diagnosis of food allergy in their stride, treating it as a challenge they will approach with a 'can do' attitude and, consequently, experience minimal anxiety. Many others (myself included), sit somewhere in the middle, determined to approach their child's allergies with a positive attitude, trying hard not to over-focus on the allergies, but at certain times becoming anxious about the challenges the condition presents.

Anxiety associated with food allergies is often cyclical in nature (conforming to a pattern of behaviour that has been defined in studies of families coping with chronic illness).[5, 6] With the initial diagnosis, there tends to be a peak in anxiety, as parents question what it means. As families come to terms with the diagnosis, researching and learning more about the condition, they adapt to a new way of life and their anxiety levels even out. The anxiety is then likely to peak again under certain circumstances: for example, an allergic reaction; a period of change, such as a child starting school or going on their first camp; or a child being diagnosed with an additional medical condition, for instance asthma. The family then needs to adapt to that change or learn from that challenge in order for their anxiety levels to again stabilise.

While this pattern of anxiety is to be expected, the authors of a recently published paper, 'Addressing the psychological needs of families of food-allergic children' in *Current Allergy and Asthma Reports*,[7] observe that some families find it impossible to re-stabilise their anxiety levels, and consequently remain in a highly anxious state. When this happens, sometimes driven by a distorted perception of the real dangers faced by the food-allergic child, it can lead to extreme vigilance, and the restricting of normal child and family activities in an attempt to protect the child. This can then have a negative impact on the child's normal growth and development. The authors refer to this as an 'overresponding' pattern of adaptation.

Parents of food-allergic children interviewed for this book commonly reported a swinging pattern in regard to their anxiety, describing their family as moving backwards and forwards between a 'crisis' and 'non-crisis' mode of operating (this pattern has also been previously identified in studies of families coping with chronic illness).[8, 9]

Olivia Keene confirms that a pattern of swinging emotions is to be expected. 'The swing, initially, while a family is adapting to a diagnosis, is going to be quite strong, and then it will slow over a period of time.

It will depend on how resilient a family has been in the past over other events, too; predisposing factors will affect how a family will adapt, and how they integrate food allergies and the associated risks into their life. The swinging reflects the level of impact the allergies have on the family, so as a family becomes more used to coping and adapting, the force of the swing is going to be reduced. You are always going to get a bit of a swing, but in life that is true for anyone.'

From my own research, it seems likely that anxiety levels can also be influenced by how and when the condition is diagnosed. Parents who are introduced to food allergy by watching their child suffer an unexpected life-threatening reaction aren't given the opportunity to research the condition and adapt to a diagnosis, but rather are thrust into the peak of anxiety without warning or context.

Trauma from witnessing a child experience anaphylaxis — whether before or after medical diagnosis — may also impact on a parent's ability to manage their anxiety, either negatively or positively. In one interview, a mother who had witnessed her child experience anaphylaxis on countless occasions reported that she was now better able to manage her anxiety because, through experience, her son and family have realised that they do have the ability to cope in an emergency. Some time ago, the teenager's specialist advised the parents that they needed to accept that their son would have reactions — that despite putting risk-minimisation strategies in place, they would never be able to prevent *every* reaction. This was really helpful advice, because it shifted their focus: instead of living in fear of anaphylaxis, the teen and his family (and friends) expect it will happen from time to time, and have equipped themselves with the skills, both practical and emotional, to be able to cope when it does.

Anxiety is not all bad: it can also play a protective role in managing food allergies.[10, 11] Anxiety motivates parents to seek medical help and appropriate information about how to manage their child's condition. It can also ensure parents remain vigilant in complying with the day-to-day tasks necessary to avoid their child experiencing an allergic reaction, for example, reading food labels, preparing safe meals, carrying an Action Plan and emergency medications.

A Canadian study in 2005 — *Anaphylaxis: How do you live with it?*[12]

— found that if anxiety levels fell to a low point, the level of vigilance in parents and children also dropped, meaning they were not always cautious enough about preventing a reaction or prepared to respond in the event of anaphylaxis. However, the study also found that when levels of anxiety were described by participants as 'extremely intense', the extent of the stress and fear they experienced was 'maladaptive'.

Parents need to aim at finding a balance between reasonable, and possibly helpful, levels of anxiety while still being able to enjoy normal family life. The authors of the above-mentioned study suggest that the 'Goldilocks principle' (acknowledged in the study as a borrowed term) be used — to refer to the level of anxiety that is 'just right' for a family's best possible adjustment to living with the risk of anaphylaxis.[13] (This psychosocial study is highly recommended reading: see Endnotes, page 382, for details.)

Finding the balance

Discovering the level of anxiety that is 'just right' for your family will take time, and will also be influenced by circumstances (for example, past experiences, current stresses and individual personalities). Below is a collection of ideas — based on a mixture of feedback from parents interviewed for this book, published literature, research and personal experience — to help keep anxiety about your child's food allergies at a manageable level.

1. Encourage shared ownership of your child's food allergy

When your child is diagnosed with a food allergy, view the diagnosis as an issue the whole family needs to be involved in. If everyone in the family feels they have a role to play, you can create a trusted support network in your own home. For example, if possible, ensure both parents attend appointments with your allergy specialist so both understand what is going to be involved in managing your child's allergy. If you are a single parent, consider taking someone else with you to the appointment who is closely involved in your child's life, such as a grandparent or family friend. Make time to educate your other children about food allergies and teach them age-appropriate responsibilities that can help. For example, they could learn what foods their brother or sister can and can't eat, and develop the habit of washing their hands and face after eating a food to which their sibling is allergic.

In our family, I carry the bulk of everyday responsibility for managing Noah's food allergies, but my husband also plays an important role. For example, we have agreed that when Noah and Lucy are both invited to the same birthday party, my husband and I both go, as it is too hard for me to watch the two of them and make sure Noah doesn't eat any unsafe foods. We book Noah's allergy review appointments a long way in advance and it goes in my husband's diary as a meeting that cannot be moved. When Noah started childcare last year, my husband and I went together to meet with the centre's director, cook and Noah's teacher. My husband and I have both done anaphylaxis training and education courses and I feel at ease when my husband takes our son on an outing without me. Having someone to share the responsibility with also enables either parent to take some much-needed 'time out' every now and then.

Once you have created a safe network at home, it can then feel more manageable to start educating others. In our case, we researched and found an anaphylaxis management course in the city where Noah's grandparents live and asked them if they would like to attend. Once educated by an external source, Noah's grandparents became 'champions of the cause', and their 'can do' attitude rubbed off on other family members. From grandparents, we went on to educate aunties, uncles, cousins and family friends. Nearly all have been supportive and want to help, but it has happened gradually.

Educating others is an ongoing job, but in the very beginning, start in your own home: with the help of other close family members, you will gain confidence to increase your support network.

2. Be prepared — and organised

The risk of an allergic reaction can never be eliminated, and environments can never be controlled, but ensuring you put risk-minimisation strategies in place and are prepared in the event of a reaction can help parents to feel empowered and less anxious about managing their child's allergies.

Put aside some time to sit down and write a checklist of all the things you still need to do to manage your child's food allergies. If you are a list-maker by nature, you may even benefit from jotting down all the things you are already doing — you might be surprised by just how much you have achieved. The checklist you create can be reviewed and updated on a regular basis, as what needs to be done will change over time.

Transferring some of the worries from your mind to a piece of paper can be a useful outlet and prevent a 'backlog' of worries from developing. At our house, I have created a 'food allergy drawer' in our office space, where I keep my own checklist, copies of documentation from Noah's doctors, copies of information supplied to Noah's kindergarten, a copy of our kindergarten's anaphylaxis policy, information sheets from our specialist and dietitian, scripts for his eczema creams, our EpiPen trainer, my collection of Anaphylaxis Australia newsletters and anything else related to Noah's food allergies. I have found that in creating a small physical space devoted to food allergy, I am able to put firm boundaries around my 'worry time'.

When a new challenge arises, I set aside time to prepare for it and do so in our office. For example, I was feeling anxious in the lead-up to Noah starting kindergarten, so I made a checklist of all the things I needed to do before his first day. These included meeting with his teacher, ordering a new medic alert bracelet (he had just outgrown his), taking an updated photo for his Action Plan and so on. Just before Noah started kindergarten, I allocated more time to follow up everything on my checklist, again retreating to our office. In doing so, I felt a lot less anxious and, importantly, I didn't allow my worries to take over family time or space. I lessened my anxiety by being organised and prepared and was then able to focus on sharing in Noah's excitement about starting kindergarten (with worry being at the back of my mind instead of front and centre).

As parents, we can't control our child's allergies, but we can be in control of how the allergies are managed.

3. Communicate openly as a family
Often it is easier said than done, but in most situations in life where anxiety is involved, open communication can make an enormous

difference. When you are experiencing negative emotions, getting them out in the open is good for everyone around you; if you keep them to yourself, they will only magnify over time. For example, you might snap at your partner or child over an innocent comment such as, 'What's for dinner?', when what you really need to communicate is that you are feeling frustrated that you are the only one taking responsibility for everyone's meal preparation, which involves seemingly endless grocery shopping and reading of food labels. When you communicate your feelings and raise concerns early in the piece, it is much easier to discuss things calmly and look at finding solutions to worries rather than waiting until a situation reaches breaking point.

4. Become better at communicating about your child's allergies to others

Research confirms what many parents of food-allergic children will tell you: a lack of support and understanding from others about their child's food allergy is one of the biggest factors that can hinder a family's ability to cope.[14]

In some cases, parents have to accept that certain people will never understand food allergy because they just don't want to, but in many cases, others don't 'get it' because of the way the message is being communicated.

So how should a parent communicate their child's food allergies to others? Olivia Keene suggests that honesty is always the best policy, and if you are feeling anxious about your child's allergies, you should say so.

'It has been estimated that over 90 per cent of communication is non-verbal. So while a parent is communicating educational material about food allergy in a verbal way, all the non-verbal communication (for example, body language and the tone, pace and volume of their voice) is around their anxiety. Other people — including the child, teachers and other parents — don't know how to handle that, because the parent's anxiety is being pushed towards them. And they are thinking, "Wow, what do I do with all of this?" So they might then label you: "You're neurotic."

'It helps if parents can have the awareness to label their anxiety before that happens. For example, they might say, "This has been traumatic because Tom did go through a severe reaction, and we're still coming to terms with that. And the best way you can support us, while we are still quite anxious, is to [do X, Y and Z] …" So name your anxiety and give people around you the opportunity to support you, without getting egos or who's "right or wrong" involved.'

Olivia Keene also points out that people's concern over 'getting it wrong' when a food-allergic child is in their care can further contribute to an overall atmosphere of fear and lead to an increase in isolation for a child with food allergies.

'Many "non-allergy" parents and teachers may hold back from offering additional support to children with food allergies due to fear of doing the wrong thing. This then continues the contagious nature of anxiety. Reassuring others that you know they will do their best and you appreciate their support increases the likelihood that they will be confident to offer help in the future.'

My husband and I have learned that when we offer information to others, starting with small bits of simple information works best. Once people become interested and, importantly, *unafraid* of your child's allergy, they are often keen to learn more. Also, keep your expectations of others realistic: if parents of food-allergic children make it too complicated or taxing for family and friends to help, their requests won't be heard.

5. Find answers to your questions

Sometimes anxiety can stem from not having enough or correct information. When Noah was first diagnosed with food allergies as an infant, every time he had a touch reaction — usually hives from others kissing him or forgetting to wash their hands before giving him a cuddle — I was worried that he was at risk of a serious reaction. The presence of hives was enough to unnerve me. However, once I talked to our specialist about the issue I felt much better. He referred me to a study that had been done on the relevance of casual skin contact with peanut butter and the risk of severe allergic reactions. Once I understood that it was extremely unlikely Noah would experience anaphylaxis from touching an allergen, I felt far less anxious. (More about touch reactions can be found on page 71.) This was in the very early days of Noah's diagnosis, and I had much to learn. Since this time, Noah has had countless bouts of hives, most of which have been in response to 'invisible' or trace allergens on surfaces — for example, crawling on carpet in a holiday apartment, playing on climbing equipment at the park, sitting at a seemingly clean café table. We now expect that these skin reactions will happen from time to time and we focus on being prepared to deal with them when they do (by always carrying his medications as well as wipes). I no longer expect a skin reaction will be anything more than a skin reaction if he has not ingested his allergen, and this makes a big difference to my anxiety levels.

If you are concerned or fearful about any aspect of your child's food allergies, always seek clarification from your child's GP or allergy specialist to ensure the information you receive is accurate and specific to your child's allergies.

6. Schedule medical appointments in advance of predictable periods of change

Some periods of increased anxiety are predictable, for example, when a child is starting childcare, school or high school, or your child is nearing an age where they want to start going out with their friends on their own. While a certain level of anxiety is inevitable and, as we have already mentioned, even helpful, ensuring you have access to accurate and timely information in advance of developmental milestones can help keep anxiety at a manageable level.

We have scheduled Noah's next appointment with our allergy specialist for 3 months before he starts school. Having access to our specialist at this time will ensure we have the opportunity to request any paperwork we may need, including an up-to-date signed Action Plan, a review of any new medical conditions that may have developed, and also allow time for a food challenge before school if — fingers crossed — any of his skin prick test results suggest he may have outgrown an allergen by then.

This appointment won't eliminate our anxiety, but it will help, because we can talk to our doctor about any specific worries we have by then, and ensure all the medical information I hand over to Noah's new school will be up to date.

7. Ask yourself, 'What am I feeling anxious about?'

When you are feeling anxious about a particular situation, it can be helpful to ask yourself, 'What am I feeling anxious about?'

In some cases, anxiety is a result of a parent not taking care of something they need to address. For example, if your child has recently started school and you have not made an appointment to discuss your child's allergies with the teacher, your anxiety is probably warranted. In this case, anxiety is playing a helpful role, motivating you to phone your child's teacher and make an appointment to discuss how your child's allergy will be managed.

Another example is preparing for your child to go on a school camp. Perhaps you have run through all the safety precautions with your child's teacher but you are still feeling anxious because you have no idea who will be preparing your child's meals and how knowledgeable they are about food allergies. Again, anxiety is warranted, and may motivate you to call the camp caterers.

Questioning and understanding the trigger for an increase in anxiety is especially helpful. In these examples, anxiety is playing a 'protective role', motivating a parent to take appropriate action. In taking action, the parent is often minimising the risk of their child experiencing an allergic reaction and lessening their anxiety in the process.

Olivia Keene also suggests parents try using a useful tool she calls the 'mind whiteboard'. If you are lying awake in bed at night feeling anxious and unable to sleep, try picturing a whiteboard in your mind. On your 'whiteboard', list three of the things you are worried about. Then go through each item, one at a time, and think of a practical solution to resolve each concern. For example, a worry might be: 'I'm anxious about my daughter going to a birthday party on the weekend.' The solution might be: 'Tomorrow I am going to call the host of the party and talk to her about my daughter's food allergies.' Each time you come up with a solution, wipe the problem off your whiteboard. It sounds simple because it is. The process of taking action, or at least taking a step towards resolving a worry, will increase your sense of empowerment and decrease your anxiety — and hopefully means you will also get a good night's sleep.

8. Keep your child's allergies in perspective and be positive

While it is impossible to take the emotion out of statistics, it is still important to remember that the majority of allergic reactions to food are mild. And while the rate of food-related anaphylaxis appears to be increasing,[15] fatalities remain rare,[16, 17] suggesting that current education around risk-minimisation strategies and emergency treatment of anaphylaxis is proving effective.

Remember that thousands of Australian children with food allergies safely go to childcare and school every day, enjoy birthday parties, travelling and eating out. Food allergies can be successfully managed.

Adopting a positive attitude has been associated with parents feeling empowered in managing food allergy. According to one study, a positive attitude 'translated into a lack of self-pity, an emphasis on coping and agency rather than deprivation or anxiety, and striving for an optimal balance between vigilance and normal daily living'.[18] In simple terms, parents with positive attitudes had lower levels of anxiety.

Most parents are acutely aware of the challenges food allergy has presented their family, but has it also provided any opportunities or gifts? For example, we have a great relationship with our GP thanks to Noah's numerous food-allergy and eczema-related consults; Noah has an excellent diet and is a good eater thanks to helpful information from a paediatric dietitian; I now enjoy cooking and am much better at it; our whole family eats more healthily since his diagnosis; we have a closer relationship with staff at his kindergarten than we otherwise might have had; I have had the opportunity to meet positive and inspiring people since joining Anaphylaxis Australia. Acknowledging what you have been able to gain out of a challenging situation can also help in maintaining a positive outlook.

Many parents interviewed for this book acknowledged positive side effects of their child having food allergies, including healthy eating habits (in some cases) as well as their child being independent, resilient and possessing social skills and confidence. While no parent would ever wish for their child to have a food allergy, it can help to see the 'up' side.

9. Take time out on a regular basis

Parenthood is one of the most exhilarating experiences in life, but also one of the most exhausting. A large part of parenting is about giving, and making time for you to give back to yourself is essential.

Many parents of children with food allergies spend so much time managing their children's health that their own can start to suffer, especially during periods of increased stress. Making time for yourself — during which you don't have to think about food allergies or the needs of anyone else but you — is important in managing stress.

Arrange for your children to be cared for by a trusted minder — your partner, relatives, friends, a babysitter — and book in a massage, exercise, meditation, dinner out with friends, a movie or whatever it is that makes you feel relaxed and happy.

Don't view time out as an indulgence; it's a necessity. When parents are feeling rested and renewed from their own form of time out everyone in the family benefits.

10. Join an education and support group

When a child has just been diagnosed with food allergy, you can feel very alone, especially if friends and family have not yet been educated in how to offer support and understanding. Joining an education and support group, such as Anaphylaxis Australia — **www.allergyfacts.org.au** — can help you to cope and develop a positive outlook.

Joining a support group does not mean you will sit in a circle and talk about what is wrong with your child and your life: in fact, quite the opposite. Joining a support group offers you the opportunity to meet other parents who are facing similar challenges. A support group can reassure you that you are not alone and that many of the emotions you are experiencing are perfectly normal.

Belonging to a support group also means you can get involved in making a positive difference, for example, helping in food-allergy awareness campaigns and contributing to fundraising activities. Importantly, joining Anaphylaxis Australia also provides you with access to ongoing food-allergy education in the form of a fantastic printed newsletter, science-based information about research developments, food industry news, product recall alerts, access to education seminars and information evenings and reasonably priced education resources to help you with educating those involved in your child's life. Anaphylaxis Australia has members in all states and territories of Australia.

One caveat about *any* support group for food allergy should be offered. A recent research study of families with food-allergic children who were members of consumer support organisations reported that parents valued such organisations 'as sources of practical information and emotional support, but viewed advice which did not acknowledge their individual circumstances and heightened anxiety from contact with other anxious parents as being unhelpful'.[19]

What does this mean? Every family has different emotional needs and concerns and every child with food allergies must receive medical advice specific to their condition from their own specialist. If a member of a support organisation informally offers you advice or an opinion on food allergy based on their own experience, it may not be correct or it may not apply to your child.

Seeking professional help

While it is perfectly normal for parents of food-allergic children to experience a range of negative emotions, if you feel as though you are not coping, you may need to seek professional help.

In many cases, it takes a crisis before parents realise they need help, but it is preferable to get on top of things early. Many parents discover it is a relief to talk to someone else about their child's food allergy because they feel as though it has been overtaking all of their conversations with their partner and friends. Talking to a psychologist can 'free up some space' so parents can enjoy talking about other things with everyone else in their life.

Parents often wonder when they should seek outside help, but there is no simple answer. It is encouraging that just as more people are starting to visit their GP regularly to stay on top of their physical health, more people are also starting to visit psychologists to help manage stress and family problems. You do not have to reach breaking point before seeking help.

As a general rule, if your day-to-day functioning or enjoyment of life is being affected by your child's food allergies, you should consider professional help. In addition, Olivia Keene says the following signs can also indicate a parent may need to seek professional help:

- Withdrawal (social or emotional) from partner, family, friends and work colleagues
- Emotional symptoms (including anxiety, anger, sadness) that are interfering with your ability to function and participate fully in your life
- Changes in behaviour that are out of character for you
- If you are over-focusing or becoming obsessed with your child's issues or needs
- Experiencing difficulty in owning or expressing your own emotions as separate from your child's
- Disturbances in basic body functioning and body rhythms (eating, sleeping, frequent illness)

Visiting your GP is the ideal starting point for finding a psychologist — for you or your child. Psychologists train and specialise in different fields, and your GP will be able to refer you to a psychologist with experience relevant to your situation.

The Australian Psychological Society has a website where you can search for a registered psychologist by area of specialty and location. Visit **www.psychology.org.au**

Fees charged for consultations vary depending on individual practitioners; however, the Australian Psychological Society does publish a schedule of recommended fees on their website. Medicare and health insurance rebates are available for a range of psychological services, and these are also explained on the website.

Visit: **www.psychology.org.au/community/fees_rebates**

If you are worried about the cost of professional care, some psychologists do bulk bill (and are often linked with bulk-billing GP practices). In some cases, if patients are unable to afford the upfront fee, some psychologists allow patients to only pay the 'gap' between the cost of a consult and their Medicare rebate. Some psychologists also offer special rates for concession-card holders. Spacing out sessions over a longer period of time is also an option. Don't let financial stress deter you from seeking help; ask your GP to help you find appropriate *and* affordable care.

Other contacts to consider in accessing further help include your Maternal and Child Health Nurse or your child's school counsellor.

If you or your child are seeking immediate and urgent counselling, call:

Lifeline: 13 11 14

Kids help line: 1800 55 1800

If you are seeking an ambulance in a medical emergency, call 000.

Have you visited the MoodGYM?

MoodGYM is an interactive website developed by the Centre for Mental Health Research at the Australian National University. The website is designed to help users recognise and overcome problem emotions and provides information about how to develop good coping skills for the future.

The screening tests offered on the website can be helpful in identifying symptoms of depression and anxiety. (It should be noted, however, that the website is intended for information purposes only and is not intended as a substitute for diagnosis or treatment by an appropriate health professional.)

Visit: **www.moodgym.anu.edu.au**

Post-traumatic stress disorder symptoms following anaphylaxis

The symptoms of anaphylaxis are dramatic, and the event itself can be traumatic. In some cases, a post-traumatic response in either a parent or a child may follow anaphylaxis. A post-traumatic response is when someone experiences a prolonged reaction to a stressful event, and this continues to seriously disrupt their life.

Symptoms of post-traumatic stress disorder are associated with:

● Intrusive thoughts or memories about the event
● Avoidance (avoiding things that remind you of the event)
● High levels of arousal (for example, inability to sleep, anxiety)
● Symptoms of anxiety

Olivia Keene explains a common post-traumatic stress disorder symptom in parents in relation to anaphylaxis. 'What a parent is looking back on is: "I almost lost my child", so every time they are in an environment where their child may be exposed to their allergen, they are actually thinking back to that past experience. This means they are going to over-react, because they aren't reality-checking. For example, at a birthday party with their child, they might be going back in their mind to the traumatic experience of almost losing their child, when what is in front of their eyes is their child at a birthday party, not in a hospital bed. But their brain often doesn't know the difference, because their memory might be producing the same emotion or physiological arousal (heart racing, breathing fast, sweating) as if it was happening right then.'

Professional help is needed to overcome the symptoms of post-traumatic stress disorder, but it is treatable. If you think you or your child may be experiencing post-traumatic stress disorder symptoms, talk to your GP, who can assist you in accessing professional help and support.

17

Anxiety in children

It is normal for children with food allergies to experience varying levels of anxiety about their condition, including concern about being exposed to their allergen,[1] fear of an adverse reaction[2] and worry about eating away from home.[3] Anxiety levels in children with food allergies can be influenced by a wide range of factors, including their age, previous experiences of allergic reactions, level of education about their diagnosis and, importantly, the attitudes and behaviour of their parents.

As parents, we can't bullet-proof our children against anxiety. We can, however, play a pivotal role in influencing how they perceive their food allergies and — just as we need to do for ourselves — encourage them to find a balance between reasonable levels of anxiety and encouraging them to lead and enjoy a normal life.

In this chapter, we look at research findings about the quality of life of children with food allergies and then summarise how anxiety levels may vary at different stages of their development. Importantly, we also outline how the levels of anxiety experienced in children can be directly influenced by parents (both negatively and positively), and offer some practical tips for parents to help their children manage anxiety about food allergies. At the end of this chapter, we also list some of the symptoms in children and adolescents that may indicate professional help is needed.

Quality of life of children with food allergies

There is no doubt that the quality of life for a child with food allergies can be affected by their condition. Two recent studies have compared the quality of life of individuals managing food allergy with that of individuals dealing with other chronic medical conditions. One study, conducted in Canada in 2000,[4] reported that parents of peanut-allergic children detailed significantly more disruption in their daily activities and familial-social relations than parents of children with rheumatological disease.

Another study, conducted in Great Britain in 2003,[5] found that children with peanut allergy reported significantly higher anxiety about eating, especially when eating away from home, and about the possibility of an adverse reaction, than children with insulin-dependent diabetes. Overall, this study concluded that children with peanut allergy had a lower quality of life than children with diabetes — and quality of life appeared to be related to anxiety.

The news isn't all bad, however. Children with peanut allergy in the 2003 study did report feeling safe if they carried their emergency medications and were also positive about eating at familiar restaurants.[6] This is a really encouraging finding, because it implies that the better the condition is *managed* (through minimising risks, education and being prepared in the event of an allergic reaction), the better a child's emotional adjustment may be, resulting in lower levels of anxiety. The study also suggested that the anxiety experienced by children with peanut allergy may play a positive role, encouraging allergen avoidance and better compliance with emergency management plans.

Anxiety and fears at different stages of development

As with parents, the pattern of anxiety in older children can be cyclical (as described on page 316); however, a child's anxiety levels will also vary according to their cognitive, social and emotional development.

In infants and toddlers, food allergies are largely managed by parents and carers and, during these early years, they are not yet cognitively aware of the potential implications and severity of the condition. While young children can and do experience anxiety and fears, for example, separation anxiety or feeling scared when the household vacuum cleaner is switched on, they are not yet fully capable of consciously experiencing or taking ownership of anxiety about their food allergies. (Children of any age, however, may be affected by anxiety transferred from their parents: see pages 334–35 for more information.)

As children mature, their awareness about their condition increases as 'their emotional responses and self-management strategies evolve', according to one research study.[7] For example, my own son, at 4 years of age, now understands he has allergies because he has allergic reactions from time to time and is able to remember what they feel like; he understands that he often has to eat foods different from his friends at kindergarten and is conscious of his responsibilities, such as washing his hands before eating and asking adults if food is safe for him to eat. He also understands he needs to wear a special allergy alert bracelet to make sure others don't feed him the wrong foods, and he recognises that this makes him a little bit different from his friends. However, while he is increasingly learning more about his allergies and taking on responsibilities for managing them, he still has no concept that his allergies can be life-threatening.

According to the 2005 Canadian study referred to in the previous chapter, the anxiety and fears of children and parents in regard to food allergies are most intense between the ages of 6 and 11, when a child's independence and comprehension of the dangers steadily increase, but they do not yet have all the skills they need to effectively self-manage their condition.[8]

This finding is supported by another research study published in 2008, which reports that 'clinical experience suggests that an increase in anxiety develops in some children with food allergy at around age 7, as their cognitive development allows them to appreciate the possibility of serious reactions and as they move toward more independent functioning at school and with peers'.[9]

As children move into adolescence, it is well known that the risks associated with food allergy increase in line with teenagers developing autonomy and engaging in risk-taking behaviour.[10] However, fears and concerns about food allergies in the teenage years appear to change. One study found that while parents of teens considered fear of a fatal reaction in their child the most difficult issue, teens were primarily concerned about social isolation. The study concluded that teens may be at higher risk for fatal food-allergic reactions because they are impacted more by the social ramifications of their condition as opposed to *fear* of reactions.[11] (Food allergy in the teenage years is discussed in detail in Chapter 13, page 265.)

While more research is needed, it appears the level of anxiety experienced in relation to food allergy varies at different stages of development in children and adolescents, and that the fears and concerns they experience also shift significantly over time.

Anxious parents ... anxious children

While it is normal for children to feel anxious about their food allergies at different stages of their development, the levels of anxiety experienced can also be directly influenced by parents.

Children have a unique ability to both watch and feel whatever is going on in their environment. The behaviour and emotions of parents are constantly under surveillance by children: even if you think you are hiding an issue from them, their 'antennae' will usually detect that something is occurring beneath the surface. For example, if parents are experiencing relationship problems, children don't have to hear raised voices to understand that something is going on. They can tell by the interactions, or lack thereof, between Mum and Dad, that there is tension in the house.

In research studies, anxiety in children has been positively associated with anxiety in both mothers and fathers, and fearfulness in children has also been associated with mothers who express fears in front of their children.[12] What does this mean? Children learn by example.

Even though it may be unintentional, parents are constantly transmitting messages to their children about food allergy through their own attitudes and behaviour. Psychologist Olivia Keene explains how the culture parents allow to develop around food allergies will impact on how a child perceives their condition. 'If every time food allergy is mentioned, Mum and Dad are saying, "Arrrggghh" — communicating stress and anxiety — children will learn that this is the emotional response to food allergy. Likewise, if parents have normalised food allergy within their family's culture, this is what children will model their response upon.

'The more we can upskill parents to deal with anxiety the better because, on an emotional level, kids will take their cues from Mum and Dad, particularly in the early years.'

This doesn't mean parents have to conceal their anxiety, but it does mean taking responsibility for emotions rather than handballing them to the child.

'If parents are anxious about their child's food allergy, it helps if they can be open about owning their anxiety, rather than making it the young person's,' says Olivia Keene. 'For example, a parent might say to their child, "You had a reaction when you were young, your mouth was swollen and you were really unwell, and I felt really distressed. So when I think of you going to a party on your own, I feel a bit anxious about making sure that doesn't happen again." The child needs to be able to recognise that the anxiety belongs to the parent, not them.

'It is important for parents to use "I" statements as much as possible when talking about their emotions in the family. If you have a feeling, accept that it is yours. Avoid saying, "You make me feel ..." as this unwittingly makes your child (or your partner) responsible for your emotions. Taking ownership of emotions is very empowering, because as soon as you are able to own a feeling you then have the potential to change it.'

Children don't need to be protected from their parents' emotions. In fact, when a parent labels an emotion and takes ownership of it, they are teaching their child that they can do the same thing.

'Parents can teach their children by example how to regulate emotions,' says Olivia Keene. 'This is fantastic, because it can help to restore balance — by making it clear which emotions belong to which family member.'

As parents, we need to understand and accept that anxiety is contagious and then work hard to separate the emotions of our family members. Which emotions actually belong to us and which emotions belong to our child? If we can label and accept responsibility for our anxiety, it means our children then only have to be responsible for theirs.

Anxiety or behaviour problems?

It is not uncommon for a parent to jump to the conclusion that behavioural problems in their child are linked to anxiety about food allergy, especially in younger children. Yet this is not always the case. In her work as a psychologist, Olivia Keene has observed that more often than not children with food allergies turn out to be experiencing garden-variety behaviour issues for all sorts of reasons.

'An example is a parent who reports that their child is only eating one food; so the child is excluding everything else from their diet. The parent may tell us this is a result of their child feeling severely anxious about the allergy. But when the child presents to us, we see tantruming, acting out, fighting or other behaviour which is not actually anxiety.

'What can happen is that when there is so much focus on what food a child can and can't have, the child will dig their heels in and potentially take over the whole family with their behaviour. Sometimes parents will tiptoe around behavioural issues because they think it is about anxiety and don't want to put into place consequences for what they think is anxiety.'

In these circumstances, Olivia Keene says, it is essential for parents to re-establish normal patterns of parenting.

'If there is an issue that a parent or child is anxious about, that tends to be what parents will focus on. The more attention a parent gives the issue, in this case food allergy, the bigger it will become. And while the parent is focusing on food allergy, they may not be doing normal parenting. For example, if a child is tantruming, a parent shouldn't be afraid to let the child know that the tantrum is not okay, and there is a consequence. If a child is worried about something, that is okay, but the behaviour itself is not. Parents need to work out: what is about the food allergy, what is about the parents' own anxiety, what is about the child's anxiety — and then, finally, what are the actual behaviours that have developed around all of these factors? Parents then need to re-implement appropriate parenting.

'A lot of the feedback we receive from parents is, "Oh, thank God," as if they have been waiting for someone to give them permission to run the household like a normal family, to separate issues and put appropriate boundaries in place. They are also relieved to discover lots of parents have children who are a bit under-confident at school, or fussy eaters, and it's not always directly related to food allergy.'

While parents can't control their child's allergies, they *do* have control over their parenting skills. Realising this can bring a sense of relief and help restore balance to family life.

Helping your children find a balance

The goal for children in dealing with anxiety about food allergies is the same as it is for their parents: to find a balance between manageable (and possibly even helpful) levels of anxiety and a sense of normalcy.

The emotional needs of children coping with food allergies will vary, and what works for some families may not necessarily work for others. Below is a collection of ideas — based on a mixture of feedback from parents interviewed for this book, published literature, research and personal experience — to consider in supporting your child to find the balance that is 'just right' for them.

1. Educate your child about how to manage their food allergies

As mentioned at the beginning of this chapter, the better the condition of food allergy is managed, the better a child's emotional adjustment may be, resulting in lower levels of anxiety. The key to successfully managing food allergies is education.

Educate your child about how to manage their allergies: teach them to understand what foods they can and can't eat, how to interpret food labels, how to communicate their food allergies to others, and to carry their Action Plan and medical kit at all times, as well as all the other practical measures relevant to your child's diagnosis.

Understand that educating your child about their allergies is an ongoing commitment. Make time to talk to your child about their allergies on a regular basis, offering age-appropriate information combined with reassurance. For example, after the initial diagnosis (if your child is old enough to understand), explain what their allergy means but also tell them what your family will do to keep them safe.

As you continue to educate your child, give careful consideration to the way in which you communicate new information. Wherever possible, set aside time to discuss new issues in a positive and calm manner rather than talking about food allergies at every opportunity. For example, if your child is going on their first school camp, make time to talk to your child on their own. Let them know what they will need to do to stay safe, but also reassure them by outlining the steps you have taken to support them while on camp, such as talking to their teacher and calling the caterers. Having a detailed but calm conversation also offers the opportunity for your child to ask questions and tell you if they have any worries.

Providing children with education in a positive manner, combined with support, will go a long way towards alleviating any fears or anxiety they may be experiencing.

A range of age-appropriate education resources is available at **www. allergyfacts.org.au**

2. Encourage self-responsibility

Support your child from a young age to be involved in taking responsibility for their food allergies. As your child grows, increase their responsibilities so they can gradually develop the skills and confidence to be able to self-manage their allergies in the teenage years. If children feel involved in their allergy management, and confident they are prepared in the event of an allergic reaction, it can help to lessen anxiety levels.

According to Anne Muñoz-Furlong, co-founder of the Food Allergy and Anaphylaxis Network in the US, 'Empowering a child to participate in food-allergy management strategies will yield a confident child who is less likely to make mistakes or take unnecessary risks and who can rebound after an allergic reaction.'[13]

It is natural for parents to want to take care of their child, doing as much for them as they possibly can; however — as covered in Chapter

15, Resilience in children — children learn best through experience. Encourage young children to remember to wash their hands before eating and not to share food. When your child can read, ask them to check labels and tell you whether or not a food is safe for them to eat. When you eat out, let your child talk to staff so they can practise communicating their allergies to others. Think about the ways in which you currently take responsibility for your child's food allergies and whether or not you can hand over, or at least share, some of these responsibilities with your child.

3. Ensure your child has access to accurate information about their diagnosis

It is just as important for children to have access to accurate information about their diagnosis as it is for their parents. Not having enough or correct information about their allergies can sometimes lead to a child's imagination taking over, resulting in anxiety.

A child's fears may be rational or perceived, but either way they will feel very real to the child. Your child needs support in the form of accurate, age-appropriate information. For example, children need to understand that simply being in the same room as their allergen does not mean they are going to have an allergic reaction. Likewise, if they have skin contact with their allergen, they may experience a local reaction, but as long as they don't ingest their allergen, there is no need to panic and expect that a life-threatening reaction is about to take place (see 'Touch reactions', page 71).

Olivia Keene encourages parents to understand that the age of their child should influence how much information they are offered in regard to their food allergies. 'If parents give a really young child too much information about their allergy they are not going to understand it, and it may even frighten them. With adolescents, their ability to put information together is obviously a lot higher. Parents need to strike a balance of giving children of any age factual information, but not overdoing it; parents can't expect children to have the same thirst for knowledge about food allergies that they might have. Most children need to know how food allergies will affect them in the here and now. In simple terms, this means understanding: what to do to avoid a reaction, how to recognise the symptoms of an allergic reaction and what to do if they think they are having an allergic reaction.'

If you notice your child seems overly anxious about a particular aspect of their allergy, talk to your child and try to identify their concerns. Once you understand what is bothering them, you can then help them to access the information they need to keep their allergy in perspective.

Involving a neutral party to provide the information needed — especially in older children — can also help, for example, your GP, allergy specialist or paediatric dietitian (if concerns are related to diet or eating behaviours).

4. Foster an ongoing relationship between your child and their allergy specialist

A positive relationship between a doctor and a child can often go a long way towards decreasing a child's fear and anxiety about their condition. Our allergy specialist began directing questions to Noah from the age of 2, and we understand it is our role to let Noah respond, even though our natural urge is to jump in with adult answers.

Over the past few years, even though Noah dislikes his skin prick test, he has not been fearful of our specialist and likes seeing him. By encouraging a positive relationship in these early years, we hope Noah will feel at ease in asking his doctor questions or telling him anything he feels anxious about when he is older. Our allergy specialist has a very positive and pragmatic approach to managing Noah's food allergies, and each visit is an education opportunity for Noah, reinforcing to him that his allergies are being well managed and that he will hopefully outgrow at least some of them when he is a 'big lad'.

Of course, parents still need to have adult conversations with their child's allergy specialist and ensure their questions and concerns are addressed, but make a conscious effort to allow your child to have some air-time, too.

5. Acknowledge the uncertainty surrounding food allergy

Children need to understand that uncertainty is part of food allergy and that no one can 'fix it' for them. Avoid offering blanket and unrealistic statements to children, for example, 'It's going to be okay' or 'You'll be fine', because as parents, we can't always guarantee this is going to be the case. If unrealistic expectations are established and the child then experiences an allergic reaction, it may result in a breakdown in trust, with the child becoming anxious about future reactions.

'Parents need to acknowledge the uncertainty surrounding their child's allergy and work on reaching a point where the family and the child can cope with this,' explains Olivia Keene. 'For example, a parent might say to their child: "We don't always know when an allergic reaction will happen, but when it happened last time, we had a plan in place; you remembered to stay calm and you coped really well."'

Children can learn to deal with the uncertainty of food allergy if they are reassured that there is a plan in place for when things go wrong, and are encouraged to understand that they have the internal strength to cope with whatever comes their way. (Also see Chapter 15, Resilience in children, page 306.)

6. Don't let allergies define a child's life

Food allergies represent only one component of your child's life and you need to make sure there is room for everything else. If parents place too much attention on a child's allergies, the significance will be magnified and the child may be left with the distorted perception that food allergies define their life. Over time, this can lead to a child resenting their food allergies or feeling anxious about the restrictions the condition has placed on their life.

Children need to be educated about their allergies, but the subject doesn't have to be emphasised at every opportunity. Olivia Keene recommends parents put boundaries in place to ensure 'allergy time' does not hijack childhood activities.

'Once a family has a plan in place for managing their child's allergies, they need to put boundaries around this. For example, if there is a medical appointment coming up, or issues that need to be addressed, make one particular time where the matters are reviewed and discussed. Don't let food allergies swamp family time that could be spent doing other things. Ensure a range of activities are happening in the family environment rather than over-focusing on the allergy.'

7. Participation and inclusion

Social isolation has been identified by adolescents as the most difficult aspect of food allergy.[14] One of the best ways for a child with food allergies to believe that they can lead a normal life is by parents allowing them to do just that. This means children being encouraged to participate and enjoy regular family and childhood activities.

Previous chapters detail lots of practical suggestions on how children with food allergies can be included in all sorts of activities and social events. Parents need to plan ahead and be creative, not only to allow attendance but to also ensure inclusion.

If children understand that food allergies don't have to stop them from enjoying life they are less likely to feel resentful of their allergies and more likely to adopt a positive outlook.

As discussed in Chapter 15, Resilience in children, participation and inclusion in normal activities also enables children to encounter challenges in relation to their food allergies so they can learn how to cope with, and grow from, these experiences.

The role of allergy-friendly play groups

Allergy-friendly play groups can be a blessing, allowing parents to enjoy a supportive environment and enabling children with allergies to play independently. One study has confirmed that children with peanut allergy feel reassured by knowing other children experience the same problems as them.[15] However, they may not be a great fit for all children with food allergies.

Olivia Keene has found that in *some* cases, children feel as though parents are imposing friendships on them based on their food allergies: so rather than the friendship being about two children connecting and wanting to spend time together, it's about the parents feeling comfortable that their children can play at one another's houses. If the focus is on food allergy as opposed to friendship, it doesn't help to normalise allergies for the child.

This is not to say allergy-friendly play groups can't be wonderful, they can be — I love nothing better than play dates with a friend of ours whose children have food allergies; they provide a welcome break from worrying about Noah being exposed to his allergens — but parents need to be honest with themselves and their children about the reason for attending, and allow children to foster their own friendships in whatever environment they are in.

8. Remember, children are listening

Whenever you are talking about food allergies to anyone — friends, family, teachers, café staff — be conscious of the messages your child may be picking up on.

For example, if your child hears you criticising how their teacher is managing food allergies, or overhears you complaining about their teacher to others, your child may become anxious and interpret your criticism as meaning school is no longer a safe place for them to be.

If you are in a café where staff are not being helpful about catering for your child's needs, and you react with anger and create a scene, your child may take home the message that food allergies are embarrassing.

Another example many parents are probably guilty of (myself included) is venting to other parents at play group (or some other social situation) about how food allergies impact upon your life. If your child overhears your comments, they may worry that they are personally responsible for your anxiety.

It's normal for parents to want to vent and complain at times, but try not to do so when your child is within earshot. It is important to be honest with your children about their allergies, but you also need to filter some of your responses to ensure your child doesn't receive unintended messages.

9. Don't instil fear in your child or their carers about food allergies

Media coverage has raised awareness about food allergy and the associated risks, but to some extent it has also added to an atmosphere of fear and anxiety via headlines such as 'Danger at the dinner table', 'When food can be fatal', 'Bureaucrats ban peanut butter over deadly smell'. In an attempt to make others take your child's allergies seriously, it can be tempting at times to adopt a 'headline' approach, for example, 'My child will die if they eat egg.' While food allergies need to be taken seriously and can be life-threatening, telling others your child will die if they eat a certain food is only likely to frighten anyone who cares for your child. Fear can be paralysing, so others may then feel too afraid to take responsibility for your child.

Not for a second is this to suggest parents should conceal that their child is at risk of a life-threatening reaction, but be aware that whatever approach you adopt in educating others will dictate the response. If you attempt to educate through fear, you will create fear.

The same applies when educating children about their allergy. If a parent frequently tells their child, 'You will die if you eat peanuts', for example, their intentions may be good — wanting their child to take the condition seriously — but their child may become frightened and anxious, and develop a distorted perception of the real risk of a life-threatening reaction.

Be honest when you explain food allergies to your child and others, but don't employ scare tactics.

10. Model a positive attitude

'Can-do families create can-do children,' says Olivia Keene. If parents adopt a positive attitude about their child's food allergies, children will learn by example.

Focus on what your child *can* eat, how they *can* be included in social situations, and share with them information about positive developments in research into cures and treatments for food allergies. Also remember to give your child positive messages about their capacity to handle themselves around others. Reinforce their skills and strengths to encourage self-confidence and optimism about their ability to manage their allergies.

A positive attitude is a great defence against anxiety.

Seeking professional help for your child

It is normal for children to have temporary worries and fears. For instance many young children are afraid of the dark, strangers or thunderstorms; older children may feel stressed about upcoming school exams or social situations. However, when worries and fears are ongoing, seem out of proportion to the particular situation a child is fearful about, or interfere with a child's participation and enjoyment of life, professional help may be needed. If anxiety is ongoing and left untreated, it can become a chronic condition.

Olivia Keene says the following signs can also indicate a child or young person may need to seek professional help:

- Withdrawal (social or emotional) from family and friends
- Emotional symptoms (including anxiety, anger, sadness) that is interfering with their ability to function and participate fully in life (for example, missing school)
- Inability to enjoy things in life
- Changes in behaviour that are out of character for your child
- Disturbances in basic body functioning and body rhythms (eating, sleeping, frequent illness)

As detailed in Chapter 16, Anxiety in parents, visiting your GP is the ideal starting point for finding a psychologist. See pages 327–29 for more information on how to access professional help for your child.

If you or your child are seeking immediate and urgent counselling, call:

Lifeline: 13 11 14

Kids help line: 1800 55 1800

If you are seeking an ambulance in a medical emergency, call 000.

Siblings without food allergies

Siblings of food-allergic children can also feel affected by the condition. Siblings may feel resentful that allergies are taking up too much of their parents' time, or that the allergic child is receiving more than their fair share of attention, for example, in the form of home-made cakes and special time with parents around medical appointments. At times they may feel anxious that their sibling is at risk of or has suffered a serious allergic reaction and, in some cases, may think it's just not fair that they have to miss out on certain foods because their brother or sister has an allergy. In addition, if parents place too much responsibility onto a sibling for keeping their food-allergic brother or sister safe, the sibling may become anxious.

According to Olivia Keene, it is important that siblings are invited to play a balanced role in supporting their brother or sister in managing their allergy, and parents also need to ensure that the family does not over-focus on the allergy.

'It's helpful if the whole family can approach the allergies as a team. Allowing siblings to come up with their own ideas in how they can support their brother or sister is a good idea. It also comes back to the issue of balance: not making family time about allergies, and ensuring everyone in the family has a voice. If allergies are always being discussed over the dinner table it becomes energy-sapping and, indirectly, this says to the sibling that they have to be discussing the allergy in order to be heard.'

Some parents interviewed for this book said they make an effort to spend one-on-one time with all of their children to ensure each child feels special (sometimes taking their non-allergic children to a café or fast-food outlet and allowing them to eat whatever they want). In general, however, very few parents interviewed had encountered siblings of food-allergic children feeling adversely affected. In fact, many parents commented that in some ways the allergy was a positive for siblings, who had become especially empathetic and caring because of their brother or sister's allergies, and they enjoyed being charged with special responsibilities to help keep their brother or sister safe (for example, knowing how to dial '000' in an emergency, knowing what symptoms to look out for, washing their hands and faces after eating, remembering the EpiPen and reading food labels).

The 'why me?' question

Q My 6-year-old daughter is allergic to wheat and peanuts. Most of the time she is accepting of her allergies and not worried about having to eat different foods from her friends. This week, however, on our way home from school, she started crying and told me she hates her food allergies. 'Why did this happen to me?' she asked, and I don't know what to tell her.

A As children mature, they become increasingly aware of ways in which they are the same as or different from their friends. When a child becomes concerned about being different in some way, they are often in the process of trying to integrate this difference — in this case food allergy — into who they are as a person.

Olivia Keene says encouraging children to understand that it is normal for people to have all kinds of differences is important.

'Try to help your child identify other people who have to do things a little bit differently, too. So not just about allergies, but anything that might make someone different. For example, some people ride a bike to school, some are dropped off by their parents and others walk. Some kids wear red hats, others wear blue.

'Normalising and celebrating difference among children is really helpful in this situation. Exploring diversity and how all people are different can be done in a fun and powerful way through creative means, for example, storytelling, play and reading books. There are some great children's books available that focus on children who are different: exploring your child's own point of difference through a character in a story (third person), can make it easier for a child to then relate to their point of difference.'

Olivia Keene also recommends that, wherever possible, parents re-direct 'why' questions, which are often disabling — and endless — to more useful 'what', 'when', 'where' and 'how' questions, which tend to be active and enabling. In this situation, for instance, instead of answering your child's 'Why me?' question, you could redirect the question by asking her, '*What* do you find hardest about your food allergies?' You could then follow this with another active and enabling question, for example, '*What* do you think you could do differently that might make life a bit easier?' In this way, you are encouraging your daughter to begin finding her own solutions. If your daughter isn't sure about what she could do differently, offer some gentle coaching around possible strategies, but let your daughter decide which ideas she wants to put into action.

Children can ask the 'Why me?' question from a very young age. When Noah recently asked me, 'But why can't *I* drink cow's milk?' I responded by telling him that lots of people can't eat certain foods for all kinds of reasons. I reminded him that Nana can't eat gluten, Aunty Anita can't drink cow's milk and Daddy couldn't eat eggs when he was a boy but he can now. Inside Noah's head, at the age of 4, it seemed he was worrying all of a sudden that maybe he was the only one in the world not allowed to drink cow's milk (the only one of his allergens he seems to mind missing out on), and that wasn't fair. He was very happy to learn there were lots of people in the world who couldn't or didn't want to drink cow's milk and a whole lot of other foods.

When you talk to your daughter, try to establish if there is anything in particular she is angry or worried about in regard to her allergies — does she feel as though she is the only one in the world with an allergy, does she feel she is somehow to blame for her allergy, has someone been teasing her, did something happen at school on this particular day to trigger your daughter's response? If you can find out where your child's sudden sense of injustice is stemming from, it might also help you to respond.

While it is important to encourage your child to be open about her feelings and offer an understanding response, try not to react with pity, or encourage a 'poor me' attitude. Help your child to understand that food allergy is only one small component of her life.

Part 4

Food allergy in the future

18

Allergy prevention

Most parents who have a child with food allergy are desperate to know if there is anything they can do to prevent the condition from developing in their other children (or future children). Unfortunately, there are no black-and-white answers as yet.

The prevention of allergic disease, including food allergy, remains an active and exciting area of research. A broad range of studies has already been conducted, some producing very promising results, but there is still a long way to go before doctors can present any solid recommendations to parents.

Over the course of time, new research will probably continue to home in on emerging and changing trends in the development of allergic disease in children which, in turn, may change the thinking of doctors and scientists. This is all part of the process of eventually uncovering the right answers.

At the moment, doctors generally take the approach of sharing with parents the latest information based on current research. That way, parents can make decisions (in conjunction with their doctor) about allergy prevention strategies that are as informed as possible at the time, and *possibly* reduce the likelihood of their child developing allergic diseases — but there are no guarantees.

In this chapter, we outline factors that have been identified as placing a child 'at risk' of developing allergic diseases (such as asthma, eczema, hayfever and food allergies) and then provide an overview of current suggestions from the Australasian Society of Clinical Immunology and Allergy (ASCIA) worth considering to try to reduce the risk of allergic diseases developing in 'at risk' children. We also include a summary of other approaches to allergy prevention which have either been used in the past or are currently being researched but remain *unproven*.

In essence, the research shows that there are very few interventions that have been proven to prevent allergic disease. As such, many of the current recommendations regarding infant feeding are practical approaches to promote the general wellbeing of the mother and baby. Some earlier recommendations regarding the delayed introduction of solids have been removed because they are not based on conclusive scientific evidence.

Bear in mind that this chapter discusses strategies that may help to prevent allergic diseases, that is, to stop allergic disease from happening. If you suspect your child may already have a food allergy — or any allergic disease (for example, eczema) — you should see your doctor for advice specific to your child. The information in this chapter is *not* about treating allergic disease.

We would like to acknowledge the role of the Australasian Society of Clinical Immunology and Allergy (ASCIA) in providing the latest information on allergy prevention. Throughout this chapter, frequent reference is made to 'Primary Allergy Prevention in Children: Updated Summary of a Position Statement of the Australasian Society of Clinical Immunology and Allergy 2007',[1] and 'Allergy Prevention in Children' (2009).[2] We also provide a link to ASCIA's Infant Feeding Advice (see page 355). For more information, visit **www.allergy.org.au**

Risk factors for developing allergic disease

When scientists are conducting research into possible allergy prevention measures, they usually study families considered 'at risk' of developing allergic diseases. Two main factors have been identified as increasing the risk of allergic diseases developing:

- Genetic predisposition:[3] Any child can develop allergic disease; however, babies born into atopic families (so-called if a parent or sibling has a history of allergic disease) do have a greater risk of developing allergies
- Cigarette smoke:[4] Exposure to cigarette smoke increases the risk of respiratory symptoms

Suggestions which may be helpful in preventing the development of allergic diseases in children

As parents, we can't do anything to change the genetic risk of our children developing allergic diseases, but we may have some sway over a range of environmental factors.

Below we provide an overview of current suggestions from the Australasian Society of Clinical Immunology and Allergy[5, 6] that *may* help to reduce the risk of allergic diseases from developing in 'at-risk' children. Be aware that there is no guarantee that any steps taken will result in your child not developing an allergic disease. You should always discuss any questions or concerns in regard to allergy prevention with your allergy specialist. (Also see 'A very important reminder', page 360.)

- **Breastfeed for at least 6 months**
  Where possible, breastfeed your baby for at least 6 months. Breastfeeding *may* reduce the risk of allergic diseases in the early years of life; however, more research is needed to understand the protective role of breastfeeding in preventing allergic disease later in life.[7] Breastfeeding is suggested on the basis that it is known to have a range of beneficial effects in addition to any potential protection against allergy.

- **If not breastfeeding or if you are supplementing, use hydrolysed formulas**
  If you can't breastfeed your baby, or supplementary formula feeds are needed, partially hydrolysed formula (commonly referred to as 'Hypoallergenic' or 'HA' formula) is recommended over conventional cow's-milk based formula for the first 4–6 months of life.[8] Partially hydrolysed formulas have been shown to have protective effects in infants considered at high risk of developing allergic disease.[9] Check with your doctor if partially hydrolysed formula is suitable for your infant. Several brands of partially hydrolysed formula are available in supermarkets and pharmacies; they are usually labelled as 'hypoallergenic' and you do not need a prescription.

If your baby already has a medically diagnosed cow's milk allergy, then partially hydrolysed formula should *not* be used unless you have received specific medical advice that recommends this.

- **No smoking during pregnancy and do not expose children to cigarette smoke**

  Smoking during pregnancy impacts on the lung development of the child[10] and has also been linked with wheezing in early childhood.[11, 12] Do not smoke during pregnancy and do not expose your child to passive smoke, especially in confined spaces.

- **Introduce solid foods from 4–6 months of age**

  There is 'no current convincing evidence' to suggest that delaying the introduction of any solid foods beyond 4–6 months of age will protect against the development of allergic disease.[13, 14] (Also see page 356, 'Avoidance of potentially allergenic foods'.)

Infant feeding advice available from ASCIA

The Australasian Society of Clinical Immunology and Allergy (ASCIA) has recently released practical and helpful Infant Feeding Advice. The advice is relevant for all families, including those where other children have allergies; it is a brilliant resource for parents.

Visit: **www.allergy.org.au/content/view/350/287/**

Approaches to allergy prevention which remain unproven

Over the years, doctors and parents have tried all sorts of measures in the quest to prevent allergies. A range of these is discussed below. All of these remain unproven, although some are still being studied.

- **Mothers restricting diet during pregnancy**

  Excluding common allergens (for example, cow's milk, egg, peanut or seafood) from your diet during pregnancy is unlikely to reduce the risk of your child developing allergic disease.[15, 16] Dietary restrictions during pregnancy may have an adverse effect on the nutrition of the mother and baby,[17] and are not recommended.

- **Mothers restricting diet during breastfeeding**

  Restricting your diet while breastfeeding is not currently recommended as a measure for preventing the development of allergic disease.[18] However, if your baby does have atopic eczema and shows symptoms of being allergic, avoiding specific allergens while breastfeeding may, in some cases, reduce the severity of eczema.[19] Removing foods from your diet should only be done under medical supervision, so talk to your doctor about whether or not dietary restriction while breastfeeding is recommended. (Keep in mind that a lot of babies have eczema, and often it is not exacerbated by food.)

- **Avoidance of potentially allergenic foods**

  Doctors used to recommend avoidance of potentially allergenic foods, such as cow's milk and egg, until at least 12 months of age. It is now clear that there is no conclusive evidence to support delaying the introduction of these foods beyond 6 months.[20, 21]

  Research studies are currently examining whether early and regular exposure to common allergens may actually reduce the risk of allergic disease, including specific food allergies, from developing. (See 'Learning Early About Peanut Allergy [LEAP] Study, page 358.)

- **The use of probiotics in pregnancy and infants**

  There has been a range of studies looking at the role of probiotics ('good bacteria') in preventing the development of allergic disease, and the results have been varied.[22] Further studies are needed, looking at the strain of probiotic used as well as dosage and timing of administration.[23] The use of probiotics in preventing the development of allergic disease is not currently recommended.[24, 25]

- **The use of fish oils during pregnancy**

  Again, more studies are needed in this area. Currently there is no evidence that consuming fish oils during pregnancy will reduce the risk of allergic disease.[26]

- **Pet exposure**

  There is no evidence to suggest that removing pets from your home will reduce the risk of allergic disease from developing. In fact, some studies suggest that exposure to pets in the first year of life may even have a protective effect against some allergic diseases,[27] but more research is needed — so choosing to have a pet for the purpose of allergy prevention is not recommended either!

If your child already has an allergic disease and is allergic to your pet, then removing the pet may be helpful. Discuss this with your doctor before making any decisions.

● **Avoidance of house dust mite**

There is no compelling evidence to suggest that avoiding dust mite exposure either during pregnancy or infancy will reduce the risk of allergic diseases from developing.[28]

Immunotherapy for allergy prevention

Immunotherapy (or 'desensitisation') is currently used to treat medically diagnosed allergies to specific allergens, for example, dust mite, pollens and bee and wasp venom.

Immunotherapy involves introducing small and incrementally increasing doses of an allergen to the allergic patient with the aim of decreasing their sensitivity to the allergen over time.

Studies are now underway looking at the role of immunotherapy in reducing the risk of progressive allergic diseases from developing as well as trying to reduce the severity of allergic diseases. This is referred to as 'secondary prevention'. Early research findings suggest that using immunotherapy in children with hayfever may reduce the risk of asthma and new sensitivities from developing later in life.[29] This is a promising area of research.

Learning Early About Peanut Allergy (LEAP) Study

Until recently, it was thought that delaying the introduction of highly allergenic foods into the diets of 'at risk' infants may help in the prevention of allergy, and that even if that strategy failed, it would not do any harm. The reasoning was that giving an infant's immune system time to mature before exposing it to allergens might be beneficial and that exposure at a young age could cause allergic sensitisation.

Scientists now suspect that delaying the introduction of common allergens may have no impact on preventing the development of allergy. Furthermore, in order for the body to develop tolerance to an allergen, it may need to be exposed to it regularly during the early years of life. It is too soon for any advice to be offered to parents about early introduction of common allergens into the diets of 'at risk' infants; however, research is ongoing and will hopefully produce some very helpful results in the near future.

One study currently examining the best strategy to prevent peanut allergy in young children is the LEAP study in the UK. The LEAP study is looking at a large number of infants considered at high risk of developing peanut allergy, and they are adhering to either an avoidance or consumption strategy. Those in the avoidance group are avoiding the consumption of peanut-containing products until the age of 3, while those in the consumption group are consuming a peanut-containing snack three times a week. Scientists are aiming to determine whether avoidance or consumption works best in preventing peanut allergy by examining the proportion of children from each group who develop peanut allergy by the age of 5.

For more information, visit **www.leapstudy.co.uk**

Parental guilt about child's food allergy

Q My 18-month-old son has just been diagnosed with peanut allergy. I craved and ate peanut butter all through my pregnancy with him and feel so guilty I may have caused his peanut allergy. Am I to blame?

A You are definitely not to blame. Currently there is no evidence to suggest there is any risk of a child developing a peanut allergy if the mother eats peanuts or peanut-containing products during pregnancy. Likewise, there is no evidence to suggest a mother restricting her diet in any way during pregnancy reduces the risk of *any* allergic diseases.

The current position of the Australasian Society of Clinical Immunology and Allergy is that food avoidance during pregnancy and breastfeeding is not recommended[30, 31] and, in fact, restricting the diet of a mother-to-be can pose a risk of the mother and fetus missing out on appropriate nutritional requirements.

Maternal diet during pregnancy and breastfeeding is a common cause of guilt in many mothers of food-allergic children, and sometimes both parents feel guilty for passing on 'atopic' genes to their children. As a parent, we like to take responsibility for whatever happens to our child, but in the case of food allergies, no one is to blame, regardless of what food your child happens to be allergic to.

Remember that no one yet knows why food allergies are occurring or increasing, or how to prevent them. It may be helpful to talk openly to your partner about any feelings of guilt you are experiencing and really try to accept that no one is to blame. Try not to focus on why your child has a peanut allergy but rather how you can help your child manage his allergy and live as normal a life as possible. Talk to your doctor about your feelings if you need further reassurance or help, and consider joining a support group where you can share your thoughts and emotions with other parents in the same situation.

A very important reminder

A final reminder: there are no fail-proof recommendations, as yet, about how to prevent allergies from developing in your children.

Research into a wide range of areas about allergy prevention is ongoing, so information and recommendations for allergy prevention are likely to change. To keep up to date with the latest information on allergy prevention, visit the website of the Australasian Society of Clinical Immunology and Allergy at **www. allergy.org.au**

Always talk to your doctor before undertaking any allergy prevention strategies to ensure you receive up-to-date advice specific to your individual circumstances.

19

Future treatments

Treatment of food allergy is currently limited to strict avoidance of foods (and any other products) which contain an allergen, in addition to food-allergy sufferers and their carers becoming educated about how to recognise and treat an allergic reaction if it does occur through accidental exposure. In the future, however, it is hoped that a range of treatment options will become available. Future treatment options will probably be chosen on an individual basis, depending on the type and severity of the allergy.

The research around food allergy treatments and therapies is wide-ranging and promising. In this chapter we provide brief summaries of a select range only — the list of therapies included here is by no means exhaustive.

A word of warning: the therapies mentioned below, while exciting, are taking place in a research setting only and under strict medical supervision. None of these therapies are available in clinical practice to treat food allergy as yet.

Do not try to apply any of these therapies to your own child at home.

Potential therapies and cures

Immunotherapy

Immunotherapy ('desensitisation'), as described in the previous chapter on page 357, is currently used to treat medically diagnosed allergies to specific allergens, for example, dust mite, pollens and bee and wasp venom. Immunotherapy involves introducing small and incrementally increasing doses of an allergen to an allergic patient with the aim of building their tolerance to the allergen over time. Theoretically, this has the potential to cure the person of that allergy. The successful treatment of some types of allergic rhinitis (hayfever) has added scientific proof to this theory.

In researching immunotherapy for food allergy, three main routes of administration have been (and continue to be) explored.

1. Subcutaneous immunotherapy (Allergy shots)

Early immunotherapy studies using allergy shots (where the allergen is injected under the skin) in patients with peanut allergy found that tolerance to peanut could be induced. However, a significant number of participants suffered severe allergic reactions during the therapy. Doctors agreed that the frequency of severe reactions using subcutaneous immunotherapy was unacceptably high[1,2] so this method was discontinued. In the future, subcutaneous immunotherapy may be reconsidered if the method can be combined with anti-IgE therapy (see page 363), so that patients can tolerate small doses of their allergen without experiencing severe reactions.

2. Sublingual immunotherapy

Sublingual immunotherapy involves patients placing an allergen extract beneath their tongue for a set period of time (usually for 2 minutes) and then spitting it out or swallowing it. The safety record of sublingual therapy for non-food allergens (for example, pollens) is very good and has produced promising results, so scientists have been busy applying the same method in food-allergy research. In a 2005 study of sublingual immunotherapy for hazelnut,[3] 23 participants received either hazelnut extract or a placebo (a substance containing no medication; it is used as a control in research studies) for 8–12 weeks. In the food challenge conducted following treatment, the group receiving the hazelnut extract recorded a significant increase in their tolerance to hazelnut compared to those in the placebo group. A more recent study in Italy in 2007 used sublingual immunotherapy in children allergic to milk, egg, cod, wheat and apple and reported a success rate of tolerance in more than 85 per cent of participants.[4] While these results offer hope, it is early days, and more research is needed to see whether the tolerance induced is long term or whether the therapy needs to be continued in order to maintain tolerance. It may be that this therapy helps to reduce the risk of severe allergic reactions in some people by increasing the amount they can ingest safely before they develop a reaction. Another outcome could be that the therapy needs to be taken long term to maintain tolerance and is therefore not a cure.

3. Oral immunotherapy

Oral immunotherapy involves patients swallowing and ingesting tiny amounts of their food allergen. In general, the results of studies have been varied (and not without risk) but considered encouraging. Recently, however, some very promising outcomes have emerged from experimental studies in the UK and the US.

In a UK study published in 2009,[5] four children with peanut allergy were initially given a 5 milligram serving of peanut flour, and this dosage was incrementally increased over a 6-month period until they could tolerate more than 800 milligrams (the equivalent of five peanuts). While the treatment is not a cure, researchers are hopeful that if the children continue to take their daily maintenance dose, they should maintain their tolerance, providing protection from a severe reaction in the event of accidental exposure.

In a US study published in 2009,[6] also on peanut allergy, nine out of 33 children participating in the study have been on oral maintenance doses of peanut for more than 2.5 years and four have now been taken off the maintenance dose and are regularly eating peanuts. This treatment remains experimental, and considerably more research is needed before the treatment can be offered to patients, but it does offer hope that treatment may become available in the near future. (Potential drawbacks of the therapy, however, include the risk of anaphylaxis during treatment and the logistics of running such a therapy in hospitals that are already stretched for resources.)

Again, it cannot be overemphasised that you should never try this at home with your child.

Anti-IgE therapy

Briefly recapping information from Chapter 1, IgE stands for immunoglobulin E. This is a type of protein which is also known as an antibody — a substance the body produces in order to protect against infection. This antibody circulates through the blood.

In IgE-mediated food allergy, the immune system produces IgE antibodies to particular proteins found in a food. These IgE antibodies then attach to mast cells as well as other cells in the body. When a food-allergy sufferer ingests a food or product containing their allergen, the allergen attaches to the IgE antibodies on cells and triggers an allergic response.

Scientists have recently engineered 'anti-IgE', a chemical agent designed to bind to IgE antibodies floating in the blood. When anti-IgE binds with IgE, it reduces the level of IgE antibodies circulating in the body, and interrupts the chain of events that results in an allergic reaction.

Clinical trials of anti-IgE therapy have focused on peanut allergy, with treatment involving patients receiving regular injections of an anti-IgE agent. In an early study, the administration of one anti-IgE agent (TNX-901) resulted in the majority of participants (approximately 75 per cent) increasing their threshold for sensitivity to peanut. Participants were not cured of their allergy, but could tolerate a larger amount of allergen than previously before experiencing allergic symptoms (increasing from approximately half a peanut to almost nine peanuts). In other words, participants have gained protection against inadvertent exposure to peanut. This approach did not work in all patients, and some had no change in their threshold of sensitivity. It was not possible to predict from this study who was more likely to be protected using this drug.[7, 8]

In a later study, another anti-IgE agent (Omalizumab) was trialled in patients with peanut allergy. Unfortunately, the study had to be discontinued because of safety concerns over challenging some patients orally with peanut. The data produced were too limited to draw conclusions, but the results were consistent with the anti-IgE agent potentially increasing tolerance to peanut.[9]

There are drawbacks associated with the therapy — including the need for regular injections of the anti-IgE agent, the fact that it is expensive and that it doesn't work for all patients — however, it may play a significant role in protecting patients from experiencing anaphylaxis while undergoing food allergen immunotherapy. (See 'Immunotherapy', page 361.) Research is ongoing.[10]

Baked egg and milk trials

Research studies have recently found that the majority of children with egg allergy may be able to eat limited quantities of foods containing baked egg, and the majority of children with cow's milk allergy may be able to eat food containing extensively heated cow's milk.

The proteins in egg trigger allergic reactions. Extensive heating, such as in baking, is thought to break down the protein and lessen the likelihood of the protein triggering an allergic reaction. A study published in 2007 found that 77 per cent of study participants with confirmed egg allergy were able to tolerate limited amounts of baked egg in their diet.[11] This was followed by a study in Greece, published in 2008,[12] in which children were daily given small and increasing amounts of baked egg in the form of cake for 6 months. More than 90 per cent of children were able to tolerate the cake. Furthermore, at the end of 6 months, children were challenged to whole egg and more than 95 per cent had no reaction (and were subsequently followed up to confirm they had outgrown their egg allergy). This has given rise to the hypothesis that consumption of baked egg in children with egg allergy may improve the likelihood of a child outgrowing their allergy to whole egg. This theory will continue to be explored in controlled trials.

Similarly, it has been hypothesised that children with cow's milk allergy may also be able to tolerate extensively heated milk products. A study published in 2008[13] involving 100 participants with cow's milk allergy found that 75 per cent could tolerate extensively heated cow's milk. Those who could tolerate baked milk were found to have significantly smaller skin prick wheals after 3 months than before they started regularly consuming heated milk. As with egg, research continues, looking at whether or not the consumption of extensively heated milk can improve the likelihood of a child outgrowing their allergy to cow's milk.

The baked egg and milk studies are potentially very exciting because if a significant number of children with egg and/or milk allergy can consume their allergen when baked, it will greatly improve the quality of life of many families. Think of all the new foods that could be added to a child's diet! Then there's the reduction in anxiety, the relief at being able to allow children to enjoy eating birthday cakes and, potentially, speed up the time it takes for a child to become tolerant to these allergens.

Again, it must be cautioned that baked egg and heated milk trials take place in hospital under strict medical supervision. Baked egg and extensively heated milk can trigger severe allergic reactions, and parents should *not* try this at home.

Adrenaline administration

While scientists and doctors are hopeful that a cure will one day be found for food allergies, for now, adrenaline remains the best immediate treatment in the event of anaphylaxis. Unfortunately, a delay in, or failure to, administer adrenaline has been found to be a significant contributing factor in fatalities from food-induced anaphylaxis — possibly due to a fear of administering a 'needle'[14] and the inconvenience of carrying a bulky autoinjector.

Research is currently underway to investigate better ways to administer adrenaline. One non-injectable alternative being researched is a sublingual tablet — a fast-disintegrating tablet that is placed under the tongue. The tablet has been tested in rabbits and was found to be effective.[15] Clinical trials are the next step, to see if it is a safe and effective way to administer adrenaline to humans.

Interestingly, Intelliject, a company in the US, is developing the 'epiCard': a compact adrenaline auto-injector about the length and width of a credit card in shape, and the thickness of a compact mobile phone. The device also features step-by-step audio instructions on how to use the device in an emergency. The product has not received FDA approval in the US, so it is not yet available. Even so, it is encouraging for parents to know that companies are working on developing new ways of administering adrenaline that may mean patients are more likely to carry adrenaline at all times and be able to use it effectively and quickly in the event of anaphylaxis.

Traditional Chinese medicine

Western medical research methodologies and protocols are currently being applied to traditional Chinese medicine, with scientists examining herbal formulas that hold promise for food-allergy treatment.[16]

Traditional Chinese medicine does not define a specific treatment for food allergy; however, herbal formulas are used in treating gastrointestinal problems which involve symptoms similar to those of food allergy.[17] With this knowledge, scientists have recently developed a special herbal formula called FAHF-2 (Food Allergy Herbal Formula; the '2' represents that the initial formula has been refined and this is the second version). FAHF-2 has been used in research studies with peanut-allergic mice and has been found to block peanut-induced anaphylaxis for up to 5 weeks after therapy; it has also been found to induce peanut tolerance in peanut-allergic mice.[18]

Clinical trials with FAHF-2 in humans are underway in the US,[19] and it is hoped that a herbal remedy may be available for allergy specialists to use in treating food-allergic patients in the future.

The barrier function of skin and allergy

The outer skin of our body acts as a physical barrier against the outside environment.[20] If the barrier function of skin is compromised, the skin could be more vulnerable to allowing allergens into the body — and possibly letting water escape. If allergens are penetrating the skin, it may be that allergic sensitisation is occurring — that is, the allergen is entering the body via the skin, activating immune cells to produce IgE and then preparing the immune system to react to the allergen in the future — which can lead to the development of allergic disease. Recently, scientific interest has centred on an essential component of skin called filaggrin, a protein which forms part of the skin barrier. Researchers have discovered that a filaggrin

continued

gene is abnormal in some people. Some patients with an abnormal filaggrin gene have defective skin barriers, and an abnormal filaggrin gene has been linked to chronic eczema.

Research findings are not conclusive as yet. Patients with a normal filaggrin gene may still develop eczema, and some patients with a defective filaggrin gene do not develop eczema. However, the focus on the role of the skin as a barrier against allergic sensitisation is an important development.[21] Supporting this research is a previous UK study of children with atopic dermatitis who were exposed to topical creams containing peanut protein. In this study, these children showed an increased risk of becoming sensitised to peanut.[22]

Research into the role of the barrier function of skin and the development of allergic disease continues.[23, 24, 25, 26]

Keeping up to date with new developments

Q My teenage daughter is allergic to peanut, and when we last visited her allergy specialist, admittedly over 4 years ago now, he told us it was likely her allergy would be lifelong. I have read some media reports about potential peanut allergy cures and am keen to learn more. What is the best way to keep up to date with new developments in potential treatments and cures for peanut allergy?

A Even though your daughter's allergy to peanut may be considered lifelong (until a cure is found!) it really is important that she keeps seeing her allergy specialist in the teen years. If your daughter has not had a reaction to peanut for some time, seeing her specialist will reinforce that the condition is real. It will also help in educating your daughter about making responsible decisions around her allergy and make sure she is confident in using her EpiPen in an emergency. In addition, an allergy specialist can be a good source of information about the latest research and development around potential treatments and cures for peanut allergy. There is a lot of 'misinformation' about allergy treatments and cures, so it is imperative that you talk to a qualified person to ensure you are receiving current and credible information.

In between appointments, you can keep up to date with new developments by joining Anaphylaxis Australia Inc (AAI). AAI produces a science-based newsletter that regularly includes articles on new developments in treatments and cures for food allergy. Visit **www.allergyfacts.org.au** to find out how to become a member. In addition, also visit the website of the Australasian Society of Clinical Immunology and Allergy, which features a regularly updated section dedicated to patient information. Visit **www.allergy.org.au**

Resist the urge to 'Google' allergy treatments and cures: information about any aspect of allergy needs to come from a credible and trustworthy source.

There are other therapies in trial not covered in this chapter, including various other forms of immunotherapy. Allergy treatments and cures will be an exciting area of development in the next 5–10 years.

APPENDIX 1

Allergy-friendly cookbooks

A range of allergy-friendly recipe books is available which can provide a really useful and practical starting point for feeding your food-allergic child. A small list of recent Australian and New Zealand titles is included below for your reference.

- *The New Zealand Food Allergy Cookbook* by Allergy New Zealand, Hodda Moa 2007
- *Fast Ideas: Safe Recipes for Kids* by Denise King, Ilhan Food Allergy Foundation 2006
- *Allergy-Safe Family Food* by Suzanna Paxton, HarperCollins*Publishers* 2009
- *Allergies: Egg, Nut & Dairy* (Health for Life series) by Jody Vassallo, Fortiori 2005

Once you get the hang of cooking without your child's allergens, you will soon find it easy to adapt regular recipes. Also remember that paediatric dietitians can assist in providing allergen-free recipes and, importantly, help with behavioural issues around eating.

Paediatric dietitian Barbara Dennison also suggests enlisting the help of a grandparent. Old-fashioned cookbooks can be a wonderful source of simple recipes based on fresh ingredients. Inviting a grandparent to hunt down some suitable recipes for your family helps them to learn and be involved in the management of food allergy.

Anaphylaxis Australia Inc is another fantastic source of allergy-friendly recipes. The AAI member newsletter features allergy-friendly recipes in every edition and a range of allergy-friendly cookbooks is also available for sale from AAI. Visit **www.allergyfacts.org.au** for more information.

Remember: Always check the label of every food product every time you use it.

APPENDIX 2

Copy of ASCIA Action Plan for Anaphylaxis

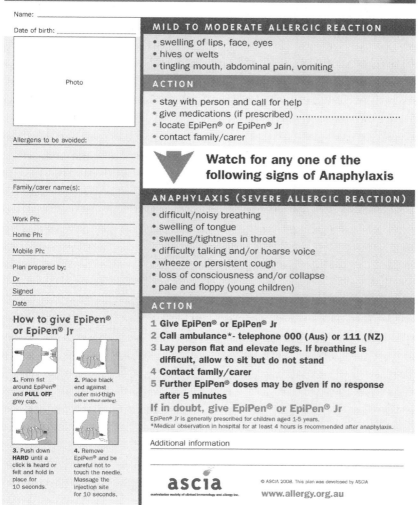

ACTION PLAN FOR
Anaphylaxis

Name: _____

Date of birth: _____

Photo

Allergens to be avoided: _____

Family/carer name(s): _____

Work Ph: _____

Home Ph: _____

Mobile Ph: _____

Plan prepared by:

Dr _____

Signed _____

Date _____

How to give EpiPen® or EpiPen® Jr

1. Form fist around EpiPen® and **PULL OFF** grey cap.

2. Place black end against outer mid-thigh (with or without clothing).

3. Push down **HARD** until a click is heard or felt and hold in place for 10 seconds.

4. Remove EpiPen® and be careful not to touch the needle. Massage the injection site for 10 seconds.

MILD TO MODERATE ALLERGIC REACTION

- swelling of lips, face, eyes
- hives or welts
- tingling mouth, abdominal pain, vomiting

ACTION

- stay with person and call for help
- give medications (if prescribed) ....
- locate EpiPen® or EpiPen® Jr
- contact family/carer

Watch for any one of the following signs of Anaphylaxis

ANAPHYLAXIS (SEVERE ALLERGIC REACTION)

- difficult/noisy breathing
- swelling of tongue
- swelling/tightness in throat
- difficulty talking and/or hoarse voice
- wheeze or persistent cough
- loss of consciousness and/or collapse
- pale and floppy (young children)

ACTION

1 **Give EpiPen® or EpiPen® Jr**
2 **Call ambulance*- telephone 000 (Aus) or 111 (NZ)**
3 **Lay person flat and elevate legs. If breathing is difficult, allow to sit but do not stand**
4 **Contact family/carer**
5 **Further EpiPen® doses may be given if no response after 5 minutes**

If in doubt, give EpiPen® or EpiPen® Jr

EpiPen® Jr is generally prescribed for children aged 1-5 years.
*Medical observation in hospital for at least 4 hours is recommended after anaphylaxis.

Additional information _____

_____

ascia
australasian society of clinical immunology and allergy inc.

© ASCIA 2008. This plan was developed by ASCIA

www.allergy.org.au

ASCIA Action Plans for Anaphylaxis and Allergic Reactions are reproduced with permission from the Australasian Society of Clinical Immunology and Allergy (ASCIA). These are available to download from the ASCIA website **www.allergy.org. au/content/view/10/3/** or can be ordered as hard copies by emailing **education@ allergy.org.au**

APPENDIX 3

Copy of ASCIA Action Plan for Allergic Reactions

ACTION PLAN FOR
Allergic Reactions

Name: _____

Date of birth: _____

Photo

Allergens to be avoided:
_____
_____
_____
_____

Family/carer name(s):
_____

Work Ph: _____
Home Ph: _____
Mobile Ph: _____

Plan prepared by:
Dr _____
Signed _____
Date _____

MILD TO MODERATE ALLERGIC REACTION

- swelling of lips, face, eyes
- hives or welts
- tingling mouth, abdominal pain, vomiting

ACTION

- stay with person and call for help
- give medications (if prescribed) ....
- contact family/carer

▼ **Watch for any one of the following signs of Anaphylaxis**

ANAPHYLAXIS (SEVERE ALLERGIC REACTION)

- difficult/noisy breathing
- swelling of tongue
- swelling/tightness in throat
- difficulty talking and/or hoarse voice
- wheeze or persistent cough
- loss of consciousness and/or collapse
- pale and floppy (young children)

ACTION

1. **Call Ambulance if there are any signs of anaphylaxis - telephone 000 (Aus) or 111 (NZ)**
2. **Lay person flat and elevate legs. If breathing is difficult, allow to sit but do not stand**
3. **Contact family/carer**

Additional information _____
_____
_____
_____

ascia
australasian society of clinical immunology and allergy inc.

© ASCIA 2008. This plan was developed by ASCIA
www.allergy.org.au

ASCIA Action Plans for Anaphylaxis and Allergic Reactions are reproduced with permission from the Australasian Society of Clinical Immunology and Allergy (ASCIA). These are available to download from the ASCIA website **www.allergy.org. au/content/view/10/3/** or can be ordered as hard copies by emailing **education@ allergy.org.au**

ENDNOTES

Introduction by Alison Orman

1 Mandell D, Curtis R, Gold M, Hardie S, 'Anaphylaxis: How do you live with it?', *Health and Social Work* 2005; 30 (4): 325–35.
2 Australasian Society of Clinical Immunology and Allergy (ASCIA), 'Patient Information: Food Allergy', may be accessed online at www.allergy.org.au/content/view/167/140/

Chapter 1

1 Australasian Society of Clinical Immunology and Allergy (ASCIA), 'Patient Information: Food Allergy', may be accessed online at www.allergy.org.au/content/view/167/140/
2 Allen KJ, Hill DJ, Heine RG. 4. Food allergy in childhood. *The Medical Journal of Australia Practice Essentials – Allergy*, 2006; 185 (7) 394.
3 Motala C, Lockey R, 'Food Allergy', may be accessed online at: www.worldallergy.org/public/allergic_diseases_center/foodallergy/
4 Australasian Society of Clinical Immunology and Allergy (ASCIA), 'Health Professional Information: Diagnosis and management of food hypersensitivity in childhood', may be accessed online at: www.allergy.org.au/content/view/166/1/
5 Sampson HA, 'Food allergy. 1. Immunopathogenesis and clinical disorders', *Journal of Allergy and Clinical Immunology* 1999; 103 (5): 718.
6 Allen KJ, Hill DJ, Heine RG.
7 Sporik R, Hill D, 'Allergy to peanut, nuts, and sesame seed in Australian children', *British Medical Journal* 1996; 313:1477–78.
8 The International Study of Asthma and Allergies in Childhood (ISAAC) Steering Committee, 'Worldwide variation in prevalence of symptoms of asthma, allergic rhinoconjunctivitis, and atopic eczema: ISAAC', *Lancet* 1998; 351: 1225–1232.
9 Australasian Society of Clinical Immunology and Allergy (ASCIA), 'Report by Access Economics Pty Ltd: The economic impact of allergic disease in Australia: not to be sneezed at', November 2007.
10 ASCIA, 'Report by Access Economics Pty Ltd.'
11 ASCIA, 'Patient Information: Food Allergy'.
12 Poulos LM, Waters AM, Correll PK, Loblay RH, Marks GB, 'Trends in hospitalisations for anaphylaxis, angiodema, and urticaria in Australia, 1993–1994 to 2004–2005', *Journal of Allergy and Clinical Immunology* 2007; 120 (4): 878–84.
13 Liew WK, Williamson E, Tang MLK, 'Anaphylaxis fatalities and admissions in Australia', *Journal of Allergy and Clinical Immunology* 2009; 123 (2): 434–442.
14 Grundy J, Matthews S, Bateman B, Dean T Arshad SH, 'Rising Prevalence of allergy to peanut in children: Data from 2 sequential cohorts', *Journal of Allergy and Clinical Immunology* 2002; 110 (5): 784–9.
15 Sicherer SH, Muñoz-Furlong A, Sampson, HA, 'Prevalence of seafood allergy in the United States determined by a random telephone survey', *Journal of Allergy and Clinical Immunology* 2004; 114 (1): 159–65.
16 Sicherer SH, Furlong TJ, Muñoz-Furlong A, Burks AW, Sampson HA, 'Prevalence of peanut and tree nut allergy in the US determined by a random digit dial telephone survey', *Journal of Allergy and Clinical Immunology* 1999;103(4): 559–62.
17 Kjellman NI, 'Prediction and prevention of atopic allergy', *Allergy* 1998; 53:67–71.
18 Zeiger R, Heller S, Mellon M, Halsey J, Hamburger R, Sampson H, 'Genetic and environmental factors affecting the development of atopy through age 4 in children with atopic parents: a prospective randomised study of food allergen avoidance', *Pediatric Allergy and Immunology* 1992; 3:110–27.

[19] Prescott SL, Tang MLK, 'The Australasian Society of Clinical Immunology and Allergy position statement: Allergy prevention in children', 2004, may be accessed online at: www.allergy.org.au/content/view/28/1/

[20] Kjellman NI.

[21] von Mutius E, Martinez FD, Fritzsch C, Nicolai T, Reitmeir P, Thiemann H-H, 'Skin test reactivity and number of siblings', *British Medical Journal* 1994; 308: 692–695.

[22] von Mutius E, Martinez FD, Fritzsch C, Nicolai T, Roell G, Thiemann H-H.

[23] Krämer U, Heinrich J, Wjst M, Wichmann HE, 'Age of entry to day nursery and allergy in later childhood', *The Lancet* 1999; 353: 450–54.

[24] Riedler J, Braun-Fahrländer C, Eder W, Schreuer M, Waser M, Maisch S, Carr D, Schierl R, Nowak D, von Mutius E (the ALEX Study Team), 'Exposure to farming in early life and development of asthma and allergy: a cross-sectional survey', *The Lancet* 2001; 358 (9288): 1129–1133.

[25] Kabesch M, Lauener RP, 'Why Old McDonald had a farm but no allergies: genes environments, and the hygiene hypothesis', *Journal of Leukocyte Biology* 2004; 75: 383–87.

[26] Kemp A, 'Allergy prevention — what we thought we knew', T*he Medical Journal of Australia* 2003; 178, 254.

[27] Sicherer SH, Muñoz-Furlong A, Sampson HA, 'Prevalence of peanut and tree nut allergy in the United States determined by means of a random digit dial telephone survey: A 5-year follow-up study', *Journal of Allergy and Clinical Immunology* 2003; 112 (6): 1203.

[28] Grundy J, Matthews S, Bateman B, Dean T, Arshad SH, 'Rising prevalence of allergy to peanut in children: Data from 2 sequential cohorts', *Journal of Allergy and Clinical Immunology* 2002; 110 (5): 784.

[29] Rancé F, 'Mustard allergy as a new food allergy', *European Journal of Allergy and Clinical Immunology*, 2003; 58: 287.

[30] Dalal I, Binson R, Reifen R, Amitai Z, Shohat T, Rahmani S, Levine A, Ballin A, Somekh E, 'Food allergy is a matter of geography after all: sesame as a major cause of severe IgE-mediated food allergic reactions among infants and young children in Israel', *European Journal of Allergy and Clinical Immunology*, 2002; 57: 364–65.

[31] Dalal I et al., p 364.

[32] Beyer K, Morrow E, Li XM, et al., 'Effects of cooking methods on peanut allergenicity', *Journal of Allergy and Clinical Immunology* 2001; 107 : 1077–81.

[33] Sampson HA, 'Clinical Practice: Peanut Allergy', *The New England Journal of Medicine*; 2002; 346 (17):1294–95.

[34] Kramer MS, Kakuma R, 'Maternal dietary antigen avoidance during pregnancy or lactation, or both, for preventing or treating atopic disease in the child', *Chochrane Database Systematic Reviews* 2006, Issue 3, Art. No.: CD000133, DOI: 10.1002/145651858.CD000133.pub2

[35] Dioun AF, Harris SK, Hibberd PL, 'Is maternal age at delivery related to childhood food allergy?' *Pediatric Allergy and Immunology* 2003; 14: 307–11.

[36] Eggesbø M, Botten G, Stigum H, Samuelson SO, Brunekreef B, Magnus P, 'Cesarian delivery and cow milk allergy/intolerance', *Allergy* 2005; 60: 1172–73.

[37] Weidinger S, O'Sullivan M, Illig T, Baurecht H, Depner M, Rodriguez E, Ruether A, Klopp N, Vogelberg C, Weiland SK, McLean WH, von Mutius E, Irvine AD, Kabesch M, 'Filaggrin mutations, atopic eczema, hay fever, and asthma in children', *Journal of Allergy and Clinical Immunology* 2008; 121 (5): 1203–09.

[38] Hesselmar B, Aberg N, Aberg B, Eriksson B, Björkstén B, 'Does early exposure to cat or dog protect against later allergy development?' *Clinical and Experimental Allergy* 1999; 29 (5), 611–17.

[39] Boyle RJ, Tang ML, 'Can allergic disease be prevented prenatally?', *Allergy* 2006; 61: 1423–31.

[40] Untersmayr E, Jensen-Jarolim E, 'The role of protein digestibility and antacids

on food allergy outcomes', *Journal of Allergy and Clinical Immunology* 2008; 121 (6):1301–8.

[41] Kull I, Bergström A, Melén E, Lilja G, van Hage M, Pershagen G, Wickman M, 'Early-life supplementation of vitamins A and D, in water-soluble form or in peanut oil, and allergic diseases during childhood', *Journal of Allergy and Clinical Immunology* 2006; 118 (6): 1299–1304.

[42] Milner JD, Stein DM, McCarter R, Moon RY, 'Early infant multivitamin supplementation is associated with increased risk for food allergy and asthma', *Pediatrics*, 2004; 114: 27–32.

[43] Prescott SL, Björkstén B, 'Probiotics for the prevention or treatment of allergic diseases', *Journal of Allergy and Clinical Immunology* 2007; 120 (2): 255–62.

Chapter 2

[1] Australasian Society of Clinical Immunology and Allergy (ASCIA), 'Health Professional Information: Diagnosis and management of food hypersensitivity in childhood', October 2007, may be accessed online at: www.allergy.org.au/content/view/166/1/

Chapter 3

[1] Sicherer SH, Sampson HA, 'Peanut Allergy: Emerging concepts and approaches for an apparent epidemic', *Journal of Allergy and Clinical Immunology* 2007;120 (3): 493.

[2] Sporik R, Hill DJ, Hosking CS, 'Specificity of allergen skin testing in predicting positive open food challenges to milk, egg and peanut in children', *Clinical and Experimental Allergy* 2000; 30: 1540–46

[3] Allen KJ, Hill DJ, Heine RG, '4, Food allergy in childhood', *The Medical Journal of Australia Practice Essentials – Allergy*, 2007; 29.

[4] Sampson H, 'Food Allergy. Part 2: Diagnosis and management', *The Journal of Allergy and Clinical Immunology*, 1999; 103 (6). p 983.

[5] Lin MS, Tanner E, Lynn J, Friday GA Jr, 'Nonfatal systemic allergic reactions induced by skin testing and immunotherapy', *Annals of Allergy*, 1993; 71 (6):557–62.

[6] Liccardi G, D'Amato G, Walter Canonica G, Salzillo A, Piccolo A, Passalacqua G, 'Systemic reactions from skin testing: literature review', *Journal of Investigational Allergology Clinical Immunology* 2006; 16 (2): 75–78.

[7] Robinson M, Smart J, 'Allergy testing and referral in children', *Australian Family Physician*, 2008; 37 (4) 212.

[8] Robinson M, Smart J.

[9] Sampson H, 'Utility of food-specific IgE concentrations in predicting symptomatic food allergy', *The Journal of Allergy and Clinical Immunology* 2001; 107 (5): 891–96.

[10] Bock SA, Sampson HA, Atkins FM, Zeiger RS, Lehrer S, Sachs M, et al., 'Double-blind, placebo-controlled food challenge as an office procedure: A manual', *Journal of Allergy and Clinical Immunology* 1988; 82 (6):986–97.

[11] Australasian Society of Clinical Immunology and Allergy (ASCIA), 'Position Paper, Unorthodox Testing and Treatment for Allergic Disorders', November 2007, may be accessed online at: www.allergy.org.au/content/view/322/271/

[12] ASCIA, 'Position Paper, Unorthodox Testing and Treatment for Allergic Disorders', reproduced with permission from ASCIA.

Chapter 4

[1] Australasian Society of Clinical Immunology and Allergy (ASCIA), 'Patient Information: Food Allergy', July 2008, may be accessed online at: www.allergy.org.au/content/view/167/1/

Chapter 5

[1] Simons FER, 'First-aid treatment of anaphylaxis to food: focus on epinephrine', *Journal of Allergy and Clinical Immunology* 2004; 113 (5): 837–44.

[2] Simons, FER, 'First-aid treatment of anaphylaxis to food'.

[3] Australasian Society of Clinical Immunology and Allergy (ASCIA), www.allergy.org.au/images/stories/anaphylaxis/Action_Plan_anaphylaxis_personal.pdf

[4] ASCIA Action Plan.

[5] Braganza SC, Acworth JP, Mckinnon DRL, Peake JE, Brown AFT, 'Paediatric emergency department anaphylaxis: Different patterns from adults', *Archives of Disease in Childhood*, 2006; 91: 159–163.

[6] Simons FER, '9. Anaphylaxis', *Journal of Allergy and Clinical Immunology* 2008; 121 (2): S402–S404.

[7] Heddle RJ, 'Anaphylaxis to stings and bites', *The Medical Journal of Australia Practice Essentials – Allergy* 2006; 185 (5) 17.

[8] Wainstein BK, Kashef S, Ziegler M, Jelley D, Ziegler JB, 'Frequency and significance of immediate contact reactions to peanut in peanut-sensitive children', *Clinical and Experimental Allergy* 2007; 37 (6), 839–45.

[9] Wainstein BK, et al., p 839.

[10] Klein JS, Yocum MW, 'Underreporting of anaphylaxis in a community emergency room', *Journal of Allergy and Clinical Immunology* 1995; 95 (2): 637–38

[11] Simons FER, 'Anaphylaxis, killer allergy: Long-term management in the community', *Journal of Allergy and Clinical Immunology* 2006; 117 (2): 367–77.

[12] Simons FER, Frew AJ, Ansotegui IJ, Bochner BS, Golden DBK, Finkelman FD, Leung DYM, Lotvall J, Marone G, Metcalfe DD, Muller U, Rosenwasser LJ, Sampson HA, Schwartz LB, van Hage M, Walls AF, 'Risk assessment in anaphylaxis: current and future approaches,' *Journal of Allergy and Clinical Immunology* 2007; 120 (1): S2–S24.

[13] Lieberman, P, Camargo CA, Bohlke Kari, Jick Hershel, Miller RL, Sheikh Aziz, Simons FER, 'Epidemiology of anaphylaxis: findings of the American College of Allergy, Asthma and Immunology Epidemiology of Anaphylaxis Working Group,' *Annals of Allergy, Asthma and Immunology* 2006; 97 (5): 596–602.

[14] Simons FER, 'Anaphylaxis, killer allergy'.

[15] Lieberman P et al.

[16] Boros CA, Kay D, Gold MS, 'Parent reported allergy and anaphylaxis in 4173 South Australian children', *Journal of Paediatrics and Child Health* 2000; 36, 36–40.

[17] Australasian Society of Clinical Immunology and Allergy (ASCIA), 'Position Paper, Guidelines for prevention of food anaphylactic reactions in schools, preschools and childcare', 2004, updated 2007, may be accessed online at: www.allergy.org.au/pospapers/anaphylaxis.htm

[18] Poulos LM, Waters AM, Correll PK, Loblay RH, Marks GB, 'Trends in hospitalizations for anaphylaxis, angiodema, and urticaria in Australia, 1993–1994 to 2004–2005', *Journal of Allergy and Clinical Immunology* 2007; 120 (4): 878–84.

[19] Gupta R, Sheikh A, Strachan D, Anderson HR, 'Increasing hospital admissions for systemic allergic disorders in England: Analysis of national admissions data', *British Medical Journal.* 2003; 327: 1142–1143.

[20] Gupta R, Sheikh A, Strachan DP, Anderson HR, 'Time trends in allergic disorders in the UK', *Thorax* (online) 2006; 000: 1–6.

[21] Brown SGA, Mullins RJ, Gold MS, '2. Anaphylaxis: diagnosis and management', *The Medical Journal of Australia Practice Essentials – Allergy*, 2006; 185 (5) 283–89.

[22] Moneret-Vautrin DA, Morisset M, Flabbee J, Beaudouin E, Kanny G, 'Epidemiology of life-threatening and lethal anaphylaxis: a review', *Allergy* 2005; 60 (4) 443–451.

[23] Stark BJ, Sullivan TJ, 'Biphasic and protracted anaphylaxis', *Journal of Allergy and Clinical Immunology* 1986; 78:76–83.

[24] Brown SGA et al.

[25] Douglas DM, Sukenick E, Andrade WP, Brown JS, 'Biphasic systemic anaphylaxis: An inpatient and outpatient study', *Journal of Allergy and Clinical Immunology* 1994; 93 (6): 977–85.

[26] Simons FER, '9. Anaphylaxis'.

[27] Sampson HA, 'Anaphylaxis and emergency treatment', *Pediatrics* 2003; 111 (6): S1601–08.

[28] Simons FER et al., 'Risk assessment in anaphylaxis: current and future approaches'.

[29] EpiPen Jr Product Information (Aust R 42980), may be accessed online at: http://secure.healthlinks.net.au/content/csl/pi.cfm?product=cspepipj10905

[30] Australasian Society of Clinical Immunology and Allergy (ASCIA), 'Guidelines for EpiPen® prescription', 2004, may be accessed online at: www.allergy.org.au/images/stories/anaphylaxis/ASCIA_EpiPen_prescription_guidelines.pdf

[31] Information in the PBS Schedule about EpiPen, may be accessed online at: www.pbs.gov.au/html/consumer/product/restrictions?publication=GE&code=8698T&brand=EpiPen

[32] Gold MS, Sainsbury R, 'First aid anaphylaxis management in children who were prescribed an epinephrine autoinjector device (EpiPen)', *Journal of Allergy and Clinical Immunology* 2000; 106 (1): 171–76.

[33] Kim JS, Sinacore JM, Pongracic JA, 'Parental use of EpiPen for children with food allergies', *Journal of Allergy and Clinical Immunology* 2005; 116 (1): 164–68.

[34] Kim JS, Sinacore JM, Pongracic JA.

[35] Simons FER et al., 'Risk assessment in anaphylaxis: current and future approaches'.

[36] Simons FER, 'Anaphylaxis, killer allergy'.

[37] Yunginger JW, Sweeney KG, Sturner WQ, Giannandrea LA, Teigland JD, Bray M, Benson PA, York JA, Biedrzycki L, Squillace DL et al, 'Fatal food-induced anaphylaxis', *The Journal of the American Medical Association* 1988; 260 (10): 1450–52.

[38] Sampson HA, Mendelson L, Rosen J, 'Fatal and near-fatal anaphylactic reactions to food in children and adolescents', *New England Journal of Medicine* 1992; 327 (6): 380–84.

[39] Sampson HA, 'Anaphylaxis and emergency treatment'.

[40] Australasian Society of Clinical Immunology and Allergy (ASCIA), 'Patient Information: Anaphylaxis', December 2007, may be accessed online at: www.allergy.org.au/content/view/178/1/

[41] Sampson HA, 'Anaphylaxis and emergency treatment'.

[42] Sampson HA, 'Anaphylaxis and emergency treatment'.

[43] Australian Society of Clinical Immunology and Allergy (ASCIA), 'Health Professional Information: Anaphylaxis', December 2007, may be accessed online at: www.allergy.org.au/content/view/160/1/

[44] Castells M, Horan R, Sheffer A, 'Exercise-induced anaphylaxis', *Current Allergy and Asthma Reports* 2003; 3 (1): 15–21.

[45] ASCIA, 'Health Professional Information: Anaphylaxis'.

[46] Castells M, Horan R, Sheffer A, 'Exercise-induced anaphylaxis'.

[47] Sampson HA, 'Anaphylaxis and emergency treatment'.

[48] Simons FER, 'First-aid treatment of anaphylaxis to food'.

Chapter 6

[1] Allen KJ, Hill DJ, Heine RG, '4. Food allergy in childhood', *The Medical Journal of Australia Practice Essentials – Allergy* 2006; 185 (7) 394.

[2] Sporik R, Hill D, 'Allergy to peanut, nuts, and sesame seed in Australian children', *British Medical Journal* 1996; 313:1477–78.

[3] Høst, A, 'Frequency of cow's milk allergy in Childhood', *Annals of Allergy Asthma and Immunology* 2002; 89 (6 Supplement 1): 33–37.

4 Skripak JM, Matsui EC, Mudd K, Wood RA, 'The natural history of IgE-mediated cow's milk allergy', *The Journal of Allergy and Clinical Immunology* 2007; 120 (5): 1172–77.

5 Nowak-Wegrzyn A, Bloom KA, Sicherer SH, Shreffler WG, Noone S, Wanich N, Sampson HA, 'Tolerance to extensively heated milk in children with cow's milk allergy', *Journal of Allergy and Clinical Immunology* 2008; 122 (2): 342–47.

6 Høst A, Halken S, 'A prospective study of cow milk allergy in Danish infants during the first 3 years of life: clinical course in relation to clinical and immunological type of hypersensitivity reaction', *Allergy* 1990; 45: 587–96.

7 Skripak JM, Matsui EC, Mudd K, Wood RA.

8 Hill DJ, Firer MA, Ball G, Hosking CS, 'Natural history of cows' milk allergy in children: immunological outcome over 2 years', *Clinical and Experimental Allergy* 1993; 23: 124–31.

9 Kemp AS, Hill DJ, Allen KJ, Anderson K, Davidson GP, Day AS, Heine RG, Peake JE, Prescott SL, Shugg AW, Sinn JK, 'Guidelines for the use of infant formulas to treat cow's milk protein allergy: an Australian consensus panel opinion', *Medical Journal of Australia* 2008; 188 (2): 109–112.

10 Australasian Society of Clinical Immunology and Allergy (ASCIA), 'Patient Information: Food allergy: other foods', may be accessed online at: www.allergy.org. au/content/view/183/1/

11 Werfel SJ, Cooke SK, Sampson HA, 'Clinical reactivity to beef in children allergic to cow's milk', *Journal of Allergy and Clinical Immunology* 1997; 99 (3): 293–300.

12 Fiocchi A, Restani P, Riva E, Mirri GP, Santini I, Bernardo L, Galli CL, 'Heat treatment modifies the allergenicity of beef and bovine serum albumin', *Allergy* 1998; 53 (8): 798–802.

13 Kemp AS, et al.

14 Nowak-Wegrzyn A et al.

15 Sicherer SH, Sampson HA, 'Food Allergy', *Journal of Allergy and Clinical Immunology* 2006; 117 (2): S470–75.

16 Eggesbø M, Botten G, Halvorsen R, Magnus P, 'The prevalence of allergy to egg: a population-based study in young children', *Allergy* 2001; 56 (5): 403–11.

17 Wood RA, 'The natural history of food allergy', *Pediatrics* 2003; 111 (6): 1631–37.

18 Savage JH, Matsui EC, Skripak JM, Wood RA, 'The natural history of egg allergy', *Journal of Allergy and Clinical Immunology* 2007; 120 (6): 1413–17.

19 Sampson H, 'Food Allergy. Part 2: Diagnosis and management', T*he Journal of Allergy and Clinical Immunology* 1999; 103 (6): 981–89.

20 Aickin R, Hill D, Kemp A, 'Measles immunisation in children with allergy to egg', *British Medical Journal* 1994; 309: 223–5.

21 Australian Society of Clinical Immunology and Allergy (ASCIA) 2008, 'Peanut, tree nut and seed allergy info bulletin', may be accessed at: www.allergy.org.au/images/ stories/aer/infobulletins/pdf/aer_peanut_tree_nut_seed_allergy_jun08.pdf

22 Bock SA, Muñoz-Furlong A, Sampson HA, 'Fatalities due to anaphylactic reactions to foods', *Journal of Allergy and Clinical Immunology* 2001; 107 (1): 191–93.

23 Skripak JM, Matsui EC, Mudd K, Wood RA.

24 Sampson H, 'Food Allergy. Part 2'

25 Sicherer SH, Burks AW, Sampson HA, 'Clinical features of acute allergic reactions to peanuts and tree nuts in children', *Pediatrics* 1998;102: e6.

26 Sicherer SH, 'Clinical implications of cross-reactive food allergens', *Journal of Allergy and Clinical Immunology* 2001; 108 (6): 881–90.

27 Smith WB, Gillis D, Kette FE, 'Lupin: a new hidden food allergen', *Medical Journal of Australia*, 2004; 181 (4): 219–20.

28 Moneret Vautrin DA, Guerin L, Kanny G, Flabbee J, Fremont S, Morisset M, 'Cross-allergenicity of peanut and lupine: the risk of lupine allergy in patients allergic to peanuts', *Journal of Allergy and Clinical Immunology* 1999; 104 (4, Part 1): 883–38.

[29] Fleischer DM, Conover-Walker MK, Matsui EC, Wood RA, 'The natural history of tree nut allergy', *Journal of Allergy and Clinical Immunology* 2005; 116 (5): 1087–93.

[30] The Children's Hospital at Westmead, 'Fact sheet on tree nut allergy', may be accessed online at: www.chw.edu.au/parents/factsheets/tree_nut_allergy.htm

[31] Fleischer DM, Conover-Walker MK, Christie L, Burks AW, Wood RA, The natural progression of peanut allergy: Resolution and the possibility of recurrence. *Journal of Allergy and Clinical Immunology* 2003; 112 (1): 183–89.

[32] The Children's Hospital at Westmead, 'Fact sheet on seafood allergy', may be accessed online at: www.chw.edu.au/parents/factsheets/seafood_allergy.htm

[33] Bernhisel-Broadbent J, Strause D, Sampson HA, 'Fish hypersensitivity. II: Clinical relevance of altered fish allergenicity caused by various preparation methods', *Journal of Allergy and Clinical Immunology* 1992; 90 (4): 622–29.

[34] Wood RA.

[35] Dannaeus A, Inganas M, 'A follow-up study of children with food allergy. Clinical course in relation to serum IgE- and IgG-antibody levels to milk, egg and fish', *Clinical and Experimental Allergy* 1981; 111 (6): 533–39.

[36] Sicherer SH, 'Clinical implications of cross-reactive food allergens'.

[37] Sampson H, 'Food Allergy. Part 2'.

[38] The Children's Hospital at Westmead, 'Fact sheet on Seafood Allergy', may be accessed online at: www.chw.edu.au/parents/factsheets/seafood_allergy.htm

[39] The Children's Hospital at Westmead, 'Fact sheet on Seafood Allergy'.

[40] Wood RA.

[41] Sicherer SH, 'Clinical implications of cross-reactive food allergens'.

[42] ASCIA, 'Patient Information: Food allergy: other foods'.

[43] Bush RK, Taylor SL, Nordlee JA, Busse WW, 'Soybean oil is not allergenic to soybean-sensitive individuals', *Journal of Allergy and Clinical Immunology* 1985; 76 (2): 242–45.

[44] Wood RA.

[45] Sampson H, 'Food Allergy. Part 2'.

[46] Wood RA.

[47] Sampson H, 'Food Allergy. Part 2'.

[48] Sicherer SH, 'Clinical implications of cross-reactive food allergens'.

[49] Sporik R, Hill D.

[50] Gangur V, Kelly, C, Navuluri L, 'Sesame allergy: a growing food allergy of global proportions', *Annals of Allergy, Asthma and Immunology*, 2005; 95 (1): 4–11.

[51] Wood RA.

[52] Australasian Society of Clinical Immunology and Allergy (ASCIA), 'Health Professional Information: Is it allergy?', may be accessed online at: http://www.allergy.org.au/content/view/344/305/

[53] World Allergy Organization (WAO), 'Allergic reactions to latex', Allergic diseases resource center, may be accessed online at: www.worldallergy.org/public/allergic_diseases_center/latexallergy/latexallergy.php

[54] WAO, 'Allergic reactions to latex'.

[55] Charous BL, Blanco C, Tarlo S, Hamilton RG, Baur X, Beezhold D, Sussman G, Yunginger JW, 'Natural rubber latex allergy after 12 years: Recommendations and perspectives', *Journal of Allergy and Clinical Immunology* 2002; 109 (1): 31–34.

[56] Australasian Society of Clinical Immunology and Allergy (ASCIA), 'Patient Information: Latex allergy', may be accessed online at: www.allergy.org.au/content/view/107/1/

[57] ASCIA, 'Patient information: Latex allergy'.

Chapter 7

[1] Carvalho NF, Kennedy RD, Carrington PH, Hall DE, 'Severe Nutritional Deficiencies in Toddlers Resulting From Health Food Milk Alternatives' (electronic article), *Pediatrics*, 2001; 107 (4): e46.

Chapter 8

[1] www.foodstandards.gov.au/aboutfsanz/index.cfm
[2] www.foodstandards.gov.au/aboutfsanz/index.cfm
[3] Food Standards Australia New Zealand, 'Quantitative Consumer Survey on Allergen Labelling: Benchmark survey 2003, NFO Donovan Research Report', FSANZ, Canberra, 2004.
[4] Joshi P, Mofidi S, Sicherer S, 'Interpretation of commercial food ingredient labels by parents of food-allergic children', *Journal of Allergy and Clinical Immunology* 2002; 109 (6): 1019–21.
[5] Food Standards Australia New Zealand, June 2006, 'Advice for Consumers: Country of Origin Food Labelling', may be accessed online at: www.foodstandards.gov.au/_srcfiles/CoOL_brochure_2006.pdf
[6] Anaphylaxis Australia Inc., 'Food Industry Update, Vital – "May be present"', Summer 2008 Newsletter.
[7] www.foodstandards.gov.au/foodmatters/foodrecalls/foodindustryrecallprotocol5thedition/consumeradvice/index.cfm
[8] www.foodstandards.gov.au/foodmatters/foodrecalls/

Chapter 10

[1] Brown SGA, Mullins RJ, Gold MS, '2. Anaphylaxis: diagnosis and management', The *Medical Journal of Australia Practice Essentials — Allergy* 2006; 185 (5) 283–89.
[2] Sicherer SH, Furlong TJ, DeSimone J, Sampson HA, 'Self-reported allergic reactions to peanut on commercial airliners', *Journal of Allergy and Clinical Immunology* 1999; 104 (1): 186–89.
[3] Burches E, Cervera R, Peláez A, 'Food-induced anaphylaxis caused by inhalation of soy protein', *The Journal of Investigational Allergology and Clinical Immunology* 2007; 17 (6): 418–19.
[4] Crespo JF, Pascual C, Dominguez C, Ojeda I, Munoz FM, Estaban MM, 'Allergic reactions associated with airborne fish particles in IgE-mediated fish hypersensitive patients', *Allergy* 1995; 50: 257–61.
[5] Casimir G, Cuvelier P, Allard S, Duchateau J, 'Life-threatening fish allergy successfully treated with immunotherapy', *Pediatric Allergy and Immunology* 1997; 8: 103–5.
[6] Crespo JF, Rodriguez J, Vives R, James JM, Reaño M, Daroca P, Burbano C, Muzquiz M, 'Occupational IgE-mediated allergy after exposure to lupine seed flour', *Journal of Allergy and Clinical Immunology* 2001; 108: 295–297.

Chapter 11

[1] Joshi P, Katelaris CH, Frankum B, 'Adrenaline autoinjector use in preschools, poster presentation', Australasian Society of Clinical Immunology and Allergy (ASCIA) 19th Annual Scientific Meeting, November 2009, journal publication is pending.

Chapter 12

1   Brown SGA, Mullins RJ, Gold MS, '2. Anaphylaxis: diagnosis and management', *The Medical Journal of Australia Practice Essentials — Allergy*, 2006; 185 (5) 283–89.

Chapter 13

1   Noone S, Muñoz-Furlong A, Sicherer SH, 'Parent and adolescent perceptions of food allergy [abstract]', *Journal of Allergy and Clinical Immunology* 2003; 111 (1): S 133.

2   Bock SA, Muñoz-Furlong AM, Sampson HA, 'Fatalities due to anaphylactic reactions to foods', *Journal of Allergy and Clinical Immunology* 2001; 107 (1): 191–93.

3   Bock SA, Muñoz-Furlong AM, Sampson HA, 'Further fatalities due to anaphylactic reactions to foods, 2001–2006', *Journal of Allergy and Clinical Immunology* 2007; 119 (4): 1016–18.

4   Liew WK, Williamson E, Tang MLK, 'Anaphylaxis fatalities and admissions in Australia', *Journal of Allergy and Clinical Immunology* 2009; 123 (2): 434–442.

5   Tang MLK, Kang LW, 'Prevention and treatment of anaphylaxis', *Paediatrics and Child Health* 2008; 18 (7): 309–16.

6   Bock SA, Muñoz-Furlong AM, Sampson HA, 'Fatalities', 191–93.

7   Sampson HA, Mendelson L, Rosen J, 'Fatal and near-fatal anaphylactic reactions to food in children and adolescents', *New England Journal of Medicine* 1992; 327 (6): 380–84.

8   Sampson MA, Muñoz-Furlong A, Sicherer SH, 'Risk-taking and coping strategies of adolescents and young adults with food allergy', *Journal of Allergy and Clinical Immunology* 2006;117 (6): 1440–44.

9   Noone S, Muñoz-Furlong A, Sicherer SH, S 133.

10 Sampson MA, Muñoz-Furlong A, Sicherer SH, 1440–44.

11 Sampson MA, Muñoz-Furlong A, Sicherer SH, 1440–44.

12 Noone S, Muñoz-Furlong A, Sicherer SH, S 133.

13 Sampson MA, Muñoz-Furlong A, Sicherer SH, 1440–44.

14 Muñoz-Furlong A, 'Daily coping strategies for patients and their families', *Pediatrics* 2003; 111 (6): 1654–61.

15 Muñoz-Furlong A, 1654–61.

16 Monga S, Manassis K, 'Treating anxiety in children with life-threatening anaphylactic conditions', *Journal of the American Academy of Child & Adolescent Psychiatry* 2006; 45 (8): 1007–10.

17 Mandell D, Curtis R, Gold M, Hardie S, 'Anaphylaxis: How do you live with it?', *Health and Social Work* 2005; 30 (4): 325–35.

18 Akeson N, Worth A, Sheik A, 'The psychosocial impact of anaphylaxis on young people and their parents', *Clinical & Experimental Allergy* 2007; 37 (8): 1213–1220.

19 Sampson MA, Muñoz-Furlong A, Sicherer SH, 1440–44.

20 Sampson HA, Mendelson L, Rosen J, 380–84.

21 Bock SA, Muñoz-Furlong AM, Sampson HA, 'Fatalities', 191–93.

22 Bock SA, Muñoz-Furlong AM, Sampson HA, 'Further', 1016–18.

23 Liew WK, Williamson E, Tang MLK, 434–442.

24 Liew WK, Williamson E, Tang MLK, 434–442.

25 Mandell D, Curtis R, Gold M, Hardie S, 325–35.

26 Sampson MA, Muñoz-Furlong A, Sicherer SH, 1440–44.

27 Maloney JM, Chapman MD, Sicherer SH, 'Peanut allergen exposure through saliva: Assessment and interventions to reduce exposure', *Journal of Allergy and Clinical Immunology* 2006; 118 (3): 719–24.

28 Maloney JM, Chapman MD, Sicherer SH, 719–24.

29 Sicherer SH, 2006, *Understanding and managing your child's food allergies*, Johns Hopkins, Baltimore, p 157.

Chapter 15

1 Grotbeng EH, 1995, 'A Guide to Promoting Resilience in Children: Strengthening the Human Spirit', Alabama University, Birmingham, Civitan International Research Center, p 2.

Chapter 16

1 Mandell D, Curtis R, Gold M, Hardie S, 'Anaphylaxis: How do you live with it?', *Health and Social Work 2005*; 30 (4): 325–35.
2 Hu W, Kerridge I, Kemp A, 'Risk, rationality, and regret: Responding to the uncertainty of childhood food anaphylaxis', *Medical Humanities* 2005; 31: 12–16.
3 Slovic P, *Informing and educating the public about risk. The Perception of Risk*, Earthscan, London, 2000: 182–91.
4 Moneret-Vautrin DA, Morisset M, Flabbee J, Beaudouin E, Kanny G. 'Epidemiology of life-threatening and lethal anaphylaxis: a review', *Allergy* 2005; 60 (4) 443–451.
5 Roland J, 1999, 'Chronic illness and family life cycle', in Carter B, McGoldrick M (eds), *The Expanded family life cycle: Individual, family, and social perspectives*, 3rd edn, pp 492–511, Allyn & Bacon, Boston.
6 Mandell D, Curtis R, Gold M, Hardie S.
7 Klinnert MD, Robinson JL, 'Addressing the psychological needs of families of food-allergic children', *Current allergy and asthma reports* 2008; 8 (3): 195–200.
8 Roland J, 492–511.
9 Mandell D, Curtis R, Gold M, Hardie S.
10 Avery NJ, King RM, Knight S, Hourihane JO'B, 'Assessment of quality of life in children with peanut allergy', *Pediatric Allergy and Immunology* 2003; 14: 378–82.
11 Klinnert MD, Robinson JL.
12 Mandell D, Curtis R, Gold M, Hardie S.
13 Mandell D, Curtis R, Gold M, Hardie S.
14 Mandell D, Curtis R, Gold M, Hardie S.
15 Poulos LM, Waters AM, Correll PK, Loblay RH, Marks GB, 'Trends in hospitalizations for anaphylaxis, angiodema, and urticaria in Australia, 1993–1994 to 2004–2005', *Journal of Allergy and Clinical Immunology* 2007; 120 (4): 878–84.
16 Brown SGA, Mullins RJ, Gold MS, '2. Anaphylaxis: diagnosis and management', The *Medical Journal of Australia Practice Essentials — Allergy* 2006; 185 (5) 283–89.
17 Moneret-Vautrin DA, Morisset M, Flabbee J, Beaudouin E, Kanny G.
18 Mandell D, Curtis R, Gold M, Hardie S.
19 Hu W, Loblay R, Ziegler J, Kemp A, 'Attributes and views of families with food allergic children recruited from allergy clinics and from a consumer organization' (Abstract), *Pediatric Allergy and Immunology*, 2008; 19 (3): 264–269.

Chapter 17

1 Monga S, Manassis K, 'Treating anxiety in children with life-threatening anaphylactic conditions', *Journal of the American Academy of Child & Adolescent Psychiatry* 2006; 45 (8): 1007–10.
2 Avery NJ, King RM, Knight S, Hourihane JO'B, 'Assessment of quality of life in children with peanut allergy', *Pediatric Allergy and Immunology* 2003; 114 (5): 378–82.
3 Avery NJ, King RM, Knight S, Hourihane JO'B.
4 Primeau MN, Kagan R, Joseph L, Lim H, Dufresne C, Duffy C, Prhcal D, Clarke A, 'The psychological burden of peanut allergy as perceived by adults with peanut allergy and the parents of peanut-allergic children', *Clinical and Experimental Allergy* 2000; 30:1135–43.

[5] Avery NJ, King RM, Knight S, Hourihane JO'B.

[6] Avery NJ, King RM, Knight S, Hourihane JO'B.

[7] Klinnert MD, Robinson JL, 'Addressing the psychological needs of families of food-allergic children', *Current Allergy and Asthma Reports* 2008; 8 (3): 195–200.

[8] Mandell D, Curtis R, Gold M, Hardie S, 'Anaphylaxis: How do you live with it? *Health and Social Work* 2005; 30 (4): 325–35.

[9] Klinnert MD, Robinson JL.

[10] Sampson MA, Muñoz-Furlong A, Sicherer SH, 'Risk-taking and coping strategies of adolescents and young adults with food allergy', *Journal of Allergy and Clinical Immunology* 2006; 117 (6): 1440–44.

[11] Noone S, Muñoz-Furlong A, Sicherer SH, 'Parent and adolescent perceptions of food allergy [abstract]', *Journal of Allergy and Clinical Immunology* 2003; 111 (1): S 133.

[12] Muris P, Steerneman P, Merckelbach H, Meesters C, 'The role of parental fearfulness and modeling in children's fear', *Behaviour Research and Therapy* 1996; 34 (3): 265–268.

[13] Muñoz-Furlong A, 'Daily coping strategies for patients and their families', *Pediatrics* 2003; 111 (6): 1654–61.

[14] Noone S, Muñoz-Furlong A, Sicherer SH.

[15] Avery NJ, King RM, Knight S, Hourihane JO'B.

Chapter 18

[1] Prescott SL, Tang MLK, Björkstén B, 'Primary allergy prevention in children: updated summary of a position statement of the Australasian Society of Clinical Immunology and Allergy 2007', *Medical Journal of Australia Practice Essentials — Allergy Monograph*: 54–58.

[2] Australasian Society of Clinical Immunology and Allergy (ASCIA), 'Patient Information: Allergy Prevention in Children', February 2009, may be accessed online at: www.allergy.org.au

[3] ASCIA, 'Patient Information: Allergy Prevention in Children'.

[4] ASCIA, 'Patient Information: Allergy Prevention in Children'.

[5] ASCIA, 'Patient Information, Allergy Prevention in Children'.

[6] Prescott SL, Tang MLK, Björkstén B.

[7] Kemp A, 'Allergy prevention — what we thought we knew', *The Medical Journal of Australia* 2003; 178, 254–55.

[8] Sicherer SH, Burks AW, 'Maternal and infant diets for prevention of allergic diseases: Understanding menu changes in 2008', *Journal of Allergy and Clinical Immunology* 2008; 122 (1): 29–33.

[9] Prescott SL, Tang MLK, Björkstén B.

[10] Prescott SL, Tang MLK, Björkstén B.

[11] Martinez FD, Cline M, Burrows B, 'Increased incidence of asthma in children of smoking mothers', *Pediatrics* 1992; 89 (1): 21–26.

[12] Prescott SL, Tang MLK, Björkstén B.

[13] Sicherer SH, Burks AW.

[14] Greer FR, Sicherer SH, Burks AW and the Committee on Nutrition and Section on Allergy and Immunology, 'Effects of Early Nutritional Interventions on the Development of Atopic Disease in Infants and Children: The Role of Maternal Dietary Restriction, Breastfeeding, Timing of Introduction of Complementary Foods, and Hydrolyzed Formulas', *Pediatrics* 2008; 121 (1): 183–191.

[15] Sicherer SH, Burks AW.

[16] Kramer MS, Kakuma R, 'Maternal dietary antigen avoidance during pregnancy or lactation, or both, for preventing or treating atopic disease in the child', *Chochrane Database Systematic Reviews* 2006, Issue 3, Art. No.: CD000133, DOI: 10.1002/145651858.CD000133.pub2.

[17] Kramer MS, Kakuma R.

[18] ASCIA, 'Patient Information: Allergy Prevention in Children'.

[19] Kramer MS, Kakuma R.

[20] ASCIA, 'Patient Information: Allergy Prevention in Children'.

[21] Sicherer SH, Burks AW.

[22] Prescott SL, Tang MLK, Björkstén B.

[23] Tang MLK, Robinson M, 'Allergy Prevention: Current recommendations and new insights', *Australian Family Physician* 2008; 37 (4) 207.

[24] ASCIA, 'Patient Information: Allergy Prevention in Children'.

[25] Prescott SL, Björkstén B, 'Probiotics for the prevention or treatment of allergic diseases', *Journal of Allergy and Clinical Immunology* 2007; 120 (2): 255–62.

[26] ASCIA, 'Patient Information: Allergy Prevention in Children'.

[27] Hesselmar B, Aberg N, Aberg B, Eriksson B, Björkstén B, 'Does early exposure to cat or dog protect against later allergy development? *Clinical and Experimental Allergy* 1999; 29 (5): 611–17.

[28] ASCIA, 'Patient Information: Allergy Prevention in Children'.

[29] Prescott SL, Tang MLK, Björkstén B.

[30] Prescott SL, Tang MLK, Björkstén B.

[31] ASCIA, 'Patient Information: Allergy Prevention in Children'.

Chapter 19

[1] Oppenheimer JJ, Nelson HS, Bock SA, Christensen F, Leung DY, 'Treatment of peanut allergy with rush immunotherapy', *Journal of Allergy and Clinical Immunology* 1992; 90 (2): 256–262.

[2] Nelson HS, Lahr J, Rule R, Bock A, Leung D, 'Treatment of anaphylactic sensitivity to peanuts by immunotherapy with injections of aqueous peanut extract', *Journal of Allergy and Clinical Immunology* 1997; 99 (6) Part 1: 744–751.

[3] Enrique E, Pineda F, Malek T, Bartra J, Basagaña M, Tella R, Castelló JV, Alonso R, de Mateo JA, Cerdá-Trias T, del Mar San Miguel-Moncín M, Monzón S, García M, Palacios R, Cisteró-Bahíma A, 'Sublingual immunotherapy for hazelnut food allergy: A randomized, double-blind, placebo-controlled study with a standardized hazelnut extract', *Journal of Allergy and Clinical Immunology* 2005; 116 (5) Part 1: 1073–79.

[4] Patriarca G, Nucera E, Pollastrini E, Roncallo C, De Pasquale T, Lombardo C, Pedone C, Gasbarrini G, Buonomo A, Schiavino D, 'Oral Specific Desensitization in Food-Allergic Children', *Digestive diseases and sciences* 2007; 52 (7): 1662–72.

[5] Clark AT, Islam S, King Y, Deighton J, Anagnostou K, Ewan, PW, 'Successful oral tolerance induction in severe peanut allergy', *Allergy* 2009 (online).

[6] Varshney P, Jones SM, Pons L, Kulis M, Steele PH, Kemper AR, Scurlock AM, Perry TT, Burks AW, 'Oral Immunotherapy (OIT) induces clinical tolerance in peanut-allergic children', *Journal of Allergy and Clinical Immunology* 2009; 123 (2) Supplement 1: S179.

[7] Leung DY, Sampson HA, Yunginger JW, Burks AW, Schneider LC, Wortel CH, Davis FM, Hyun JD, Shanahan WR, 'Effect of anti-IgE therapy in patients with peanut allergy', *New England Journal of Medicine* 2003; 348 (11):986–993.

[8] Sicherer SH, Sampson HA, 'Peanut allergy: emerging concepts and approaches for an apparent epidemic', *Journal of Allergy and Clinical Immunology* 2007; 120 (3): 491–503.

[9] Sampson HA, 'A phase II, randomized, double-blind, parallel-group, placebo-controlled, oral food challenge trial of Xolair (omalizumab) in peanut allergy (TOPS)', *Journal of Allergy and Clinical Immunology* 2007; 119 (1): S117.

[10] Watson C, Rafi A, Do L, Sheinkopf L, Katz R, 'Efficacy of Omalizumab for the treatment of food allergy', *Journal of Allergy and Clinical Immunology* 2008; 121 (2) Supplement 1: S252.

[11] Nowak-Wegrzyn AH, Sicherer SH, Shreffler WG, Thanik E, Modifi S, Noone S, Sampson HA, 'A trial of a diet containing baked egg in children with egg allergy', *Journal of Allergy and Clinical Immunology* 2007; 119 (1) Supplement 1: S194.

[12] Konstantinou G, Giavi S, Kalobatsou A, Vassilopoulou E, Douladiris N, Saxoni-Papageorgiou P, Papadopoulos NG. MD, 'Consumption of heat-treated egg by children allergic or sensitized to egg can affect the natural course of egg allergy: Hypothesis-generating observations', *Journal of Allergy and Clinical Immunology* 2008; 122 (2): 414–15.

[13] Nowak-Wegrzyn A, Bloom KA, Sicherer SH, Shreffler WG, Noone S, Wanich N, Sampson HA, 'Tolerance to extensively heated milk in children with cow's milk allergy', *Journal of Allergy and Clinical Immunology* 2008; 122 (2): 342–47.

[14] Rawas-Qalaji MM, Simons FER, Simons KJ, 'Sublingual epinephrine tablets versus intramuscular injection of epinephrine: Dose equivalence for potential treatment of anaphylaxis', *Journal of Allergy and Clinical Immunology* 2006; 117 (2): 398–403.

[15] Rawas-Qalaji MM, Simons FER, Simons KJ.

[16] Li XM, 'Traditional Chinese herbal remedies for asthma and food allergy', *Journal of Allergy and Clinical Immunology* 2007; 120 (1): 25–31.

[17] Li XM.

[18] Li XM.

[19] Li XM.

[20] Joshi P, 'Presentation to NSW Paediatric respiratory meeting', 2006.

[21] Weidinger S, O'Sullivan M, Illig T, Baurecht H, Depner M, Rodriguez E, Ruether A, Klopp N, Vogelberg C, Weiland SK, McLean WH, von Mutius E, Irvine AD, Kabesch M, 'Filaggrin mutations, atopic eczema, hay fever, and asthma in children', *Journal of Allergy and Clinical Immunology* 2008; 121 (5): 1203–09.

[22] Lack G, Fox D, Northstone K, Golding J, for the Avon Longitudinal Study of Parents and Children Study Team, 'Factors associated with the development of peanut allergy in childhood', *The New England Journal of Medicine* 2003; 348 (11): 977–985.

[23] Henderson J et al., 'The burden of disease associated with filaggrin mutations: a population-based, longitudinal birth cohort study', *Journal of Allergy and Clinical Immunology* 2008; 121 (4): 872–77.

[24] Brown SJ, Relton CL, Liao H, Zhao Y, Sandilands A, Wilson IJ, Burn J, Reynolds NJ, McLean WH, Cordell HJ, 'Filaggrin null mutations and childhood atopic eczema: a population-based case-control study', *Journal of Allergy and Clinical Immunology* 2008; 121 (4): 940–46.

[25] Weidinger S, Illig T, Baurecht H, Irvine AD, Rodriguez E, Diaz-Lacava A, Klopp N, Wagenpfeil S, Zhao Y, Liao H, Lee SP, Palmer CN, Jenneck C, Maintz L, Hagemann T, Behrendt H, Ring J, Nothen MM, McLean WH, Novak N, 'Loss-of-function variations within the filaggrin gene predispose for atopic dermatitis with allergic sensitizations', *Journal of Allergy and Clinical Immunology* 2008; 118 (1): 214–19.

[26] Palmer CNA, Irvine AD, Terron-Kwiatkowski A, Zhao Y, Liao H, Lee SP, Goudie DR, Sandilands A, Campbell LE, Smith FJD, O'Regan GM, Watson RM, Cecil JE, Bale SJ, Compton JG, DiGiovanna JJ, Fleckman P, Lewis-Jones S, Arseculeratne G, Sergeant A, Munro CS, El Houate B, McElreavey K, Halkjaer LB, Bisgaard H, Mukhopadhyay S, Irwin McLean WH, 'Common loss-of-function variants of the epidermal barrier protein filaggrin are a major predisposing factor for atopic dermatitis', *Nature Genetics* 2006; 38: 441–446.

BIBLIOGRAPHY

Articles

Aickin R, Hill D, Kemp A, 'Measles immunisation in children with allergy to egg', *British Medical Journal* 1994; 309: 223–5.

Akeson N, Worth A, Sheik A, 'The psychosocial impact of anaphylaxis on young people and their parents', *Clinical and Experimental Allergy* 2007; 37 (8): 1213–1220.

Allen KJ, Hill DJ, Heine RG, '4. Food allergy in childhood', *Medical Journal of Australia Practice Essentials — Allergy* 2006; 185 (7): 394–400.

Australasian Society of Clinical Immunology and Allergy, 'Diagnosis and management of food hypersensitivity in childhood', may be accessed online at www.allergy.org.au/content/view/166/1/

Australasian Society of Clinical Immunology and Allergy (ASCIA), 'Guidelines for EpiPen® prescription', 2004, may be accessed online at: www.allergy.org.au/images/stories/anaphylaxis/ASCIA_EpiPen_ prescription_guidelines.pdf. Information in the PBS Schedule about EpiPen, may be accessed online at: www.pbs.gov.au/html/consumer/ product/restrictions?publication=GE&code=8698T&brand=EpiPen

Australasian Society of Clinical Immunology and Allergy (ASCIA), 'Health Professional Information: Is it allergy?', may be accessed online at: www. allergy.org.au/content/view/344/305/

Australasian Society of Clinical Immunology and Allergy (ASCIA), 'Patient Information: Allergy Prevention in Children', February 2009, may be accessed online at: www.allergy.org.au

Australasian Society of Clinical Immunology and Allergy (ASCIA), 'Patient Information: Anaphylaxis', December 2007, may be accessed online at: www.allergy.org.au/content/view/178/1/

Australasian Society of Clinical Immunology and Allergy, 'Patient Information: Food allergy', may be accessed online at: www.allergy.org.au/ content/view/167/1/

Australasian Society of Clinical Immunology and Allergy (ASCIA), 'Patient Information: Food allergy: other foods', may be accessed online at: www. allergy.org.au/content/view/183/1/

Australasian Society of Clinical Immunology and Allergy (ASCIA), 'Patient Information: Latex allergy', may be accessed online at: www.allergy.org.au/ content/view/107/1/

Australian Society of Clinical Immunology and Allergy (ASCIA) 2008, 'Peanut, tree nut and seed allergy info bulletin', may be accessed at: www. allergy.org.au/images/stories/aer/infobulletins/pdf/aer_peanut_tree_nut_ seed_allergy_jun08.pdf

Australasian Society of Clinical Immunology and Allergy (ASCIA), 'Position Paper, Guidelines for prevention of food anaphylactic reactions in schools, preschools and childcare', 2004, updated 2007, may be accessed online at: www.allergy.org.au/pospapers/anaphylaxis.htm

Australasian Society of Clinical Immunology and Allergy, 'Position paper: Unorthodox testing and treatment for allergic disorders', may be accessed online at: www.allergy.org.au/content/view/322/271/

Australasian Society of Clinical Immunology and Allergy, 'Report by Access Economics Pty Ltd: The economic impact of allergic disease in Australia: not to be sneezed at', November 2007, may be accessed online at: www. ascia.org.au

Avery NJ, King RM, Knight S, Hourihane JO'B, 'Assessment of quality of life in children with peanut allergy', *Pediatric Allergy and Immunology* 2003; 14: 378–82.

Bernhisel-Broadbent J, Strause D, Sampson HA, 'Fish hypersensitivity. II: Clinical relevance of altered fish allergenicity caused by various preparation methods', *Journal of Allergy and Clinical Immunology* 1992; 90 (4): 622–29.

Beyer K, Morrow E, Li XM, et al., 'Effects of cooking methods on peanut allergenicity', *Journal of Allergy and Clinical Immunology* 2001; 107 (6): 1077–81.

Björkstén B, 'How allergenic is food? (Editorial)', *Clinical and Experimental Allergy* 2004; 34: 673–75.

Bock SA, Muñoz-Furlong AM, Sampson HA, 'Fatalities due to anaphylactic reactions to foods', *Journal of Allergy and Clinical Immunology* 2001; 107 (1): 191–93.

Bock SA, Muñoz-Furlong AM, Sampson HA, 'Further fatalities due to anaphylactic reactions to foods, 2001–2006', *Journal of Allergy and Clinical Immunology* 2007; 119 (4): 1016–18.

Bock SA, Sampson HA, Atkins FM, Zeiger RS, Lehrer S, Sachs M, et al., 'Double-blind, placebo-controlled food challenge as an office procedure: A manual', *Journal of Allergy and Clinical Immunology* 1988; 82 (6): 986–97.

Boros CA, Kay D, Gold MS, 'Parent reported allergy and anaphylaxis in 4173 South Australian children', *Journal of Paediatrics and Child Health* 2000; 36: 36–40.

Boyce JA, 'Successful treatment of cold-induced urticaria/anaphylaxis with anti-IgE (Case study)', *Journal of Allergy and Clinical Immunology* 2006; 117 (6): 1415–18.

Boyle RJ, Tang ML, 'Can Allergic disease be prevented prenatally?' *Allergy* 2006; 61: 1423–31.

Bråbäck L, Hjern A, Rasmussen F, 'Trends in asthma, allergic rhinitis and eczema among Swedish conscripts from farming and non-farming environments: A nationwide study over three decades', *Clinical Experimental Allergy* 2004; 34 (1): 38–43.

Brown A, McKinnon D, Chu K, 'Emergency department anaphylaxis: A review of 142 patients in a single year', *Journal of Allergy and Clinical Immunology* 2001; 108 (5): 861–66.

Brown SGA, Mullins RJ, Gold MS, '2. Anaphylaxis: diagnosis and management', *Medical Journal of Australia Practice Essentials — Allergy* 2006; 185 (5): 283–89.

Brown SJ, Relton CL, Liao H, Zhao Y, Sandilands A, Wilson IJ, Burn J, Reynolds NJ, McLean WH, Cordell HJ, 'Filaggrin null mutations and childhood atopic eczema: a population-based case-control study', *Journal of Allergy and Clinical Immunology* 2008; 121 (4): 940–46.

Burches E, Cervera R, Peláez A, 'Food-induced anaphylaxis caused by inhalation of soy protein', *The Journal of Investigational Allergology and Clinical Immunology* 2007; 17 (6): 418–19.

Busse PJ, Nowak-Wegrzyn AH, Noone SA, Sampson H, Sicherer S, 'Recurrent peanut allergy (correspondence)', *New England Journal of Medicine* 2002; 347 (19): 1535–36.

Caffarelli C, Petroccione T, 'False-negative food challenges in children with suspected food allergy', *The Lancet* 2001; 358: 1871–72.

Carvalho NF, Kennedy RD, Carrington PH, Hall DE, 'Severe nutritional deficiencies in toddlers resulting from health food milk alternatives (Electronic article)', *Pediatrics* 2001; 107 (4): e46.

Casimir G, Cuvelier P, Allard S, Duchateau J, 'Life-threatening fish allergy successfully treated with immunotherapy', *Pediatric Allergy and Immunology* 1997; 8: 103–5.

Castells M, Horan R, Sheffer A, 'Exercise-induced anaphylaxis', *Current Allergy and Asthma Reports* 2003; 3 (1): 15–21.

Charous BL, Blanco C, Tarlo S, Hamilton RG, Baur X, Beezhold D, Sussman G, Yunginger JW, 'Natural rubber latex allergy after 12 years: Recommendations and perspectives', *Journal of Allergy and Clinical Immunology* 2002; 109 (1): 31–34.

Clark S, Bock SA, Gaeta TJ, Brenner BE, Cydulka RK, Camargo CA on behalf of the Multicenter Airway Research Collaboration — 8 Investigators, 'Multicenter study of emergency department visits for food allergies', *Journal of Allergy and Clinical Immunology* 2004; 113 (2): 347–52.

Cohen BL, Noone S, Muñoz-Furlong A, Sicherer SH, 'Development of a questionnaire to measure quality of life in families with a child with food allergy', *Journal of Allergy and Clinical Immunology* 2004; 114 (5): 1159–63.

Colver A, 'Are the dangers of childhood food allergy exaggerated?', *British Medical Journal* 2006; 333; 494–96.

Crespo JF, Pascual C, Dominguez C, Ojeda I, Munoz FM, Estaban MM, 'Allergic reactions associated with airborne fish particles in IgE-mediated fish hypersensitive patients', *Allergy* 1995; 50: 257–61.

Crespo JF, Rodriguez J, Vives R, James JM, Reaño M, Daroca P, Burbano C, Muzquiz M, 'Occupational IgE-mediated allergy after exposure to lupine seed flour', *Journal of Allergy and Clinical Immunology* 2001; 108: 295–97.

Dalal I, Binson R, Reifen R, Amitai Z, Shohat T, Rahmani S, Levine A, Ballin A, Somekh E, 'Food allergy is a matter of geography after all: sesame as a major cause of severe IgE-mediated food allergic reactions among infants and young children in Israel', *European Journal of Allergy and Clinical Immunology* 2002; 57: 362–65.

Dannaeus A, Inganas M, 'A follow-up study of children with food allergy: Clinical course in relation to serum IgE- and IgG-antibody levels to milk, egg and fish', *Clinical and Experimental Allergy* 1981; 111 (6): 533–39.

Dioun AF, Harris SK, Hibberd PL, 'Is maternal age at delivery related to childhood food allergy?', *Pediatric Allergy and Immunology* 2003; 14: 307–11.

Douglas DM, Sukenick E, Andrade WP, Brown JS, 'Biphasic systemic anaphylaxis: An inpatient and outpatient study', *Journal of Allergy and Clinical Immunology* 1994; 93 (6): 977–85.

Douglass JA, O'Hehir RE, '1. Diagnosis, treatment and prevention of allergic disease: the basics', *Medical Journal of Australia Practice Essentials — Allergy* 2006; 185 (4): 228–33.

Du Toit G, Katz Y, Sasieni P, Mesher D, Maleki SJ, Fisher HR, Fox AT, Turcanu V, Amir T, Zadik-Mnuhin G, Cohen A, Livne I, Lack G, 'Early consumption of peanuts in infancy is associated with a low prevalence of peanut allergy', *Journal of Allergy and Clinical Immunology* 2008; 122 (5): 984–91.

Eggesbø M, Botten G, Halvorsen R, Magnus P, 'The prevalence of allergy to egg: a population-based study in young children', *Allergy* 2001; 56 (5): 403–11.

Eggesbø M, Botten G, Stigum H, Samuelson SO, Brunekreef B, Magnus P, 'Caesarian delivery and cow milk allergy/intolerance', *Allergy* 2005; 60: 1172–73.

Eigenmann PA, Sicherer SH, Borkowski TA, Cohen BA, Sampson H, 'Prevalence of IgE-mediated food allergy among children with atopic dermatitis', *Pediatrics* 1998; 101: 8–12.

Enrique E, Pineda F, Malek T, Bartra J, Basagaña M, Tella R, Castelló JV, Alonso R, de Mateo JA, Cerdá-Trias T, del Mar San Miguel-Moncín M, Monzón S, García M, Palacios R, Cisteró-Bahíma A, 'Sublingual immunotherapy for hazelnut food allergy: A randomized, double-blind, placebo-controlled study with a standardized hazelnut extract', *Journal of Allergy and Clinical Immunology* 2005; 116 (5) Part 1: 1073–79.

Fiocchi A, Restani P, Riva E, Mirri GP, Santini I, Bernardo L, Galli CL, 'Heat treatment modifies the allergenicity of beef and bovine serum albumin', *Allergy* 1998; 53 (8): 798–802.

Fleischer DM, Conover-Walker MK, Christie L, Burks AW, Wood RA, 'The natural progression of peanut allergy: Resolution and the possibility of recurrence', *Journal of Allergy and Clinical Immunology* 2003; 112 (1): 183–89.

Fleischer DM, Conover-Walker MK, Matsui EC, Wood RA, 'The natural history of tree nut allergy', *Journal of Allergy and Clinical Immunology* 2005; 116 (5): 1087–93.

Food Standards Australia New Zealand, 'Quantitative Consumer Survey on Allergen Labelling: Benchmark survey 2003', NFO Donovan Research Report, Canberra, 2004: may be accessed online at: www.foodstandards. gov.au/newsroom/publications/evaluationreportseries/allergensurveyno7/ index.cfm

Friedman N, Zeiger RS, 'The role of breast-feeding in the development of allergies and asthma', *Journal of Allergy and Clinical Immunology* 2005; 115 (6): 1238–47.

Gangur V, Kelly, C, Navuluri L, 'Sesame allergy: a growing food allergy of global proportions', *Annals of Allergy, Asthma and Immunology* 2005; 95 (1): 4–11.

Gold MS, 'EpiPen epidemic or good clinical practice? Commentary', *Journal of Paediatrics and Child Health* 2003; 39, 376–77.

Gold MS, Kemp AS, '6. Atopic disease in childhood', *Medical Journal of Australia Practice Essentials — Paediatrics* 2005; 182 (6): 298–304.

Gold MS, Sainsbury R, 'First aid anaphylaxis management in children who were prescribed an epinephrine autoinjector device (EpiPen)', *Journal of Allergy and Clinical Immunology* 2000; 106 (1): 171–76.

Gowland MH, 'Food allergen avoidance — the patient's viewpoint', *Allergy* 2001; 56 (Supplement 67): 117–20.

Greer FR, Sicherer SH, Burks AW and the Committee on Nutrition and Section on Allergy and Immunology, 'Effects of early nutritional interventions on the development of atopic disease in infants and children: The role of maternal dietary restriction, breastfeeding, timing of introduction of complementary foods, and hydrolyzed formulas', *Pediatrics* 2008; 121 (1): 183–191.

Grundy J, Matthews S, Bateman B, Dean T, Arshad SH, 'Rising prevalence of allergy to peanut in children: Data from 2 sequential cohorts', *Journal of Allergy and Clinical Immunology* 2002; 110 (5): 784–9.

Gupta R, Sheikh A, Strachan D, Anderson HR, 'Increasing hospital admissions for systemic allergic disorders in England: Analysis of national admissions data', *British Medical Journal* 2003; 327: 1142–43.

Gupta R, Sheikh A, Strachan DP, Anderson HR, 'Time trends in allergic disorders in the UK', *Thorax* (Online) 2006; 000: 1–6.

Henderson J, Northstone K, Lee SP, Liao H, Zhao Y, Pembrey M, Mukhopadhyay S, Smith GD, Palmer CN, McLean WH, Irvine AD, 'The burden of disease associated with filaggrin mutations: a population-based, longitudinal birth cohort study', *Journal of Allergy and Clinical Immunology* 2008; 121 (4): 872–77.

Hesselmar B, Aberg N, Aberg B, Eriksson B, Björkstén B, 'Does early exposure to cat or dog protect against later allergy development?', *Clinical and Experimental Allergy* 1999; 29 (5): 611–17.

Hill DJ, Firer MA, Ball G, Hosking CS, 'Natural history of cow's milk allergy in children: immunological outcome over 2 years', *Clinical and Experimental Allergy* 1993; 23: 124–31.

Hill DJ, Hosking CS, Reyes-Benito LV, 'Reducing the need for food allergen challenges in young children: a comparison of in vitro with in vivo tests', *Clinical and Experimental Allergy* 2001; 31: 1031–35.

Høst, A, 'Frequency of cow's milk allergy in Childhood', *Annals of Allergy Asthma and Immunology* 2002; 89 (6 Supplement 1): 33–37.

Høst A, Halken S, 'A prospective study of cow milk allergy in Danish infants during the first 3 years of life: clinical course in relation to clinical and immunological type of hypersensitivity reaction', *Allergy* 1990; 45: 587–96.

Hourihane J O'B, 'Community management of severe allergies must be integrated and comprehensive, and must consist of more than just epinephrine (Editorial)', *Allergy* 2001; 56: 1023–25.

Hourihane J O'B, Roberts SA, Warner JO, 'Resolution of peanut allergy: Case-control study', *British Medical Journal* 1998; 316: 1271–5.

Hu W, Kerridge I, Kemp A, 'Risk, rationality, and regret: Responding to the uncertainty of childhood food anaphylaxis', *Medical Humanities* 2005; 31: 12–16.

Hu W, Loblay R, Ziegler J, Kemp A, 'Attributes and views of families with food allergic children recruited from allergy clinics and from a consumer organization', *Pediatric Allergy and Immunology* 2008; 19 (3): 264–69.

Illi S, von Mutius E, Lau S, Bergmann R, Niggemann B, Sommerfeld C, Wahn U, 'Early childhood infectious diseases and the development of asthma up to school age: A birth cohort study', *British Medical Journal* 2001; 322: 390–95.

James JM, Burks AW, Roberson PK, Sampson HA, 'Safe Administration of the measles vaccine to children allergic to eggs', *New England Journal of Medicine* 1995; 332 (19): 1262–66.

Johansson SGO, Bieber T, Dahl R, Friedmann PS, Lanier BQ, Lockey RF, Motala C, Ortega Martell JA, Platts-Mills TAE, Ring J, Thien F, Van Cauwenberge P, Williams HC, 'Revised nomenclature for allergy for global use: Report of the Nomenclature Review Committee of the World Allergy Organization, October 2003', *Journal of Allergy and Clinical Immunology* 2004; 113 (5): 832–36.

Joshi P, Mofidi S, Sicherer S, 'Interpretation of commercial food ingredient labels by parents of food-allergic children', *Journal of Allergy and Clinical Immunology* 2002; 109 (6): 1019–21.

The International Study of Asthma and Allergies in Childhood Steering Committee, 'Worldwide variation in prevalence of symptoms of asthma, allergic rhinoconjunctivitis, and atopic eczema: ISAAC', *The Lancet* 1998; 351: 1225–32.

Kabesch M, Lauener RP, 'Why Old McDonald had a farm but no allergies: genes environments, and the hygiene hypothesis', *Journal of Leukocyte Biology* 2004; 75: 383–87.

Kalliomäki M, Salminen S, Poussa T, Arvilommi H, Isolauri E, 'Probiotics and prevention of atopic disease: 4-year follow-up of a randomized placebo-controlled trial', *The Lancet* 2003; 361: 1869–70.

Katelaris CH, Peake JE, '5: Allergy and the skin: eczema and chronic urticaria', *Medical Journal of Australia* 2006; 9: 517–22.

Kemp A, 'Allergy prevention — what we thought we knew', *Medical Journal of Australia* 2003; 178: 254–55.

Kemp A, 'Hypoallergenic formula prescribing practices in Australia', *Journal of Paediatrics and Child Health* 2006; 42: 191–95.

Kemp A, 'The EpiPen epidemic — suggestions for rational prescribing in childhood food allergy', *Journal of Paediatric Child Health* 2003; 39: 372–75.

Kemp AS, Hill DJ, Allen KJ, Anderson K, Davidson GP, Day AS, Heine RG, Peake JE, Prescott SL, Shugg AW, Sinn JK, 'Guidelines for the use of infant formulas to treat cow's milk protein allergy: an Australian consensus panel opinion', *Medical Journal of Australia* 2008; 188 (2): 109–12.

Kemp AS, Hu W, 'Food allergy and anaphylaxis — dealing with uncertainty', *Medical Journal of Australia* 2008; 188 (9): 503–04.

Kemp, AS, Mullins RJ, Weiner JM, 'The allergy epidemic: what is the Australian response?' *Medical Journal of Australia Practice Essentials — Allergy* 2006; 185 (4): 226–227.

Kim JS, Sinacore JM, Pongracic JA, 'Parental use of EpiPen for children with food allergies', *Journal of Allergy and Clinical Immunology* 2005; 116 (1): 164–68.

Klein JS, Yocum MW, 'Underreporting of anaphylaxis in a community emergency room', *Journal of Allergy and Clinical Immunology* 1995; 95 (2): 637–38.

Konstantinou G, Giavi S, Kalobatsou A, Vassilopoulou E, Douladiris N, Saxoni-Papageorgiou P, Papadopoulos NG, 'Consumption of heat-treated egg by children allergic or sensitized to egg can affect the natural course of egg allergy: Hypothesis-generating observations', *Journal of Allergy and Clinical Immunology* 2008; 122 (2): 414–15.

Kramer MS, Kakuma R, 'Maternal dietary antigen avoidance during pregnancy or lactation, or both, for preventing or treating atopic disease in the child', *Chochrane Database Systematic Reviews* 2006, Issue 3. Art. No.: CD000133. DOI: 10.1002/145651858.CD000133.pub2.

Krämer U, Heinrich J, Wjst M, Wichmann HE, 'Age of entry to day nursery and allergy in later childhood', *The Lancet* 1999; 353: 450–54.

Kull I, Wickman M, Lilja G, Nordvall SL, Pershagen G, 'Breast feeding and allergic diseases in infants — a prospective birth cohort study', *Archives of Disease in Childhood* 2002; 87: 478–81.

Kull I , Bergström A , Melén E , Lilja G , van Hage M , Pershagen G , Wickman M, 'Early-life supplementation of vitamins A and D, in water-soluble form or in peanut oil, and allergic diseases during childhood', *Journal of Allergy and Clinical Immunology* 2006; 118 (6): 1299–304.

Lack G, Fox D, Northstone K, Golding J, for the Avon Longitudinal Study of Parents and Children Study Team, 'Factors associated with the development of peanut allergy in childhood', *New England Journal of Medicine* 2003; 348 (11): 977–85.

Leung DY, Sampson HA, Yunginger JW, Burks AW, Schneider LC, Wortel CH, Davis FM, Hyun JD, Shanahan WR, 'Effect of anti-IgE therapy in patients with peanut allergy', *New England Journal of Medicine* 2003; 348 (11): 986–93.

Li XM, 'Traditional Chinese herbal remedies for asthma and food allergy', *Journal of Allergy and Clinical Immunology* 2007; 120 (1): 25–31.

Liccardi G, D'Amato G, Canonica G Walter, Salzillo A, Piccolo A, Passalacqua G, 'Systemic reactions from skin testing: literature review', *Journal of Investigational Allergology Clinical Immunology* 2006; Vol. 16 (2): 75–78.

Lieberman, P, Camargo CA, Bohlke Kari, Jick Hershel, Miller RL, Sheikh Aziz, Simons FER, 'Epidemiology of anaphylaxis: findings of the American College of Allergy, Asthma and Immunology Epidemiology of Anaphylaxis Working Group', *Annals of Allergy, Asthma and Immunology* 2006; 97 (5): 596–602.

Liew WK, Williamson E, Tang MLK, 'Anaphylaxis fatalities and admissions in Australia', *Journal of Allergy and Clinical Immunology* 2009; 123 (2): 434–42.

Lin MS, Tanner E, Lynn J, Friday GA Jr, 'Nonfatal systemic allergic reactions induced by skin testing and immunotherapy', *Annals of Allergy*, 1993; 71 (6): 557–62.

Lowe AJ, Carlin JB, Bennett CM, Abramson MJ, Hosking CS, Hill DJ, Dharmage SC, 'Atopic disease and breast-feeding — cause or consequence?' *Journal of Allergy and Clinical Immunology* 2006; 117 (3): 682–87.

Macdougall CF, Cant AJ, Colver AF, 'How dangerous is food allergy in childhood? The incidence of severe and fatal reactions across the UK and Ireland', *Archives of Disease in Childhood* 2002; 86: 236–39.

Maloney JM, Chapman MD, Sicherer SH, 'Peanut allergen exposure through saliva: Assessment and interventions to reduce exposure', *Journal of Allergy and Clinical Immunology* 2006; 118 (3): 719–24.

Mandell D, Curtis R, Gold M, Hardie S, 'Anaphylaxis: How do you live with it?', *Health and Social Work* 2005; 30 (4): 325–35.

Martinez FD, 'The coming-of-age of the hygiene hypothesis', *Respiratory Research* 2001; 2 (3): 129–32.

Martinez FD, Cline M, Burrows B, 'Increased incidence of asthma in children of smoking mothers', *Pediatrics* 1992; 89 (1): 21–26.

Milner JD, Stein DM, McCarter R, Moon RY, 'Early infant multivitamin supplementation is associated with increased risk for food allergy and asthma', *Pediatrics* 2004; 114: 27–32.

Moneret-Vautrin DA, Morisset M, Flabbee J, Beaudouin E, Kanny G, 'Epidemiology of life-threatening and lethal anaphylaxis: a review', *Allergy* 2005; 60 (4) 443–451.

Moneret-Vautrin D A, Guerin L, Kanny G, Flabbee J, Fremont S, Morisset M, 'Cross-allergenicity of peanut and lupine: the risk of lupine allergy in patients allergic to peanuts', *Journal of Allergy and Clinical Immunology* 1999; 104 (4, Part 1): 883–88.

Monga S, Manassis K, 'Treating anxiety in children with life-threatening anaphylactic conditions', *Journal of the American Academy of Child & Adolescent Psychiatry* 2006; 45 (8): 1007–10.

Motala C, Lockey R (Ed), 'Food allergy: Allergic Diseases Resource Center', may be accessed online at: www.worldallergy.org/professional/allergic_ diseases_center/foodallergy/

Mullins R, 'Paediatric food trends in a community-based specialist allergy practice, 1995–2006', *Medical Journal of Australia* 2007; 186: 618–21.

Mullins R, 'Anaphylaxis: risk factors for recurrence', Clinical Experimental Allergy 2003; 33: 1033–40.

Muris P, Steerneman P, Merckelbach H, Meesters C, 'The role of parental fearfulness and modeling in children's fear', *Behaviour Research and Therapy* 1996; 34 (3): 265–68.

Nelson HS, Lahr J, Rule R, Bock A, Leung D, 'Treatment of anaphylactic sensitivity to peanuts by immunotherapy with injections of aqueous peanut extract', *Journal of Allergy and Clinical Immunology* 1997; 99 (6) Part 1: 744–51.

NIH Expert Panel on Food Allergy Research, 'Food Allergy: Report of the NIH Expert Panel on Food Allergy Research', may be accessed online at: www3.niaid.nih.gov/topics/foodAllergy/research/ReportFoodAllergy.htm

Noone S, Muñoz-Furlong A, Sicherer SH, 'Parent and adolescent perceptions of food allergy [abstract]', *Journal of Allergy and Clinical Immunology* 2003; 111 (1): S 133.

Nowak-Wegrzyn AH, Bloom KA, Sicherer SH, Shreffler WG, Noone S, Wanich N, Sampson HA, 'Tolerance to extensively heated milk in children with cow's milk allergy', *Journal of Allergy and Clinical Immunology* 2008; 122 (2): 342–47.

Nowak-Wegrzyn AH, Sicherer SH, Shreffler WG, Thanik E, Modifi S, Noone S, Sampson HA, 'A trial of a diet containing baked egg in children with egg allergy', *Journal of Allergy and Clinical Immunology* 2007; 119 (1) Supplement 1: S194.

Nurmatov U, Worth A, Sheikh A, 'Anaphylaxis management plans for the acute and long-term management of anaphylaxis: A systematic review', *Journal of Allergy and Clinical Immunology* 2008; 122 (2): 353–61.

Palmer CNA, Irvine AD, Terron-Kwiatkowski A, Zhao Y, Liao H, Lee SP, Goudie DR, Sandilands A, Campbell LE, Smith FJD, O'Regan GM, Watson RM, Cecil JE, Bale SJ, Compton JG, DiGiovanna JJ, Fleckman P, Lewis-Jones S, Arseculeratne G, Sergeant A, Munro CS, El Houate B, McElreavey K, Halkjaer LB, Bisgaard H, Mukhopadhyay S, Irwin McLean WH, 'Common loss-of-function variants of the epidermal barrier protein filaggrin are a major predisposing factor for atopic dermatitis', *Nature Genetics* 2006; 38: 441–46.

Peat J, van-den-Berg R, Green W, Mellis C, Leeder S, Woolcock A, 'Changing prevalence of asthma in Australian school children', *British Medical Journal* 1994; 308: 1591–96.

Pereira B, Venter C, Grundy J, Clayton CB, Arshad SH Dean T, 'Prevalence of sensitization to food allergens, reported adverse reactions to foods, food avoidance, and food hypersensitivity among teenagers', *Journal of Allergy and Clinical Immunology* 2005; 116 (4): 884–92.

Poulos LM, Waters AM, Correll PK, Loblay RH, Marks GB, 'Trends in hospitalisations for anaphylaxis, angiodema, and urticaria in Australia', 1993–1994 to 2004–2005, *Journal of Allergy and Clinical Immunology* 2007; 120 (4): 878–84.

Prescott SL, Björkstén B, 'Probiotics for the prevention or treatment of allergic diseases', *Journal of Allergy and Clinical Immunology* 2007; 120 (2): 255–62.

Prescott SL, Tang MLK, 'The Australasian Society of Clinical Immunology and Allergy position statement: Summary of allergy prevention in children', *Medical Journal of Australia* 2005; 182 (9): 464–67.

Prescott SL, Tang MLK, Björkstén B, 'Primary allergy prevention in children: updated summary of a position statement of the Australasian Society of Clinical Immunology and Allergy 2007', *Medical Journal of Australia Practice Essentials — Allergy Monograph*: 54–58.

Primeau MN, Kagan R, Joseph L, Lim H, Dufresne C, Duffy C, Prhcal D, Clarke A, 'The psychological burden of peanut allergy as perceived by adults with peanut allergy and the parents of peanut-allergic children', *Clinical and Experimental Allergy* 2000; 30: 1135–43.

Pumphrey RSH, Gowland MH, 'Further fatal allergic reactions to food in the United Kingdom, 1999–2006', *Journal of Allergy and Clinical Immunology* 2007; 119 (4): 1018–19.

Rankin KE, Sheikh A, 'Serious shortcomings in the management of children with anaphylaxis in Scottish schools', PLoS Med 2006; 3 (8): e326.

Rancé F, 'Mustard allergy as a new food allergy', *European Journal of Allergy and Clinical Immunology* 2003; 58: 287.

Rawas-Qalaji MM, Simons FER, Simons KJ, 'Sublingual epinephrine tablets versus intramuscular injection of epinephrine: Dose equivalence for potential treatment of anaphylaxis', *Journal of Allergy and Clinical Immunology* 2006; 117 (2): 398–403.

Riedler J, Braun-Fahrländer C, Eder W, Schreuer M, Waser M, Maisch S, Carr D, Schierl R, Nowak D, von Mutius E (the ALEX Study Team), 'Exposure to farming in early life and development of asthma and allergy: a cross-sectional survey', *The Lancet* 2001; 358: 1129–33.

Roberts G, Lack G, 'Diagnosing peanut allergy with skin prick and specific IgE testing', *Journal of Allergy and Clinical Immunology* 2005; 115 (6): 1291–6.

Roberts G, Lack G, 'Relevance of inhalational exposure to food allergens', *Current Opinion in Allergy and Clinical Immunology* 2003; 3 (3): 211–15.

Robertson CF, Dalton MF, Peat JK, Haby MM, Bauman A, Kennedy JD, Landau LI, 'Asthma and other atopic diseases in Australian Children (Australian arm of the International Study of Asthma and Allergy in Childhood)', *Medical Journal of Australia* 1998; 168: 434–38.

Robertson CF, Roberts MF, Kappers JH, 'Asthma prevalence in Melbourne schoolchildren: Have we reached the peak?', *Medical Journal of Australia* 2004; 180: 273.

Robinson M, Smart J, 'Allergy testing and referral in children', *Australian Family Physician* 2008; 37 (4): 210–13.

Rona, RJ, Keil T, Summers C, Gislason D, Zuidmeer L, Sodergren E, Sigurdardottir ST, Lindner T, Goldhahn K, Dahlstrom J, McBride D, Madsen C, 'The prevalence of food allergy: A meta-analysis', *Journal of Allergy and Clinical Immunology* 2007; 120 (3): 638–46.

Said M, Weiner JM, 'May contain traces of ...: Hidden food allergens in Australia (Editorial)', *Medical Journal of Australia* 2004; 181 (4): 183–84.

Sampson HA, 'A phase II, randomized, double-blind, parallel-group, placebo-controlled, oral food challenge trial of Xolair (omalizumab) in peanut allergy (TOPS)', *Journal of Allergy and Clinical Immunology* 2007; 119 (1): S117.

Sampson HA, 'Anaphylaxis and emergency treatment', *Pediatrics* 2003; 111 (6): 1601–08.

Sampson HA, 'Clinical Practice: Peanut Allergy', *New England Journal of Medicine* 2002; 346 (17): 1294–9.

Sampson HA, 'Food Allergy', *Journal of Allergy and Clinical Immunology* 2003; 111 (2): S540–47.

Sampson HA, 'Food allergy. 1. Immunopathogenesis and clinical disorders', *Journal of Allergy and Clinical Immunology* 1999; 103 (5): 717–28.

Sampson HA, 'Food allergy. Part 2: Diagnosis and management', *Journal of Allergy and Clinical Immunology* 1999; 103 (6): 981–89.

Sampson HA, 'Food sensitivity and the pathogenesis of atopic dermatitis', *Journal of the Royal Society of Medicine* 1997; 90 (Supplement 30): 3–9.

Sampson HA, 'The evaluation and management of food allergy in atopic dermatitis', *Clinics in Dermatology* 2003; 21: 183–92.

Sampson HA, 'Use of food-challenge tests in children (Commentary)', *The Lancet* 2001; 358: 1832–33.

Sampson HA, 'Utility of food-specific IgE concentrations in predicting symptomatic food allergy', *Journal of Allergy and Clinical Immunology* 2001; 107 (5): 891–96.

Sampson HA, Mendelson L, Rosen J, 'Fatal and near-fatal anaphylactic reactions to food in children and adolescents', *New England Journal of Medicine* 1992; 327 (6): 380–84.

Sampson HA, Muñoz-Furlong A, Bock SA, Schmidt C, Bass R, Chowdhury BA, *et al*, 'Second symposium on the definition and management of anaphylaxis: Summary report — Second National Institute of Allergy and Infectious Disease/Food Allergy and Anaphylaxis Network symposium', *Journal of Allergy and Clinical Immunology* 2006; 117 (2): 391–97.

Sampson HA, Muñoz-Furlong A, Campbell RL, Adkinson FN, Bock SA et al, 'Symposium on the definition and management of anaphylaxis: Summary report', *Journal of Allergy and Clinical Immunology* 2005; 115 (3): 584–92.

Sampson MA, Muñoz-Furlong A, Sicherer SH, 'Risk-taking and coping strategies of adolescents and young adults with food allergy', *Journal of Allergy and Clinical Immunology* 2006; 117 (6): 1440–44.

Savage JH, Matsui EC, Skripak JM, Wood RA, 'The natural history of egg allergy', *Journal of Allergy and Clinical Immunology* 2007; 120 (6): 1413–17.

Schaub B, Lauener R, von Mutius E, 'The many faces of the hygiene hypothesis', *Journal of Allergy and Clinical Immunology* 2006; 117 (5): 969–77.

Sheikh A, Alves B, 'Hospital admissions for acute anaphylaxis: Time trend study', *British Medical Journal* 2000; 320: 1441.

Sicherer SH, 'Clinical implications of cross-reactive food allergens', *Journal of Allergy and Clinical Immunology* 2001; 108 (6): 881–90.

Sicherer SH, 'Food allergy', *The Lancet* 2002; 360: 701–10.

Sicherer SH, Bock AS, 'An expanding evidence base provides food for thought to avoid ingestion in managing difficult dilemmas in food allergy', *Journal of Allergy and Clinical Immunology* 2006; 117 (6): 1419–22.

Sicherer SH, Burks AW, 'Maternal and infant diets for prevention of allergic diseases: Understanding menu changes in 2008', *Journal of Allergy and Clinical Immunology* 2008; 122 (1): 29–33.

Sicherer SH, Burks AW, Sampson HA, 'Clinical features of acute allergic reactions to peanuts and tree nuts in children', *Pediatrics* 1998; 102: e6.

Sicherer SH, Furlong TJ, DeSimone J, Sampson HA, 'Self-reported allergic reactions to peanut on commercial airliners', *Journal of Allergy and Clinical Immunology* 1999; 104 (1): 186–89.

Sicherer SH, Furlong TJ, Maes HH, Desnick RJ, Sampson HA, Gelb BD, 'Genetics of peanut allergy: A twin study', *Journal of Allergy and Clinical Immunology* 1999; 103 (4): 559–62.

Sicherer SH, Furlong TJ, Muñoz-Furlong A, Burks AW, Sampson HA, 'Prevalence of peanut and tree nut allergy in the US determined by a random digit dial telephone survey', *Journal of Allergy and Clinical Immunology* 1999; 103 (4): 559–62.

Sicherer SH, Leung YM, 'Advances in allergic skin disease, anaphylaxis, and hypersensitivity reactions to foods, drugs, and insects', *Journal of Allergy and Clinical Immunology* 2007; 119 (6): 1462–69.

Sicherer SH, Muñoz-Furlong A, Sampson HA, 'Prevalence of peanut and tree nut allergy in the United States determined by means of a random digit dial telephone survey: A 5-year follow-up study', *Journal of Allergy and Clinical Immunology* 2003; 112 (6): 1203–07.

Sicherer SH, Muñoz-Furlong A, Sampson HA, 'Prevalence of seafood allergy in the United States determined by a random telephone survey', *Journal of Allergy and Clinical Immunology* 2004; 114 (1): 159–65.

Sicherer SH, Sampson HA, 'Food allergy', *Journal of Allergy and Clinical Immunology* 2006; 117 (2): S470–75.

Sicherer SH, Sampson HA, 'Peanut allergy: emerging concepts and approaches for an apparent epidemic', *Journal of Allergy and Clinical Immunology* 2007; 120 (3): 491–503.

Simons ECW, Muñoz-Furlong A, Furlong TJ, Sicherer SH, 'Management of food-induced anaphylaxis by caregivers and medical professionals: a survey', *Journal of Allergy and Clinical Immunology* 2006; 117 (Supplement 1): S134–5.

Simons FER, 'Anaphylaxis', *Journal of Allergy and Clinical Immunology* 2008; 121 (2): S402–07.

Simons FER, 'Anaphylaxis, killer allergy: Long-term management in the community', *Journal of Allergy and Clinical Immunology* 2006; 117 (2): 367–77.

Simons FER, 'First-aid treatment of anaphylaxis to food: focus on epinephrine', *Journal of Allergy and Clinical Immunology* 2004; 113 (5): 837–44.

Simons FER, Frew AJ, Ansotegui IJ, Bochner BS, Golden DBK, Finkelman FD, Leung DYM, Lotvall J, Marone G, Metcalfe DD, Muller U, Rosenwasser LJ, Sampson HA, Schwartz LB, van Hage M, Walls AF, 'Risk assessment in anaphylaxis: current and future approaches', *Journal of Allergy and Clinical Immunology* 2007; 120 (1): S2–S24.

Simons FER, Gu X, Silver NA, Simons KJ, 'EpiPen Jr versus EpiPen in young children weighing 15 to 30 kg at risk for anaphylaxis', *Journal of Allergy and Clinical Immunology* 2002; 109 (1): 171–75.

Simonte SJ, Ma S, Mofidi S, Sicherer SH, 'Relevance of casual contact with peanut butter in children with peanut allergy', *Journal of Allergy and Clinical Immunology* 2003; 112 (1): 180–82.

Skolnick HS, Conover-Walker MK, Koerner CB, Sampson HA, Burks W, Wood RA, 'The natural history of peanut allergy', *Journal of Allergy and Clinical Immunology* 2001; 107 (2): 367–74.

Skripak JM, Matsui EC, Mudd K, Wood RA, 'The natural history of IgE-mediated cow's milk allergy', *Journal of Allergy and Clinical Immunology* 2007; 120 (5): 1172–77.

Smart JM, Kemp AS, 'Increased Th1 and Th2 allergen-induced cytokine responses in children with atopic disease', *Clinical Experimental Allergy* 2002; 32: 796–802.

Smith WB, Gillis D, Kette FE, 'Lupin: a new hidden food allergen', *Medical Journal of Australia* 2004; 181 (4): 219–20.

Spergel JM, 'Atopic march: link to upper airways', *Current Opinion in Allergy and Clinical Immunology* 2005; 5: 17–21.

Sporik R, Hill DJ, Hosking CS, 'Specificity of allergen skin testing in predicting positive open food challenges to milk, egg and peanut in children', *Clinical and Experimental Allergy* 2000; 30: 1540–46.

Sporik R, Hill DJ, 'Allergy to peanut, nuts, and sesame seed in Australian children', *British Medical Journal* 1996; 313: 1477–78.

Stark BJ, Sullivan TJ, 'Biphasic and protracted anaphylaxis', *Journal of Allergy and Clinical Immunology* 1986; 78: 76–83.

Strachan DP, 'Hay fever, hygiene, and household size', *British Medical Journal*, 1989; 299: 1259–60.

Tang MLK, Kang LW, 'Prevention and treatment of anaphylaxis', *Paediatrics and Child Health* 2008; 18 (7): 309–16.

Tang MLK, Robinson M, 'Allergy prevention: Current recommendations and new insights', *Australian Family Physician* 2008; 37 (4) 204–08.

Thien FCK, '3. Drug hyersensitivity', *Medical Journal of Australia Practice Essentials — Allergy* 2006; 185 (6) 333–38.

Untersmayr E, Jensen-Jarolim E, 'The role of protein digestibility and antacids on food allergy outcomes', *Journal of Allergy and Clinical Immunology* 2008; 121 (6): 1301–8.

Vadas P, Perelman B, 'Activated charcoal forms non-IgE binding complexes with peanut proteins', *Journal of Allergy and Clinical Immunology* 2003; 112 (1): 175–9.

Vickers DW, Maynard L, Ewan PW, 'Management of children with potential anaphylactic reactions in the community: a training package and proposal for good practice', *Clinical and Experimental Allergy* 1997; 27: 898–903.

von Mutius E, Martinez FD, Fritzsch C, Nicolai T, Roell G, Thiemann H-H, 'Prevalence of asthma and atopy in two areas of West and East Germany', *American Journal of Respiratory and Critical Care Medicine* 1994; 149; 358–64.

von Mutius E, Martinez FD, Fritzsch C, Nicolai T, Roell G, Thiemann H-H, 'Skin test reactivity and number of siblings', *British Medical Journal*, 1994; 308: 692–95.

Wainstein BK, Kashef S, Ziegler M, Jelley D, Ziegler JB, 'Frequency and significance of immediate contact reactions to peanut in peanut-sensitive children', *Clinical and Experimental Allergy* 2007; 37 (6): 839–45.

Weidinger S, Illig T, Baurecht H, Irvine AD, Rodriguez E, Diaz-Lacava A, Klopp N, Wagenpfeil S, Zhao Y, Liao H, Lee SP, Palmer CN, Jenneck C, Maintz L, Hagemann T, Behrendt H, Ring J, Nothen MM, McLean WH, Novak N, 'Loss-of-function variations within the filaggrin gene predispose for atopic dermatitis with allergic sensitizations', *Journal of Allergy and Clinical Immunology*, 2008; 118 (1): 214–19.

Weidinger S, O'Sullivan M, Illig T, Baurecht H, Depner M, Rodriguez E,

Ruether A, Klopp N, Vogelberg C, Weiland SK, McLean WH, von Mutius E, Irvine AD, Kabesch M, 'Filaggrin mutations, atopic eczema, hay fever, and asthma in children', *Journal of Allergy and Clinical Immunology* 2008; 121 (5): 1203–09.

Weiland SK, Bjorksten B, Brunekreef B, Cookson WOC, von Mutius E, Strachan DP and the International Study of Asthma and Allergies in Childhood Phase II Study Group, 'Phase II of the International Study of Asthma and Allergies in Childhood (ISAAC II): Rationale and methods', *European Respiratory Journal* 2004; 24: 406–12.

Weiner JM, 'Allergen injection immunotherapy', *Medical Journal of Australia Practice Essentials — Allergy* 2006; 185 (4): 234.

Werfel SJ, Cooke SK, Sampson HA, 'Clinical reactivity to beef in children allergic to cow's milk', *Journal of Allergy and Clinical Immunology* 1997; 99 (3): 293–300.

Weston S, Halbert A, Richmond P, Prescott SL, 'Effects of probiotics on atopic dermatitis: a randomized controlled trial', *Archives of Disease in Childhood* 2005; 90: 892–97.

Wood RA, 'The natural history of food allergy', *Pediatrics* 2003; 111 (6): 1631–37.

Wrobel JP, O'Hehir RE, Douglass Jo A, 'Food allergy in adults', *Australian Family Physician* 2008; 37 (4): 222–26.

Yu JW, Kagan R, Verreault N, Nicolas N, Lawrence J, St. Pierre Y, Clarke A, 'Accidental ingestions in children with peanut allergy', *Journal of Allergy and Clinical Immunology* 2006; 118 (2): 466–72.

Yunginger JW, Sweeney KG, Sturner WQ, Giannandrea LA, Teigland JD, Bray M, Benson PA, York JA, Biedrzycki L, Squillace DL et al., 'Fatal food-induced anaphylaxis', *The Journal of the American Medical Association* 1988; 260 (10): 1450–52.

Zeiger RS, Heller S, Mellon MH, Forsythe AB, O'Connor RD, Hamburger RN, Schatz M, 'Effect of combined maternal and infant food-allergen avoidance on development of atopy in early infancy: A randomized study', *Journal of Allergy and Clinical Immunology* 1989; 84 (1): 72–89.

Books

— Barber, Marianne S., 2001, *The Parents' Guide to Food Allergies: Clear and complete advice from the experts on raising your food-allergic child*, Owl Books, New York

— Coss, Linda Marienhoff, 2004, *How to Manage Your Child's Life Threatening Food Allergies: Practical Tips for Everyday Life*, Plumtree Press, California

— Sicherer, Scott H., 2006, *Understanding and managing your child's food allergies*, Johns Hopkins, Baltimore

— Wood, Robert A, with Kraynak J., 2007, *Food Allergies for Dummies*, Wylie Publishing, Inc., New York

ACKNOWLEDGMENTS

This book is the result of a collaboration of many wonderful medical and health professionals, organisations and individuals who so generously contributed their time, knowledge and expertise.

Dr Preeti Joshi, specialist Paediatrician in Allergy and Immunology in the Department of Allergy and Immunology at The Children's Hospital at Westmead, Sydney, has been the best co-author I could ever hope for: helping me to understand complex medical concepts, answering questions during countless hours of interviews and hundreds of email queries, as well as reviewing and fine-tuning all copy. Dr Joshi understands, first-hand, what the parents of food-allergic children are experiencing. Her warmth and empathy for food-allergic patients and their families, in addition to her professional expertise and positive outlook, is inspiring.

The support and enthusiasm of Maria Said, President of Anaphylaxis Australia Inc, has been resolute from the day we first spoke about this book. Maria is a tireless and optimistic leader who has made a positive difference in the lives of so many Australian families living with food allergies. Maria's assistance with research for this book and scrupulous review of all copy was invaluable.

Barbara Dennison, paediatric dietitian at The Children's Hospital at Westmead, Sydney, was so kind in allowing me to interview her at length and then come back to her time and again (… and again) during the writing and editing process to access her expertise on all matters related to diet. This book is all the better for her insight, attention to detail and good humour.

Special thanks to Olivia Keene, psychologist and Clinic Director of Keene Insight Child and Adolescent Specialists (Melbourne), for her extensive contribution to the chapter on teens, information on bullying and the chapters within Part 3: The emotions of food allergy. Olivia very generously allowed me to interview her on numerous occasions for hours at a time. She pointed me in the direction of research material and welcomed me to come back to her repeatedly with even more questions. I learned so much. Olivia also kindly reviewed copy and ensured that the information we included was accessible, realistic and, above all else, positive. I am very grateful.

Thank you to Lydia Buchtmann at Food Standards Australia New Zealand for her help in interpreting the FSANZ Code, answering my never-ending questions and reviewing the chapter on food labelling. Lydia offered patience and dedication to ensure the information on food labelling was accurate. I thank, too, the Allergen Bureau, for their help with information about VITAL in the food labelling chapter.

I would like to thank Jill Smith, Executive Officer of the Australasian Society of Clinical Immunology and Allergy (ASCIA), for her kind assistance in granting permission to reproduce and refer to particular ASCIA resources in this book. Patient Information available on the ASCIA website (www.allergy.org.au) is essential reading for parents of food-allergic children.

Thank you to The Children's Hospital at Westmead, Sydney, for granting permission to reproduce the fish classification table on page 106.

I am grateful to the many early childhood professionals who offered me guidance and feedback on Chapter 11, Childcare and pre-school: Naomi Harris, Loata Mataitoga, Kylie Sanderson and my lovely sister, Ann-Maree Fisher, as well as Monique Webber, General Manager of Family Day Care Australia, and Family Day Care Australia directors. I am equally grateful to Jane Danvers, Karen King and Eric Patatoukos for their assistance with research for Chapter 12, The school years.

To all the families throughout Australia who so generously allowed me to interview them, thank you for your honesty and willingness to share your experiences with others: Jill Ahmed, Angela Batten, Jodie Bellchambers, Claire Bent, Geoffrey Browning, Judy Browning, Amanda Cheong-Duryea, Anne Frisby and Phil Solomon, Andrew and Merryn Gibbons, Anne-Lii Hardy, Janelle Imber, Annelise Kirkham, Emilia Lie, Tinmimi Maung, Peta Mawson, Katrina Meldrum, Juliet Nicholls, Tanya Paine, Kris Piotrowski, Kerry Pontin, Justine Sayers, Sally Voukelatos, and Barbara.

To HarperCollins, thank you for your enthusiasm to publish this book, especially Amruta Slee and Shona Martyn. Extra special thanks to Anne Reilly, for her meticulous editing and careful guidance, and to Judi Rowe for designing and typesetting the internals, Darren Holt for the cover design and Alexis Seabrook for the illustrations.

On a personal note, I thank my dear friend Dr Rowley Richards for monitoring my progress every week, and the Orman and Dekker families for your support, especially my mum and dad. Thank you to Naomi, Leah and Sheryl, as well as the wonderful staff at Noah's kindergarten, who have all helped to keep him safe, happy, loved, well-fed and, importantly, always included.

Finally, thank you to my own family — Jan, Noah and Lucy — for putting up with all the hours I have spent at the 'pooter (one of Lucy's first words) during the past few years, and for your encouragement and sense of humour.

Alison Orman

This book is a true collaboration. There are many individuals who lent their time and expertise to contribute.

Firstly Ali Orman, who is one of the most intelligent and eloquent people I have met. Ali quickly grasped scientific concepts, trawled through masses of medical literature, talked to many people and drew on her own experiences in order to write this book. She was able to encapsulate medical facts into accessible language whilst at the same time injecting warmth and compassion into her writing. Her gentle and patient approach ensured that I was organised and able to respond to most queries on time. Importantly she is also a wonderful mother and a positive person — I have enjoyed working with her and learnt much from her.

Professor Andrew Kemp — a very clever and enthusiastic doctor, who has taught me a great deal about interpreting medical literature over the last few years. Andrew read and offered advice about the first seven chapters to help ensure that all the medical facts were thoroughly checked.

Barbara Dennison, paediatric dietitian at The Children's Hospital at Westmead, Sydney, was generous with her time and knowledge. The book is richer because of her valued contribution.

The allergy and immunology staff at The Children's Hospital at Westmead and Sydney Childrens' Hospital for their shared knowledge and friendship.

The allergy patients and the families that I treat — I often learn from them and am inspired by their courage. Their experiences have helped to shape my approach to the management of food allergies.

Maria Said, President of Anaphylaxis Australia Inc, who reviewed this book and provided encouragement when it was most needed.

Amruta Slee and Anne Reilly from HarperCollins, for their guidance and encouragement.

My extended family (the Joshis and the Kumaradevas) — especially my dear parents and sisters, Shilpi and Sonal — for their interest in the book, for sharing their own experiences in managing food allergies and for keeping our children safe and happy.

My friends and the school community who have been so careful and inclusive of our daughters — much of my experience has been positive because of them.

Importantly, my wonderful husband Anand for his encouragement, generosity and tolerance for the reams of copy in our study over the last year.

My darling daughters, Maya and Anika, who have had their own journeys with food restrictions and reactions. Their positive attitudes and boundless joy in life are the motivation for my involvement with this book.

Preeti Joshi

INDEX